A Primer on International Health

Robert W. Buckingham
New Mexico State University

Allyn and Bacon

Boston • London • Toronto • Sydney • Tokyo • Singapore

To the Joffroy family of Nogales, Arizona—
A family filled with a passion for life, compassion for others,
eternal love for each other, and a living work of beauty

Vice President: *Paul A. Smith*
Publisher: *Joseph Burns*
Editorial Assistant: *Annemarie Kennedy*
Editorial Production Service: *Chestnut Hill Enterprises, Inc.*
Manufacturing Buyer: *Julie McNeill*
Cover Administrator: *Kristine Mose-Libon*

Copyright © 2001 by Allyn & Bacon
A Pearson Education Company
160 Gould Street
Needham Heights, MA 02494

Internet: www.abacon.com

Between the time Website information is gathered and published, some sites may have closed. Also, the transcription of URLs can result in typographical errors. The publisher would appreciate notification where these occur so that they may be corrected in subsequent editions.

Library of Congress Cataloging-in-Publication Data

Buckingham, Robert W.
    A primer on international health / Robert Buckingham.
        p.   cm.
    Includes bibliographical references and index.
    ISBN 0-205-19809-0
    1. World health.   I. Title.

RA441 .B83 2000
362.1—dc21

00-063953

Printed in the United States of America
10 9 8 7 6 5 4 3 2 1   05 04 03 02 01 00

Contents

Preface   v

1 *Introduction to International Health*
Robert W. Buckingham and Todd Smith   1

2 *Globalization: Toward One World*
Robert W. Buckingham, Teresa R. Ramírez,
and Linda J. Gough   18

3 *Global Environmental Health*
Edward A. Meister   32

4 *The Challenge of Global Malnutrition*
Robert W. Buckingham, Theresa H. Hollingsworth, and
Heather Lynn Smith   85

5 *Primary Health Care: The Global Response*
Robert W. Buckingham and Tracy Brannock   104

6 *Maternal and Child Health, A Global Health*
Perspective
Robert W. Buckingham, Matt Flint, Candice Borden,
and Lyndsay Graff   123

7 *Comparative National Health Care Systems*
Robert W. Buckingham, Zhaohui Zhong,
and Edward A. Meister   139

8 *Epidemiology: Methods and Global Practice*
Edward A. Meister and Robert W. Buckingham   177

9 *The Future of International Health:*
Problems and Prognosis
Robert W. Buckingham and Theresa H. Hollingsworth   204

Index   222

Preface

This book addresses the dynamic and interactive process of sharing knowledge of international health among colleagues and students. My primary mission is to offer a user-friendly text that covers crucial global health issues of the twenty-first century. Each chapter includes thought-provoking summary questions to stimulate and extend the discussion of topics that have been covered. To accompany the constantly evolving nature of international health issues, specific chapters include links to Websites to connect the reader directly to updated resources.

As commerce, international travel, and the Internet continue to accelerate the globalization of human life, health has become less of an isolated phenomenon. A new influenza virus emerging in central China can quickly spread to Europe and North America. Resistant strains of bacteria can travel across the globe in mere weeks. Global warming increases the range of disease vectors such as contagious mosquitoes, spreading malaria and other epidemics with increasing speed. Tobacco companies exporting cigarettes to developing companies add to chronic disease burdens and worsen their epidemiologic transition. And the pace of human and disease interactions continues to accelerate.

The mission of this book is to highlight the dimensions of international health and define the nature of health problems so that solutions can be found. Because they are becoming more and more global, health problems will increasingly necessitate international cooperative solutions.

A Primer on International Health book aspires to reduce human suffering and premature death. We are bound by our common humanity, and we must collectively commit ourselves to making a healthier world so that each generation can achieve the highest possible potential within the human spirit.

Acknowledgments

I want to acknowledge my editor Joe Burns, editor-in-chief at Allyn and Bacon, who graciously and patiently has helped me guide this book to completion.

I must also acknowledge the work of all contributing authors, especially Dr. Edward Meister, who bravely took on the adventure of pulling this manuscript together by a certain and impossible deadline.

I especially want to recognize and acknowledge Dr. William, whose suggestions and recommendations have made this book a better piece of work.

I also thank the following reviewers for their helpful suggestions: Chunhuei Chi, Oregon State University, and Richard St. Pierre, Pennsylvania State University.

1

Introduction to International Health

Robert W. Buckingham and Todd Smith

The next two decades will see dramatic changes in the health care and needs of the world's populations. In developed countries, epidemics of noncommunicable diseases, such as heart disease, obesity, and depression, have replaced the traditional causes of premature death—infectious diseases. At the same time, developing nations struggle with the inequality of health care resources; their main enemies continue to be malnutrition and infectious diseases.

International health, then, encompasses two different spectrums of public health: There are diseases that occur due to lack of resources in the poverty-stricken nations, and then there are the diseases of the developed nations—diseases that are directly attributable to the development of fast food, high fat/low fiber diets, and a demanding, stressful lifestyle. Many factors come into play and weave a complex mosaic of health challenges, successes, and constant new problems to overcome. However, international health is difficult to define in a simple manner because it encompasses such vastly different subjects. This textbook will look at international health in terms of an historical perspective of health, globalization of international health, and environmental conditions around the world. It will also discuss epidemiology and diseases that affect the world, nutritional challenges around the world, primary health care and health education as it exists in the international realm, the impact of health education on maternal/child health, a comparison of national health systems, and finally, the future of world health. These facets of international health are intended to provide an overview of health issues that face the world today.

The Definition of Health

According to the World Health Organization, health is defined as "a state of complete physical, mental, and social well-being and not merely the absence of disease or infirmity" (WHO, 1995). However, health is somewhat an elusive term to define. The biggest controversy in coming to a unique definition is the "social well-being" component of the WHO definition. What does "social well-being" actually mean? For some people it could simply mean being content in everyday life. For others, "social well-being" could mean not only being content, but also having a feeling of balance in relation to daily activities and people who interact with them during the day.

The rise of health promotion has led to the elaboration of the original WHO definition of health, which can be simplified to the extent to which an individual or a group is able to realize aspirations and satisfy needs and to change or cope with the environment (Last, 1998). Health is an essential part of everyday life; however, it is not the object of living but rather a concept that stresses social and personal resources as well as physical capabilities.

Studying International Health

Why should we study international health? It provides a global perspective of the international community environments, characteristics, political power structures, and states of physical, mental, and social health. Moreover, health in the international community encompasses factors that go far beyond traditional definitions of physical and mental health. These factors include adequate food, sanitary water, housing, income, employment, education, and safety for all people. The purposes, then, of studying international health are (1) to gain a global perspective of communities, (2) to assess and evaluate the international health status in order to effectively identify and respond to prioritized health problems and needs, and (3) to provide a future direction in developing international health policies and in setting higher standards to effectively target the world population with health resources and efforts. In addition, through knowledge it is possible to raise social consciousness and thereby inspire communities to take active roles in abating the disparity in the health status of the world population.

Each country brings its own set of unique problems and challenges to the stage of international health, and each country presents different health concerns and priorities of health care. For example, third world countries, also called developing countries, deal with health problems such as diarrheal diseases, extreme poverty, lack of immunizations, and poor or inadequate natural resources that have to be shared among large populations.

Developed countries are characterized by problems such as obesity, atherosclerosis (build up of plaque in the arteries), high blood pressure, and coronary heart disease. These can be the result of the abundance of natural resources, a lack of exercise, the lack of proper health education and poor diet, or a combination of these. When considering the overall health of a country, two factors are of considerable importance—the infant mortality rate (IMR) and the size of the population. Infant mortality rate (which will be looked at in detail in Chapter 4) is the single most important determinant in accessing the health status of a nation. Population is also important when looking at the health of a country. As the population increases, natural resources, as well as other resources, decrease. In other words, population has a direct correlation to depletion of resources.

The importance, for the student, of studying international health can be summed up in one statement—increasing knowledge and awareness on world issues and diseases. Besides the obvious goal of increasing self-knowledge, there are many other important reasons to study international health. One is that world health affects all of us. For example, the global problem of AIDS/HIV affects every nation regardless of whether the country is developed. The problem in more developed countries is that health is taken for granted, and not many people are concerned with health issues in underdeveloped countries. However, one must realize that international issues are intertwined, and that more developed countries have an obligation to provide assistance to less fortunate nations.

Another reason to study international health is the problem of poverty. Poverty and malnutrition affect every country. With poverty often comes a lack of resources—whether medical care, insurance, or education—and in these circumstances the poor state of health of a country is extremely visible. Malnutrition correlates directly with poverty. Deaths due to preventable diseases and the premature deaths of children and women in their reproductive years are often poverty-related. Most of these concerns are present in developing countries, but similar health and poverty concerns can exist in rich nations. An example would be the increasing rate of homelessness in America, which ironically is the richest country in the world.

Still another reason that international health would be of concern to the student is that it may be his or her only opportunity to learn about international issues and problems. Some devote their lives to helping people who are less fortunate than themselves. International health education provides an alternative means for students to use their knowledge. The Peace Corps (which will be discussed later), missionaries, overseas hospitals, and clinics are all ways in which people can make an international difference.

The pursuit of international health provides great career opportunities for all types of people. The international health professional must have knowledge in infectious disease control, nutrition, population dynamics, environmental health, and behavioral sciences, and—most important of all—a good background in methods of surveillance used in epidemiology as it is applied in tropical settings.

Managerial skills are equally important. Without good organization, services will not be as efficient. International health requires an unusual commitment and dedication to hard work, often in uncomfortable, even unsafe working conditions and with uncertain long-term career prospects. Organizations such as WHO and UNICEF provide career opportunities in the international health arena.

As local communities are increasingly interacting with the world community on social and economic levels, the importance of a world health view becomes immediately apparent. Historically, isolated populations were not directly affected by health conditions in other regions. However, with immigration and emigration throughout the world made possible by modern systems of transportation, populations are increasingly exposed to lifestyles and diseases that were previously unknown. These changes, coupled with moral obligations and newfound abilities to alleviate a variety of health concerns, demonstrate the importance of international health. Given this importance, this textbook will begin with an overview of the historical perspective of health.

History of International Health

Historically, lifestyles have been among the most important determinants of human health. Population movement, political change, war, and technical development have all had marked effects on the overall state of health.

First Civilizations

With the development of civilization came specialization in the division of labor, which brought about new health concerns. Among these concerns were the lack of both sanitary conditions and clean water supplies due to population density; human waste management, reservoirs and water distribution systems to meet water needs for domestic and agricultural practices; shortages of food; waterborne diseases such as cholera, typhoid fever, and leptospirosis; and vector-borne diseases such as malaria, yellow fever, and schistosomiasis (Bausch, 1990).

Newly emerging health concerns and issues of sanitation and hygiene became key factors in the development of formal rules and laws to monitor trade, water usage, and other civic functions. Between the fifth and first centuries B.C., the first codes and laws were developed in Mesopotamia, Egypt, parts of what is now India, and among Aryans. The intent was to regulate the uses of water, the disposal of human wastes, the development of agriculture, and the practice of healing by what are now recognized as the first physicians.

As the population increased, and large permanent settlements of people became established, it was inevitable that trade and travel routes also would increase. These routes enabled populations to trade items that were abundant in their region for scarce goods that were abundant elsewhere. As it became necessary to move certain commerce, particularly food items, rapidly to other cities, navigation by sea and land became more systematized and efficient. In addition to the disbursement of articles of booty or commerce throughout various regions, genes, infectious agents, and ideas were being distributed both within and between cultures (Cohen, 1989). As travel between communities increased, the spread of infectious and contagious diseases as well as the growing areas in which these diseases were found became important issues for ancient societies. Moreover, as navigational means developed, more regions became accessible, and the threat of new diseases became increasingly apparent.

Development of Medicine

India. The history of Indian medicine is divided into two periods. The first, the Vedic period, dates up to 800 B.C. Vedas were composed of collections of Indian religious texts and descriptive outlines of rituals and practices, as well as explanations for the philosophies developed behind these practices for control of demons. In Vedas, a great number of ailments were described and recorded to enable the development of a remarkable acumen for prognosis.

The Brahmanic period (800 B.C. to 1000 A.D.) took the Indian spiritual order of thought as outlined in the Vedas and generated a complex system of medicine that has remained intact to the present. This system specified a code of ethics, a theoretical configuration of medical knowledge, and practices concerning the treatment of patients. Doctors in India were taught a code of ethics to be followed in their practices. These doctors learned that they should treat each patient as if he were a son, which engendered great amounts of pressure on the doctor to make a fast prognosis in order to avoid taking on a patient who would later die or was not capable of being cured. In making a prognosis, a careful history was noted, including the patient's origin and travel route, diet, duration of disease, and hygiene. Great emphasis was placed on diet, hygiene, and mental preparation of both the physician and the patient. Diagnosis was made by listening to the sounds of the breath and entrails, observing color of the eyes, tongue, and skin, feeling the pulse, and even tasting the urine for the characteristic sweetness of diabetes (Arnold, 1993).

Foods during this period were endowed with mystical properties. In fact, there is documentation of 760 plants, herbs, and spices that were used primarily for their medicinal qualities, and diets were specified for different castes. Medicines were given by mouth, enema, inhalation, nose drops, eye drops, ear drops, smoke, and ointments. Steam treatment, sweat baths, dry cupping, and bloodletting were also commonly practiced (Bausch, 1990).

Indian surgical practices varied widely and included bone setting, removal of bladder stones, and cesarean sections. Over 100 different surgical instruments were used, many of which have survived to the present. The Indian theoretical system of medical thought was also very developed: It was believed that the body had triad energies, manifested as wind (breath), bile, and phlegm. These energies, when out of balance, produced the outer appearance and manifestation of disease. Therefore, imbalance was treated with substances and practices that utilized and produced opposing qualities to restore balance. It was also believed that the body was composed of six basic elements: chyle, blood, flesh, fat, bone marrow, and sperm. Any increase or decrease of these elements was thought to produce a wide range of disorders.

China.　The oldest ancient civilization, China, also had a complex and advanced system of thought and writings that accompanied its medical practices. The first of these writings dates from 3322 B.C., when Emperor Hu-Fsi was in power. He introduced his people to a broad range of practices such as how to keep domestic animals, how to fish, how to cook, and how to get married. He is also responsible for the development of the fundamental philosophy of yin and yang, the conceptual principles of opposites. Furthermore, Hu-Fsi invented nine different shapes of needles for the treatment of disease (Li, 1992). After Hu-Fsi, Emperor Shen-Nung reigned circa 2700 B.C. and established the fundamental theory and practice of acupuncture. In addition, he discovered medicinal properties and uses for various food and mineral substances. Two hundred years later (circa 2500 B.C.), Emperor Huang-ti wrote the *Neiching*, a book about the existence and treatment of internal diseases. These writings contributed to the cementing of medical theory and practice into a body of knowledge that is more easily defined and therefore more easily modified than the oral traditions and the passing of information down through apprentices used in the primitive hunter-gatherer societies.

In Chinese philosophy, the body was viewed as a sort of microcosmic universe. Its internal affects and dysfunctions are directly related and interconnected with affects existing in the outer world. According to this philosophy, the universe is composed of two basic opposing energies: yin (the female energy also associated with moon, sweet foods, solid organs, passivity, and night) and yang (the male energy representing sun, salty foods and meat, hollow organs, activity, and day). In addition, there are five basic elements (wood, fire, earth, metal, and water) associated with five planets, five directions, five seasons, five colors, five sounds, and five organs in the human body (Ackerknecht, 1995). Disease was thought to be a disharmony between these interrelated functions of five.

Diagnosis was made primarily by observing the body. These observations included the pulse (more than fifty different types), the tongue, breathing, the eye, and other outwardly manifested body indicators. Using elaborate definitions and categories in the philosophically based system of medicine, accurate prognoses were made for many diseases, including variations within each disease. In the writings of Emperor Shen-Nung, of the 365 medicines (many of which have been established today as empirical remedies), 46 are extracted minerals, 252 are plants, and 67 are found in animal sources. Surgery was never developed, due to a deep belief that mutilations acquired in life are brought with a person into the afterlife (Ackerknecht, 1995). Acupuncture was developed as a means to correct specific dysfunctions occurring in the body.

Other Civilizations. Many ancient civilizations such as the Aztecs, Incas, Mayans, Peruvians, and other early people inhabited what now is North America. The established medicine among these cultures was so developed that the early explorers wrote to their leaders in their home country that there was no need for them to send physicians. However, the ability to translate the primary sources of care from these cultures is lacking. The little that is known is derived mainly from writings of the early Spanish, who invaded the Americas and wrote down information given to them by their pupils and slaves. It is known that the King of Spain sent a scholar to the Americas in order to study their well-developed medicine (Ackerknecht, 1995). However, little remains of his writings.

In the Peruvian civilizations and also generally throughout the Americas, surgical technology was more developed than in the primitive cultures of the Old World. North American Indians knew of laxatives, diuretics, emetics, antipyretic drugs, and even digitalis. South American Indians developed the use of cocaine, quinine, curare emetine, and numerous other drugs (Bausch, 1990). The medicinal use of a variety of plants was a common and developed practice. The Aztecs alone used over 1,200 medicinal plants, often grown in large botanical gardens (Venzmer, 1972). It is likely that the Europeans learned about and first grew botanical gardens after observing the ones found in the Americas. There is also evidence of organized public health systems. For example, the Incas, a well-organized and powerful state of people, conducted an annual health ceremony in which large-scale cleaning occurred in homes. For those unable to do the cleaning themselves, help was provided.

Greece.   Ancient Greece was located in a geographically central port for trade, commerce, and travel. Minoans arrived and brought with them the concept of hygiene as related to health practices and healing temples. The Egyptians sailed across the Mediterranean and shared their observations regarding pharmacology and surgical techniques. Mesopotamia (present-day Iraq and Iran) provided ideas for new medicinal uses of common herbs and plants, and formulas to extract their essential healing properties (Bausch, 1990). These multiple influences made significant contributions to the strong cultural dialogues in Greece. Exposure to different cultural and governmental systems enabled Greece to focus on the issues of how best to analyze people in order to benefit society as a whole. Greece was, relative to other civilizations during that period, a very wealthy, culturally literate society. The exposure to different cultures, coupled with the multiplicity of political thought, expression, and debate created by new philosophies, caused the focal point of the Western society to decisively shift away from religion and superstition.

During this period, Hippocrates was a predominant medical figure, primarily because of the profound influence his writings and school had on the further development of medicine. His approach was based on the observation and experience that he utilized in the prognosis of disease and the treatment of his patients. The two most significant contributions made by Hippocrates were his conception of ethics and his utilization of the concept of pathogenesis, or constitution of the patient (Venzmer, 1972).

Ethically, Hippocrates' main concern was for the patient—to heal the patient, not simply the malady, which was very similar to the ethical practices of India. Hippocrates believed that the key role of the physician was to aid the body in its own natural healing process. He believed that the constitution of each patient was different, and it was the physician's task to obtain as much information relating to this constitution as possible. Hippocrates believed that the knowledge of a person's pathogenesis was essential in ascertaining how the patient would respond to treatment.

Hippocrates was an empiricist. It was this empiricism that allowed for the magnificent technologies and practices he developed. For this reason, he has been referred to as the Father of Western Medicine. Hippocrates' idea of the four elements (fire, water, earth, and air) was closely related to four bodily humors (blood, black bile, yellow bile, and phlegm), which were each given qualitative behavioral characteristics. An imbalance of any one element or humor created certain illnesses (an idea very similar to Indian and Chinese medical philosophies). These imbalances or illnesses were treated by exposure to foods, medications, or activities, which would stimulate the opposite behavioral characteristic and thereby restore the balance (an idea very much like the Chinese concept of chi).

Rome.   Ancient Rome was similar to Greece in that the Romans emulated many of the Greek customs and cultural traditions. Roman medicine was based on Galen's writings (100–200 A.D.) and was to be used for the next 1,500 years in the West as the basis for medicine and medical practices. It added to the anatomical knowledge in medical practice through the dissection of animals and, sometimes, humans.

The most significant landmarks of Roman development in the field of medicine were the systems of state-funded public health. As the Roman Empire began its decline, these public health and social systems became tragically underfunded, and they eventually disintegrated. The structure of Roman society was crumbling, and with it went its levels of hygiene, its public baths and hospitals, and the conditions in which the poor voting classes lived in the cities of the empire.

The Middle Ages.   With the fall of the Roman Empire, Europe passed into a millennium of scientific somnolence. In both the East and the West, highly organized spiritual communities were reborn as the focal points of society. Several of these developments are pertinent to international health. First, scientific knowledge, including medical knowledge, passed into the hands of the church in both the East and the West. Second, there was little in terms of new innovations or discoveries because so much of the collective energy was being spent in the Crusades or in just settling down into what was later known as Europe. The average life span of the well-to-do was thirty-one years, although for the common people that number was reduced to twenty-five (Glasscheib, 1964). Third, the church in the ninth century established a University in Salerno, near Naples, where Jewish, Arabian, and Christian students of medicine read and translated many different texts and introduced them to the rest of Europe. *The Regimen Sanitatis Salernitarium,* a series of humorous aphorisms on hygiene and healthful living, became the most popular text. With the invention of the printing press in fifteenth century, it became second only to the Bible in terms of number of publications in all of Europe (Wain, 1970).

The Plague and Other Epidemics

After the collapse of the Roman Empire, the Christian church became the primary source of civic organization in Europe. Politics had been surmounted. Unfortunately, the Christian church did little to organize systems to maintain sanitation. As a result, when contagious diseases arose, they were very difficult to control and easily became epidemic in proportion. The Black Death, the most destructive contagious disease of the time, became epidemic in Europe, Asia, parts of Africa, and India in the fourteenth and fifteenth centuries. In the history of the human race, this is the only point during which the population growth halted and reversed itself (Grey & Payne, 1993). The impact of this disease on social, political, agricultural, and economic systems was colossal, and the medical effects were equally significant. The disease, caused by the bacterium *Yersinia pestis*, is spread through rodents, and is transmitted to humans via fleas that bite both rodents and humans. The death toll in Europe exceeded 25 million people. In the Middle East, China, and India, tens of millions of people died.

Physicians had no idea what was going on. Galen never wrote about epidemiology, and Hippocrates was, during the Plague in Athens, largely ineffective. With a lack of any rational explanation, most doctors reverted to superstition, blaming the outbreak on the convergence of planets or, in some cases, on the Jewish culture. In a significant development the disease was discovered to be contagious and, as a result, medicine witnessed its first effort toward international disease control.

The first to implement this effort was the seaport of Venice, in 1348. Believing that the Plague was introduced via ships, Venice developed a 40-day detention period (quarantine) for all incoming vessels. Genoa, Marseilles, and other major ports soon adopted the quarantine. Although these internationally practiced restrictive measures were ineffective in reducing the epidemiological occurrence of the Plague, they established a concept to be employed frequently in subsequent centuries.

Other epidemics occurring in the late middle ages included smallpox, diphtheria, measles, influenza, tuberculosis, scabies, anthrax, and trachoma (Rosen, 1958). Ergotism, the contamination of rye by the fungus ergot, also occurred in dozens of different epidemics, killing and crippling thousands of people between the ninth and the fifteenth centuries. Leprosy, which was endemic in parts of Europe in the thirteenth and fourteenth centuries, was all but wiped out when the majority of people contaminated by leprosy died of plague. While it was not completely eradicated, the disease was never again endemic. However, it has continued to develop sporadically since that period.

Hospitals were established in Europe during the Middles Ages. During this time, these institutions were the only places specializing in care for the sick. The churches dedicated their charities to them, and church healings were chartered in this period, partly to meet the needs of returning Crusaders (Bausch, 1990).

The continual onslaught of epidemic after epidemic created a sociopolitical movement in the late Middle Ages. The governments started to pay people to maintain a certain level of sanitation within the cities. Dead animals were disposed of, the dumping of pollutants into streams and other water sources became monitored, bathing became popular, and hospitals started to stress cleanliness. Nonetheless, the life expectancy dropped and was lower than it had been in the early part of the first century B.C.

European Colonial Expansion

The period of exploration and colonization profoundly affected international health. Columbus and his crew, through their interactions with the natives of Hispanola, Haiti, and Cuba, had contracted a deadly venereal disease, syphilis. As these infected sailors celebrated their homecoming, the disease dispersed into the unknowing population of Europe. It followed in the footsteps of its host, across continents and through trade routes. Three years after Columbus set sail for the Indies, syphilis became endemic in every large city across Europe, as well as in parts of India and China. The medical community was not prepared for a disease of this proportion. However, its contagious and sexual nature was recognized, and city officials organized quarantines.

Many European attempts at colonization were decimated by disease (Bausch, 1990). The discovery of a medication to help treat malaria in the 1600s can be considered a milestone in human history. The cure, a substance known as quinine, can be found in the bark of *Cinchona officinalis,* a tree native to the forests of South America. After the discovery, the rapidly growing demand for cinchona bark led to the destruction of the tree in Peru, Bolivia, and Ecuador. The Dutch established cinchona tree plantations in Java and had a virtual monopoly of quinine production up to World War II. The Japanese developed synthetic antimalarials such as chloroquine, and the use of natural quinine reduced the devastation malaria had on its host (Bausch, 1990).

The severity of malaria in many parts of the world was a potent inhibitor of economic development. The most compelling example occurred during the building of the Panama Canal. In 1880, the Panama Canal building project was started by the French. After eight years, 300 million dollars, and almost 20,000 deaths from malaria and yellow fever, the French abandoned their effort (Bausch, 1990). The French had not allocated funds for hygiene regulation and sanitation, and, as a result, suffered great losses.

When the United States decided to continue the project of building the Panama Canal, participants were better educated and prepared than the French had been. After recognition that the mosquito is the sole vector that transmits yellow fever and malaria, mosquito extermination became a major priority. William Gorgas was hired to monitor the sanitation and to control yellow fever and malaria—a major step in the use of applied epidemiology (Bausch, 1990). The annual mortality rate for workers was reduced from 39% in 1906 to 6% in 1912 (Macleod & Milton, 1988).

Industrialization

The Industrial Revolution, which occurred from 1750 to 1830, resulted in population surges and industry intensification. Machinery was first employed in factories for mass production of articles of commerce. Competition was strict between companies. The key to success was making more and selling for less, so profit-driven factory owners paid their workers very little. The result was the stratification of society into definite classes. Crowded apartment buildings and filthy streets stretched for miles, occupied by industry workers and their children. Children were often put to work to help supplement the income of their parents, and hours were long. Working conditions were usually deplorable. Eventually, these conditions became so hazardous to the workers that laws were produced in order to regulate these business practices—seen particularly in England. Although these laws improved factory conditions somewhat, they were not substantial enough to increase overall levels of sanitation in the workplace. Outbreaks of cholera and tuberculosis resulted, as well as the continued presence of occupational toxins and the occurrence of injuries on the job.

In response, laws became stricter and regulated more diverse areas of business. Although legislation varied by country, the general trend was constant. Laws regulating maximum work hours, minimum ages for laborers, minimum wages, and environmental hygiene at the work site became sanctioned and enforced. The advent of industry brought about many changes in the scope of international health issues, specifically in the realm of regulation and sanitation. There was a strong generalized movement in public health. Health care for the poor was established in England to minimize the scope of cholera and tuberculosis epidemics. Populations were registered by the state, creating demographic data on the incidence of disease, marriage, birth, and death. The collection of these data and the creation and regulation of health sanctions were monitored by health boards organized exclusively for that purpose.

Modernization of Medicine

From prehistoric to modern times, the practice of medicine has continued to evolve greatly. Within the span of one human lifetime (from about 1840 to 1900), vague theories of miasma and divine displeasure gave way to experimentally based laboratory data regarding the genesis of infectious disease and its effects on the body. Knowledge of physiology, nutrition, and many other aspects of biomedical science also advanced during this period, with the dawn of an understanding of endocrine and metabolic function (Bausch, 1990). The rise of microbiology depended on the chemical and technological advancement provided by the Industrial Revolution. Refinements in microscope design produced the lenses of the 1880s, which are forerunners of those in use today. The chemistry of dye manufacture, which was developed for the textile industry, was incorporated into histology and bacteriology, thus allowing early scientists to glean more knowledge about the infection process. Little by little, the basis of modern medical practices was shaped (Bausch, 1990).

The study of illnesses, cures, and medicines can be understood from an historical perspective and demystified. The hunter-gatherer, farmer, city dweller, exploiter, humanitarian, and scientist still exist, as do the basic premises and problems of health that human beings have encountered from earliest civilizations (Bausch, 1990). This is why the study of health history is not only important, but also essential, for those who wish to gain a global perspective on international health.

Current International Health Concerns

The World Health Report (WHO, 1999) identified poverty as the main reason why babies are still not vaccinated on a routine basis in many parts of the world, why clean water and sanitation are not always available, why curative drugs and other treatments still remain unavailable to large numbers of people, and why mothers continue to die during childbirth. With more than 20% of the global population living in extreme poverty, it is the underlying cause of reduced life expectancy, handicaps, disability, and starvation (Fifty Facts, 1995). In addition, poverty contributes greatly to mental illness, stress, suicide, family disintegration, and substance abuse (WHO, 1999).

Despite the modern understandings of health and methods of decreasing mortality and increasing life expectancy, great disparities continue to exist among cultures. The gaps between rich and poor, the sexes, and populations continue to widen (WHO, 1995). Life expectancy in one of the world's least developed countries is 43 years, compared to 78 years in one of the world's most developed countries (Fifty Facts, 1995). This means that a rich, healthy person can live twice as long as a poor, sick person living in another region. In some developing countries, little more than the equivalent of four U.S. dollars is spent annually per person on health care, and half the world's population still lacks regular access to treatment for common diseases and to essential drugs (WHO, 1999). The inequity of life expectancies is becoming an even greater concern. In five countries, life expectancy at birth was expected to decrease by the year 2000, despite increases in all other regions. In the richest countries, life expectancy by the year 2000 was anticipated to reach 79 years, while in some of the poorest countries it would revert to levels comparable to 42 years ago. Moreover, by the year 2000 more than 45 countries were projected to have a life expectancy at birth of less than 60 years (WHO, 1999).

Global Mortality

Over the next hour alone, 1,500 people will die from an infectious disease—over half of them children under five; the rest will be working-age adults, many of whom are breadwinners and/or parents (WHO, 1999). Both of these are vital age groups that developing countries cannot afford to lose. Infectious diseases are now the world's biggest killer of children and young adults, and account for more than 13 million deaths a year—one in two deaths in developing countries (WHO, 1999). Some 39 million deaths took place in the developing world and about 12 million in developed countries from 1995 to 1998. Communicable diseases, such as tuberculosis and respiratory infections, as well as maternal, perinatal, and neonatal conditions, accounted for more than 20 million deaths (about 40% of the 51 million global deaths), 99% of which occurred in the developing world (WHO, 1999). Of these 20 million deaths due to communicable diseases, more than 16 million (about 80%) were due to infectious and parasitic diseases. Tuberculosis kills more than 7,000 people per day, totaling over 3 million deaths per year, which accounts for about 5% of the global total of deaths. It is estimated that there were 8.8 million new cases in 1995 (equal to more than 1000 new cases every hour). Malaria kills about 2 million people annually, and hepatitis B up to 1 million. Cholera has again become endemic in many countries, such as Africa, Asia, and Latin America.

In addition to other threatening communicable diseases, dengue hemorrhagic fever is now one of the most significant and rapidly rising arbovirus infections in the world. There are millions of new cases reported annually, with approximately 500,000 people needing hospital treatment, and thousands of deaths. Ebola hemorrhagic fever is also a potent killer; as humans keep migrating onto previously uninhabited land, we will encounter new diseases to which we have no resistance. Ebola virus is a prime example of this.

Parasitic diseases are increasing every day. It has been reported that onchocerciasis (river blindness) infects 18 million people in 34 countries, while dracunculiasis (Guinea-worm Disease) causes terrible suffering and disability among 3 million of the world's poorest people who have no access to safe water. Chagas disease affects 17 million people in 21 countries in Latin America and causes 45,000 deaths and 400,000 cases of heart and stomach disease annually. African sleeping sickness kills an estimated 55,000 people each year. Schistosomiasis affects 200 million people in 74 countries in the Americas, Africa, and Asia and kills perhaps 200,000 people yearly. Leishmaniasis infects about 13 million people annually, visceral leishmaniasis (kala-azar) being the most severe form. It causes 500,000 new cases and more than 80,000 deaths each year. Lymphatic filariasis (elephantiasis) affects about 100 million people annually, while ascaris causes clinical symptoms in as many as 214 million people. In addition, trichuris affects 133 million annually, and hookworm can be found in more than 96 million people (WHO, 1999).

Sexually transmitted diseases that were once thought to be under control are once again gaining ground in the face of humans' never-ending endeavors for a quick cure. An estimated 236 million people have trichomoniasis, with 94 million new cases each year. Chlamydia infections affect some 162 million people, with 97 million new cases annually. An estimated 32 million new cases of genital warts occur each year, and there are some 78 million new cases of gonorrhea. Genital herpes infects 21 million people per year, and syphilis about 19 million each year. Most of these sexually transmitted diseases can be prevented and treated effectively, but most countries are lacking both the resources and knowledge to do so. HIV continues to spread relentlessly; though people often realize the dire consequences of unsafe sex or exchanged needles, on a worldwide basis, the behavior modification that would decrease the incidence of this disease still does not occur on a regular basis. Over 13 million adults, mainly heterosexual men and women, are infected with HIV. Some 6,000 people become infected each day, and it was predicted that, by the year 2000, the cumulative total of HIV infections worldwide could reach 30 to 40 million (WHO, 1999). Furthermore, in the next 5 years, AIDS will have killed more than 8 million people, most of them young adults, with women having the largest increase of new infections. The lethal relationship between tuberculosis and HIV is making the death toll many times worse. During the next 10 years, in Asia alone, it is estimated that tuberculosis and AIDS together will kill more people than the entire population of the cities of Singapore, Beijing, Yokohama, and Tokyo combined (WHO, 1995; Fifty Facts, 1995).

Aside from the health concerns caused by infectious diseases, chronic illnesses and injuries are growing concerns in the global population. Cancer and heart disease account for about 19 million deaths annually, or about 36% of the global deaths, divided more or less equally between the developing and developed nations. The great majority of such deaths are among adults (WHO, 1995). It has been reported that every day about 600 people die, and another 33,000 are injured because of unsafe working conditions. Worldwide, 90% of workers have no access to occupational health services (Fifty Facts, 1995).

Elderly populations are rapidly becoming a more serious health concern in the world population. It has been reported that there are currently 355 million people over the age of 65. The number of people in the developing world over age 65 will increase between 200 and 400% during the next 30 years. The increase in number of older populations in the world will profoundly affect health and social services in the next century. The prevalence of chronic diseases such as stroke, dementia, and cancer is high. Furthermore, at least 165 million people in the world, most of them elderly, are estimated to have rheumatoid arthritis, and 1 in 3 women over age 50 has osteoporosis (Fifty Facts, 1995; WHO, 1995).

Who's Who in World Health

Leading the fight in international health issues is the World Health Organization (WHO). WHO's objective is the attainment by all people of the highest possible health and absence of disease. Along with the efforts of WHO there are other organizations that play a major role in international issues. The United Nations Children's Fund (UNICEF) advocates and works for the protection of children's rights, to help the young meet their basic needs and to expand their opportunities to reach their full potential. The United Nations Educational, Scientific, and Cultural Organization's (UNESCO) main objective is to contribute to peace and security in the world by promoting collaboration among nations through education, science, culture, and communication in order to further universal respect for justice, for the rule of law, and for the human rights and fundamental freedoms that are affirmed for the peoples of the world.

The United States Agency for International Development (USAID) provides economic development and assistance for the advancement of U.S. economic and political interests overseas (www.usaid.gov). Project Concern International (PCI) is a nonprofit health organization dedicated to saving the lives of children and mothers worldwide through basic medical care, nutritious food, clean water, and health education. Another organization that aids in international concerns, the Population Council, is a nonprofit organization that seeks to improve the well-being and reproductive health of current and future generations around the world and aids in achieving a humane, equitable, and sustainable balance between people and resources.

Another key international organization is the Peace Corps. CARE, one of world's largest international development and relief organizations, helped train the first Peace Corps volunteers in Latin America and became a leader in self-help development and food aid. The goal of the Peace Corps is to provide help to underdeveloped countries by people who truly care about giving aid in any way possible to the needy.

Cooperation among countries has been going on for years. The first international meeting focused on health was held in Paris in 1851. Collaboration in the twentieth century was formalized through the United Nations (UN) and its various agencies, such as WHO. In order to have worldwide cooperation in the area of health, the emphasis must shift from "international" health to "global" health. The term *international health* is used when talking about relations between states and their governments. *Global health* encompasses relations beyond governments and includes individuals and groups within societies that interact across national boundaries (Lee, 1998).

There has been some collaboration between these organizations in providing services to more needy countries. One example of this collaboration is the WHO Expanded Program on Immunization, a program that targets infants and children in developing countries. Its main objective is to provide immunizations against diseases that have been killing children and infants in those countries. These diseases include measles and diarrhea, both of which are preventable and are certainly not life-threatening in developed countries.

Addressing the World's Health Concerns

Examining past and current health issues serves to demonstrate the evolution of international health. Clearly, current trends suggest that, despite our technological advances, we must continue to strive for a healthier global community, as potential health conditions are recognized but not yet realized. By examining health from an historical perspective and recognizing both current and future trends, this book develops a unified rather than an isolated perspective. Already, the impacts of a rapidly changing and increasingly interactive global community are recognized. Global markets have crossed international barriers, and the idea of a large single community is more commonly accepted. Given this, the importance of learning from our past and planning for our future is clear. This planning can be best accomplished from an international health perspective.

This textbook provides an introduction to the vast realm of international health. It provides information on some of the most important issues that affect the world, some of which include, but are not limited to: organizations focused on international health and environmental health; the dynamic interactions between health care systems, economies, and health issues; and the concerns regarding maternal and child health, chronic and infectious disease, and nutrition. In addition, epidemiological approaches to health and the future of international health will be discussed.

TABLE 1.1   *World Wide Web Box: International Health*

1. Global Health Cooperation	Http://web.lexis-nexis.com/universe/docum
2. World Health Organization	Http://www.who.org
3. Children Worldwide	Http://www.unicef.org
4. United Nations Educational, Scientific, and Cultural Organization	Http://www.unesco.org
5. United States Agency for International Development	Http://www.usaid.gov
6. Project Concern International	Http://www.serve.com/PCI
7. Population Council	Http://www.popcouncil.org
8. Peace Corps	Http://www.care.org

Discussion Questions

1. Define health according to WHO.

2. Why is the WHO definition of health in controversy?

3. What is the purpose of studying international health?

4. What two factors are important when discussing the overall health of a nation?

5. What is the importance, for the student, of studying international health?

6. What are the skills needed in order to be an international health professional?

7. List some of the factors that have marked the state of health throughout history.

8. Starting with the Neolithic Agriculture Revolution, describe some of the health concerns that early civilizations faced.

9. Who have been the major contributors to the development of medicine? List some of their accomplishments.

10. Who was Hippocrates, and why was he a predominant medical figure?

11. What was Hippocrates' four bodily humor theory?

12. How did bubonic plague (Black Death) play a factor in the development of early civilizations?

13. List some other epidemics that occurred during the Middle Ages.

14. Who was responsible for the spread of syphilis in Europe?

15. How did the Industrial Revolution contribute to the poor standards of living?

16. What is the main reason that babies are not vaccinated?

17. List some health-related consequences of poverty.

18. What is the impact of HIV/AIDS in the world today?

19. Who are some of the major players in international health?

References

Ackerknecht, E. (1995). *A Short History of Medicine.* New York: Ronald Press Co.

Arnold, D. (1993). *Colonizing the Body: State Medicine and Epidemiology of Disease in Nineteenth-century India.* London: University of California Press.

Bausch, P. F. (1990). *Textbook of International Health* (2nd ed.). New York, Oxford: Yale University Press.

Cohen, M. N. (1989). *Health and the Rise of Civilization.* New Haven: Yale University Press.

Fifty Facts from the World Health Report. (1995). Http://www.who.org/

Glasscheib, H. S. (1964). *The March of Medicine: The Emergence and Triumph of Modern Medicine.* New York: G. P. Putnam's Sons.

Gottfried, R. (1978). *Epidemiologydemic Disease in Fifteenth Century England: The Medical Response and the Demographic Consequences.* New Brunswick, NJ: Rutgers University Press.

Gray, A. (Ed.). (1993). *World Health and Disease.* United Kingdom: Open University Press.

Grey, A., & Payne, P. (1993). *World Health and Disease.* United Kingdom: Open University Press.

Last, J. M. (1998). *Public Health and Human Ecology.* (2nd ed.). Stamford, CT: Appleton and Lange.

Lee, K. (1998). *Shaping the Future of Global Health Co-operation: Where Can We Go From Here?* London: Health Policy Unit, London School of Hygiene and Tropical Medicine.

Li, C. (1992). A Brief Outline of Chinese Medical History with Particular Reference to Acupuncture. *Perspective in Biology and Medicine* (Vol. 18, pp. 132–143).

Macleod, R., & Milton, L. (Eds.). (1988). *Disease, Medicine and Empire: Perspective on Western Medicine and the Experience of European Expansion.* New York: Routledge.

Rosen, G. (1958). *A History of Public Health.* New York: MD Publications.

Venzmer, G. (1972). *Five Thousand Years of Medicine.* Marion Koenig (translator from German). London: Macdonald and Company.

Wain, A. (1970). *A History of Perspective Medicine.* Springfield, IL: Charles C. Thomas.

WHO. (1995). *World Health Report,* 1995. Geneva, Switzerland: [Online] Available Http://www.who.org.

WHO. (1999). *World Health Report,* 1999. Geneva, Switzerland: [Online] Available Http://www.who.org.

2

Globalization: Toward One World

Robert W. Buckingham, Teresa R. Ramírez, and Linda J. Gough

A Changing World

Globalization is the process whereby the Earth is becoming part of an interconnected world. This means that new technologies have made frontiers smaller and more accessible. While access to cities and remote areas around the world is easier, societies are still complex and multifaceted. Attempting to define how globalization affects each area creates some problems. In fact, the easiest solution is to try to look at globalization as a process, one that is influenced by many aspects such as technology, politics, and economic growth.

Globalization includes the potential for people to operate at a world community level and gives rise to new systems of global governance, regionalization, decentralization, civil society, ethics, and sustainability. However, the potential for this internationalization of relations and dependencies brings about some fears and resistance. Rebound effects also have been identified, including democratic, environmental, security, and social deficits (Lubbers, 1999).

The potential to become a globalized system is directly influenced by an ideological breakthrough in which democracy is considered to be a twin of the market economy. What is known is that two causes of globalization predominate. The first identifies globalization as a direct result of technological revolution or innovation. The second cause can be identified as market ideology, the economization of life, mass consumption, and entertainment deregulation. In other words, systems identified by isolationism, dictatorial political regimes, a fragmented international order, or defensive regionalization can create a totally different atmosphere for the process of globalization (Lubbers, 1998).

There are three reactions to globalization. The first is nationalism, in which nations, communities, and countries start to lose their identity. In this process, local cultures are destroyed and regional tastes and traditions are overshadowed. The second reaction has to do with searching for a leader who in a time of crisis can act resolutely in the nation's interest. This reaction seems to appeal most to newly liberalized nations with developing political systems who are incapable of reacting effectively in the face of economic crisis. Populism, and its politics, is the third reaction against globalization. Here leaders may begin to propose forms of protectionism as a way to offset losses incurred by an embrace of competition and political change. In this reaction, globalization is made the scapegoat of domestic political ills (Annan, 1999).

Globalization is the intensification of worldwide social relations. This chapter will cover six dimensions of these changing social relations: (1) cultural: entertainment, (2) economical/political, (3) public health, (4) environmental justice, (5) technology, and (6) international development and sustainability. All of these topics help to create an understanding of the impact of globalization.

Cultural: Entertainment

The movements and interactions of globalization are now patterned and institutionalized to such an extent that local societies have to explicitly react and relate themselves to the global configurations. What does this mean to a local identity (or culture) and to local processes that would normally transpire in everyday life (Lubbers, 1998)?

Culture is defined as the way people live—the common values, assumptions, rules, and social practices that make up and contribute to personal and collective identity and security. Culture is a very dynamic idea, especially today, because it is constructed not only from local influences, but also from symbolic representations portrayed in the mass/cultural media as well. As the process of globalization unfolds, standards for a particular society no longer come from local entities. Furthermore, ideals of society do not rest upon the needs of individual communities, but instead are subject to an effort to conform to larger, more distant and removed frames of reference (Lull, 1995).

Globalized societies then have a double duty: to both oversee local priorities and keep pace with global ones. In the same sense there exists a responsibility to nurture the components of culture that shape it. However, most theorists argue that a homogeneous world culture is coming about due to the sharing by countries of commodities, money, information, and people. For example, as contact between cultures has grown with globalization, the process of dominant language killing off smaller languages has accelerated (Koop 1999; Lull, 1995).

In prehistoric times there were an estimated 10,000 to 15,000 languages spoken. Today the number of existing languages is around 6,000, and this number is expected to decrease by half in the twenty-first century. This is a very important concept because each language contains words that uniquely capture ideas, and losing words can mean losing specific ideas. Moreover, in losing a language, much of the culture is lost as well. With the growth of satellite television and the Internet, the need to communicate in a common language will increase. Hopefully, there will be a way to preserve the various native tongues as we continue to grow toward one community (Koop, 1999; Webb, 1995).

Economical/Political

There are three main events that will be discussed in this chapter in order to provide an understanding of the evolution of world commerce as we know it today. These events are the General Agreement on Tariffs and Trade (GATT), the North American Free Trade Agreement (NAFTA), and the birth of the World Trade Organization (WTO). GATT and WTO have influenced the development of world trade relations with respect to economic growth and investments and are ultimately key factors in world health and prosperity.

General Agreement on Tariffs and Trade (GATT)

In the wake of World War II, the General Agreement on Tariffs and Trade was established in order to facilitate freer trade. Since its inception, GATT has been the chief force in lowering tariff rates around the world. The globalization of the world economy has widened the scope of competition and interdependence among governments, thus more rules have been established so that all involved could benefit from fair agreements. This effort is predicated on the principle that international trade can be regulated by eliminating measures that discriminate against foreign competition (Dunning & Hamdami, 1997).

North American Free Trade Agreement (NAFTA)

Signed by Mexico, Canada, and the United States in 1993, NAFTA was designed to reduce tariff and trade barriers in order to eliminate restriction on foreign investments and capital mobility. The environmental consequences for all three countries created much controversy and debate over this agreement; however, interest in NAFTA had to do with improving or reducing poverty in Mexico by stimulating economic growth and investments (Goodstein, 1995).

Opposition to this proposal existed before the agreement was approved, and there were three prevailing arguments. The first was that poverty would not be alleviated and ultimately subsidies for corn farmers would be reduced as there was growing availability of cheap, imported grain, bringing about a net increase in unemployment. The second concern dealt with escalating pollution problems in view of Mexico's weakness in resources for environmental enforcement. Last, the opposition thought that the environmental regulations would be weakened due to trade-based challenges by foreign governments and companies. Although good effects were anticipated, there have been problems with regard to environmental pollution along the U.S.–Mexican border. In addition, subsidies on corn were removed, as Mexican growers could not compete with the imported hybrids (Goodstein, 1995; Johnston 1997).

World Trade Organization (WTO)

To reenforce trade as an important aspect of globalization, the WTO was created in 1995 and is the successor to the GATT. The objective of the organization is to help improve trade relations, and the organization lists a number of areas in which this objective is being met. The first is facilitating and administering trade agreements. It also acts as a forum for trade negotiations and in turn settles trade disputes when needed and called upon. Likewise, it serves as a reviewing body for national trade policies and assists developing countries in trade policy issues, through technical assistance and training programs. Finally, it cooperates with the efforts of other international organizations.

The World Trade Organization has the authority to override local and national decisions if there is a violation of terms of an agreement. With regard to health, it is necessary that trade of goods and services be regulated, and that equality be achieved. The importance of such organizations as WTO will continue to grow (Sassen, 1998).

Economic development and population growth have contributed greatly to current degradation of the world environment. Third world countries share some characteristics that place them in a separate category. They are less developed economically, but their economies usually depend heavily on agricultural production or the extraction of natural products.

Generally, their population numbers are very high. Moreover, these nations often contend with low levels of education, low counts of natural resources, high international debt (to developed nations or to international financial organizations), and a lack of power in the international spectrum of the economy and politics. However, extremes in this realm of underdeveloped nations are found. For instance, there are nations that are self-sufficient, very rich in resources, and very productive, whereas others rely heavily on imports of both technology and agricultural resources (Gupta, 1998).

Public Health

Globalization is becoming increasingly important in the field of public health. Transnational economic, social, and technological changes taking place in the world are associated with global health futures. When one looks at the potential consequences of globalization on the health of the world, it is clear that, by increasing trade among the different countries, we may also be at added risk for diseases and conditions not previously experienced as problems in the United States [Yach & Bettcher, 1998(a); Yach & Bettcher, 1998(b)].

Public Health Issues

Annual deaths from selected causes reflect variances in developed and developing countries. Out of eight selected causes, two reflect marked differences. The greatest difference is seen in death due to infections and parasitic disease. Seventeen million deaths are attributed to infection and parasitic disease in developing countries as opposed to 0.5 million in developed countries. Another marked difference is seen in deaths caused by chronic obstructive pulmonary disease, which accounts for 2.5 million deaths per year in developing countries and 0.39 million in developed countries (Boskin, 1995).

Another great impact pertains to infant mortality in developing countries. It is estimated that 15 million children, out of 100 million born each year, do not survive. Immunization campaigns that offer protection against six of the leading childhood diseases are estimated to reduce child mortality by 5 million. However, resources to pay for these campaigns often cover only a portion of the money needed for this goal.

In addition, diarrhea, the largest contributor to child mortality, can be alleviated through use of oral rehydration therapy. The cost of this type of therapy would amount to between $0.5 and $1 billion per year. Further, reducing the diarrheal problem would greatly help in other areas. For instance, nutritional supplementation would enable adequate nourishment to help reduce illness and to increase the ability of young people to learn and continue their educations (Repetto, 1985).

In developing countries, much more emphasis is placed on curative than on preventive measures, which greatly affects the rural, less-healthy majority. Primary care packages, which can be achieved at a cost of about $2–$4 per year, and sanitation projects are still lacking (Repetto, 1985).

World Health Organization (WHO)

The World Health Organization, the primary global health organization in the world, operates a diversity of programs from headquarters in Geneva, Switzerland. WHO's primary focus is to improve the health of all people in the world. Many of the programs supported by WHO focus on health aspects as they pertain to sustainable development and poverty. One example is the WHO program for the Promotion of Environmental Health, which addresses priority issues concerning the social environment.

WHO has established several key operating functions. The first is to give worldwide guidance in the field of health; the second is to set global standards for health; the third is to cooperate with governments in strengthening national health programs; and the last is to develop and transfer appropriate health technology, information, and standards (WHO, 1998).

WHO has made much progress in applying concepts of economic growth, health, scientific research, but much remains to be accomplished in areas such as poverty, regional conflicts and war, human rights, HIV/AIDS, and threats of other microbial agents. There are continuing efforts to alleviate conditions that are a direct consequence of poverty: These include efforts to decrease premature death by targeting health risks such as smoking, to decrease the financial burden of health care costs, and to increase access to health care (WHO, 1999b).

Pan American Health Organization (PAHO)

The Pan American Health Organization is over ninety years old and serves as the regional office for WHO for the Americas. Its fundamental purpose is to coordinate the efforts of the Americas to control disease and morbidity, and to promote the physical and mental well-being of its people. PAHO focuses on primary health care efforts as a means to reach communities with scarce resources while increasing their efficiency.

United Nations Children's Fund (UNICEF)

United Nations Children's Fund was founded in 1946 with the intent to establish international standards that protect children's rights, ensure that their basic needs are being met, and expand their opportunities to reach their full potential. UNICEF is the branch of the United Nations dealing exclusively with children on a primary health care level. Education, safe water, and sanitation are the main focus of attention in developing countries.

In order to provide a learning environment, research and evaluation are functions of UNICEF. In an ongoing human rights approach it works to improve the situation for women and children. Analysis of economic and social policy helps to monitor situations so that proper planning and action may occur.

Exportation of Lifestyle Diseases: Fast Food, Tobacco, and Biopiracy

In the last century, the ten leading causes of death in the United States have changed from infectious to noninfectious diseases. This transition has to do with control measures and lifestyle changes. Control measures—such as the use of vaccines and the production of penicillin—have decreased the rate of infectious diseases. Lifestyle change entails such factors as increases in fat consumption and tobacco use, which are correlated to the increase of noninfectious diseases—for instance heart disease and cancer. Although this trend occurs in more developed countries, it is important to understand the impact it will have in the future of developing nations (Hamann, 1994).

For instance, tobacco represents a major interest in regard to world health. In the United States, the deadliest cancer is of the lung, and smokers make up 83% of those who develop lung cancer. This should be of concern since the tobacco industry is now targeting developing nations in response to a declining market in the United States. With current smoking patterns it is estimated that around 500 million people alive today will eventually die of tobacco-related causes. This represents a double-edged sword to developing nations who are not only incurring a nicotine addiction but are also becoming dependent on the production of tobacco for their survival (Hamann, 1994; Makary, 1998; WHO, 1999b).

To make the situation worse, tobacco media campaigns in other countries are employing marketing techniques that the United States would consider illegal. For instance, no health warning labels are required on the cigarette packages. Policies and programs for the prevention and cessation of tobacco use worldwide are needed. Education, policies, and information should be made available to ensure a successful and healthy global antitobacco campaign. One event already occurs on May 31st of every year—World No Tobacco Day—which aims to educate about the health impact of smoking and the advantages of cessation (Makary, 1998; WHO, 1999a).

Biopiracy

The process of patenting in the United States has received recent attention. Patents are given very easily, and there are many loopholes in the system. According to the WTO, patents are given to inventions based on novelty and degree of utility. Although these are the criteria, recently patents have been given in the United States for medicinal herbs and plants that have been in use in other parts of the world for many years.

A major case involving patent laws and biopiracy was one that India's Council for Scientific and Industrial Research (CSIR) brought against the United States. The case involved a patent for the plant turmeric which the University of Mississippi Medical Center received in December 1993. The U.S. Patents and Trademarks Office ruled on August 14, 1998, that the patent was invalid because it was not a novel invention. The CSIR believes that these patents are given too easily because the United States is ignoring "indigenous and existing knowledge."

Most of the world's medicinal plants are located in developing countries, which lack the biotechnology to enable utilization of these potentially life-saving plant and animal-derived compounds. An international agreement negotiated in Uruguay by the WTO established TRIPS, or Trade-related Aspects of Intellectual Property Rights (Newton & Kingsnorth, 1999). TRIPS, which are compulsory for all WTO members by 2006, will have major consequences for access to medicines in developing nations (Banta, 2000). For example, medical therapy for tuberculosis with the drug ciprofloxacin costs $325.00 per month in the United States, while a generic version costs only $32.00 per month in India (Hoen, 2000). Thus, when India complies with TRIPS, it must drop local patent protection measures. The costs for treatment of tuberculosis will rise, which could have adverse health impacts. According, the pharmaceutical giant, Pfizer, has recently offered to donate the drug fluconazole (which treats AIDS-related meningitis) to South Africa. Pfizer has the patent on fluconazole and sells it for $10.00 a pill, whereas the local generic version costs six cents (Hoen, 2000).

Bioterrorism

Biological terrorism is the threat of using microbes as agents to wipe out a population. The most common and feared biological weapons today are anthrax and smallpox. Bioterrorism is dangerous because detection is almost impossible and the consequences are far more severe than those of explosives or chemicals. In the 1990s, there were 11 countries experimenting with the use of biological weaponry, not to mention numerous small protest groups (Henderson, 2000).

Anthrax occurs worldwide and is caused by *Bacillus anthracis,* which is a disease of domesticated and wild animals, mostly sheep, cattle, goats, horses, and swine. This organism is easily produced in large quantity and highly lethal if inhaled, as was experienced in 1979 in Sverdlovsk, Russia, which had the largest epidemic of inhalational anthrax of the century. A military research facility there accidentally released anthrax spore that was fatal in 66 of the 77 known cases. This accidental release did not last more than minutes but killed people within a distance of 4 km and sheep and cows up 50 km away (Henderson, 2000, Inglesby, 1999).

Smallpox was a highly infectious viral disease that was spread by respiratory discharge, killing 25%–30% of unvaccinated patients. It was eradicated in 1979. However the virus still exists in at least two laboratories in the world—the Centers for Disease Control (CDC) in Atlanta and a research institute in Moscow. The reason for storing the smallpox virus in these laboratories is to ensure that a vaccine can be made in case there is another outbreak. However, the virus is also a potential weapon for the two countries to use in war (Henderson, 2000).

Anthrax and smallpox are just two examples of organisms that are capable of killing millions. Biological warfare could conceivably kill the same number of people as nuclear bombs, but it would be less costly for several reasons: It is easy to obtain, it is easy to manufacture, and architectural structures are left standing. A major concern is the potential for dissident groups to utilize bioterrorism, as was the case in Tokyo in 1995. In late March of 1995, the Japanese cult Aum Shinrikyo released a nerve gas on the subway. This incident killed 12 people and hospitalized five thousand. Bioterrorism is an issue that many would like to ignore because of its implications (Taylor, 1996).

An effective approach to dealing with the threat of bioterrorism is proper planning. Educating the public of the health threats posed by this type of warfare represents the start of prevention. It is also necessary for local, state, and federal public health authorities to understand, prepare for, and act on biological attack by proper preparation in the detection and diagnosis of its outbreak (Center for Civilian Biodefense Studies, 2000; Henderson, 2000).

A new aspect of bioterrorism concern is "crop bioweapons," which would involve a bioterrorist releasing an anti-crop weapon upon various crops that were nationally or internationally important for feeding large populations (MacKenzie, 2000). For example, the wheat smut fungus could be released on large wheat farming regions, or whiteflies could carry viruses genetically altered to produce botulinum toxin in corn crops that is used to make beer. To address this new potential threat to the U.S. agricultural system, the United States Department of Agriculture established a counter anti-crop unit at the quarantine laboratory on Plum Island, New York.

Environmental Justice

Within the United States attempts to bring attention and action to issues of environmental equity have been slow. Consequently, what will happen when poor communities are no longer left? Such tendencies as the quest for cheap labor have resulted in taking problems into other countries. In the United States, affluent communities tend to generate more waste than poor ones. Yet, waste dumps are rarely placed among the well-to-do. An example of this is the city of Houston, Texas. African Americans represented 28% of Houston's population in the late 1970s. At that time, the majority of publicly owned landfills and municipal incinerators were in predominantly African American neighborhoods (Nadakavukaren, 1995).

Developed versus Developing Countries Waste Dumping

The probability of nuclear wastes seeping out into the environment is a constant threat. In an attempt to minimize toxicity levels and reduce migration of wastes into the environment, federal legislation in 1990 prohibited landfilling of hazardous waste unless the waste was properly treated beforehand. But chances are always present, especially in those sites that are abandoned and are no longer in operation, of leakage. In developing countries, control measures are in the beginning stages of enforcement. Legal and administrative frameworks are potential areas of future research in environmental science (Repetto, 1985).

Technology

As technology increases, so does globalization. The demand for the availability of goods and services requires state-of-the-art technology in order for information to be relayed instantly. Computers and the Internet are key players in this game, making communication much easier. Transnational companies are capable of taking orders and having an organized billing system at their fingertips, which allows for major transactions to occur in a day (Cantwell & Janne, 2000; Schiller, 1999).

Global telecommunication is dependent upon network systems. From 1990 to 1997, the number of worldwide telephone lines increase almost 60%, from 520 million to 800 million. Cellular phones and the Internet have contributed to the increase in demand for more phone lines. This also permits companies to have access to just about anywhere in the world and to do business at any time (Schiller, 1999).

The advance in technology has created a major shift in the number of people necessary for producing a product. As we move away from the industrial era there will be fewer people in the production line. The need for people to be trained in technological skills will increase so that state-of-the-art services can be provided (Cantwell & Janne, 2000; O'Reilly & Alfred, 2000; Schiller, 1999).

International Development and Sustainability

Resource Utilization

The population–resource problem is a worldwide dilemma. There are places where resources are substantial in relation to relative population (Africa and Latin America), whereas in other areas an intense dependence on agricultural practices have been created because of particular circumstances (examples are South Asia, China, and East Asia). Pressures of poverty and population growth on resources can be intense. However, abundance—more frequently than scarcity—has been the culprit of resource destruction. Some project that worldwide economic expansion in developed countries will continue to boost demand for minerals, energy resource, industrial wood, and many agricultural products (Repetto, 1985).

Two-thirds of global economic activity comes from people living in rich countries. Seventy-one percent of the world's output is consumed by people in the United States, Japan, and Western European countries, countries that account for only 15% of the world's population. Global pollution and other environmental concerns are heavily attributed to the consumption trends practiced in rich countries. Global warming, ozone depletion, acid rain, radioactive contamination, pollution of oceans, and depletion of natural resources such as water bodies are examples of the problems brought upon by increased consumption. These practices both bring about increased generation of wastes and cause a decrease in the sustainability of poor countries. Both environmental quality and the stock of natural capital have been affected by this consumption demand (Goodstein, 1995).

International trade in the twentieth century was more rapid than population growth. Many countries such as Japan, Korea, and Singapore have inadequate natural resources and have used international trade to achieve outstanding success in improving living standards. On a different spectrum, there are other poor countries that basically rely on exporting their primary sources to be able to attain access to needed imports such as fuel and food. What happens when these countries become unable to produce enough exports because of resource depletion? Unsustainable development occurs when a nation's natural capital is depleted faster than new capital is created. Sustainability would then require that a drawdown in natural capital be compensated for by investment in created capital (Goodstein, 1995; Repetto, 1985).

Social Sustainability

Societal functions or activities have consequences. But it is difficult to determine those consequences because each individual county has an individual view as to what benefits it. For instance, in the United States, the typical family—compared to 1950—owns twice as much, travels much more, and has increased per capita consumption by half.

Despite these lifestyle and consumption changes, the percentage of people reporting a "very happy" status has remained at a constant since 1957. The theory of social consumption argues that money cannot buy happiness in more affluent countries despite intense consumption practices and lifestyles. Achieving happiness may be the motivation; however, consistent survey data indicate the opposite—consistent with the theory that wealth and happiness are weakly correlated (Goodstein, 1995).

Sustainability proposes that poverty must be addressed if the deterioration of the average living standards for future generations is to be prevented. Since poverty and environmental degradation go hand-in-hand, the environmental consequences of economic growth can no longer be ignored. Economic growth does not necessarily determine living standards (Goodstein, 1995).

The biggest health threats to people in poor countries are unsafe drinking water sources and the lack of adequate sewage treatment facilities. Billions of illnesses and millions of deaths each year are attributed to water pollution. In 1990, around 1 billion people did not have access to a safe water supply, while over 1.7 billion were without adequate sanitation. When we think about the past, present, and future conditions of the world, it is inescapable that we must contemplate how resource allocation can be managed to best accommodate a sustainable world (Goodstein, 1995).

Growing populations demand more resources, more space. In turn, as more is produced, assets are depleted, the quest for more resources increases, and the environment is again compromised. As developed countries begin to grow and lose resources, the search for cheap labor and for increased production of more supplies has taken them to other areas and countries where the resources are found at cheaper costs. In turn, economic conditions of developing countries are exploited as they continue, out of economic necessity, to put an unsustainable burden on their environment.

The World Bank

The World Bank Group is an organization committed to reducing poverty and to improving living standards through sustainable growth and investment in people. This group is owned by over 180 member countries and is represented by a board of governors and a Washington-based board of directors. Each of the member countries is a shareholder, all of whom have the ultimate decision-making power in the World Bank. The World Bank ranks as the largest provider of international development assistance, granting about $20 billion in new loans every year.

With sustainable development as the goal of the World Bank Group, it supports many different activities, in addition to lending money. The focus is on assisting the poorest countries to identify their local concerns and to find ways to address them, aside from providing assistance with financing for their projects (World Bank, 2000a; World Bank, 2000b).

Beyond participating in reducing poverty and sustaining growth among poor communities, the World Bank is also committed to protecting the environment. Projects that are funded by the World Bank are tested to make sure that the funds devoted to promoting health do not harm the environment of present or future generations. Other areas of focus for projects are maternal and child health, and social services. These include, but are not limited to, reproductive health, nutrition, and early childhood development programs (World Bank, 2000c).

International Monetary Fund (IMF)

The International Monetary Fund, developed in 1946, represents 182 member countries who promote monetary cooperation, economic growth, and temporary financial assistance in order to help balance payment adjustments through surveillance and technical assistance. The need for IMF arose during the Depression, when investment and trade came to a standstill. The IMF eliminated restrictions in place during that time that stunted economic growth to enable the unrestricted conversion of one currency to another. The cooperation of the countries participating of IMF allows for the international monitoring of monetary systems.

Conclusions

Globalization has been a steady process that has synthesized bits and pieces of daily life to make it a complex phenomenon. Many definitions have been proposed; each has captured a single idea or a combination of many. Population trends such as economic and technological development, along with migration patterns, growth, and lifestyle changes all contribute to the process of globalization.

It is unclear whether globalization will bring a common culture that unifies humans while respecting differences. What is clear is that we as a species are

TABLE 2.1 *World Wide Web Sites*

1. Alternatives to Globalization	http://www.info.com.ph/~globalzn
2. Centers for Civilian Biodefense Studies	http://www.hopkins-biodefense.org
3. Centers for Disease Control	http://www.cdc.gov
4. Future Health Care	http://www.futurehealthcare.com
5. Globalization Action Center	http://www.voxcap.com
6. Globalization Studies Homepage	http://www.globalized.org
7. International Forum on Globalization	http://www.ifg.org
8. The International Institute for Sustainable Development	http://www.iisd1.iisd.ca/
9. International Monetary Fund	http://www.imf.org
10. United Nations	http://www.un.org
11. United Nations Children's Fund	http://www.unicef.org
12. World Bank	http://www.worldbank.org
13. World Health Organization	http://www.who.org
14. World Trade Organization	http://www.wto.org

moving to unprecedented levels of interconnectedness, and perhaps the seeds of global peace reside within this process of transformation.

Discussion Questions

1. What are the main forces that are driving globalization?

2. What are the key forms of globalization?

3. Discuss how globalization impacts public health.

4. For the developing world, what are the benefits and harms associated with globalization?

5. What are the ethics involved with biopiracy?

6. What are the solutions for bioterrorism?

7. Why is the WTO so controversial?

8. What role does the World Bank play in the developing world?

References

Annan, K. A. (1999). The backlash against globalism. *The Futurist* (33), 3, 27.

Banta, D. (2000). Increase in global access to essential drugs sought. *Journal of the American Medical Association*, 283(3), 321–323.

Boskin, W. (Ed.). (1995). *Readings in International Health*. Dubuque, IA: Kendall/Hunt.

Brundlant, G. H. (1999). Third Ministerial Conference on Environment and Health—Healthy Planet Forum. London: World Health Organization.

Cantwell, J., & Janne, O. (2000). The role of multinational corporations and national states in the globalization of innovatory capacity: The European perspective. *Technology, Analysis & Strategic Management*, 12(2), 243–262.

Center for Civilian Biodefense Studies. (2000). *The Centers Approach*. Johns Hopkins University Schools of Medicine and Public Health [Online] Available: Http://www.hopkins-biodefense.org/pages/center/approach.html

The Commission on Global Governance. (1999). A New World. *In Our Global Neighbourhood* [Online] Available: Http://www.cgg.ch/chap1.html

Dunning, J. H., & Hamdani, K. A. (1997). *The New Globalism and Developing Countries*. Tokyo: United Nations.

Goodstein, E. S. (1995). *Economics and the Environment*. Upper Saddle River, NJ: Prentice Hall.

Gupta, A. (1988). *Ecology and Development in the Third World*. New York: Routledge.

Hamann, B. (1994). *Disease: Idenification, Prevention, and Control*. New York: McGraw-Hill.

Henderson, D. A. (2000). *Bioterroism as a Public Health Threat*. Atlanta: Centers For Disease Control [Online] Available: Http://www.cdc.gov/ncidod/eid/vol4no3/hendrsn.htm

Hoen, E. (2000). Trade-related aspects of intellectual property rights remain a problem. *The Lancet*, 335(9214), 1528.

Inglesby, T. V., Henderson, D. A., Bartlett, J. G., Ascher, M. S., et al. (1999). Anthrax as a biological weapon: Medical and public health management. *Journal of the American Medical Association*, 281(18), 1735–1745.

Johnston, B. R. (Ed.). (1997). *Life and Death Matters: Human Rights and the Environment at the End of the Millennium*. Newbury Park, CA: Sage Publications.

Koop, D. (1999, May 16). World at Loss for Words. *Albuquerque Journal*, p. C5.

Lubbers, R. F. M. (1998). The dynamic of globalization [Online]. Available: Http://www.globlize.org/publications/dynamic.html

Lubbers, R. F. M. (1999, April 19). Lexicon Globalization [Online]. Available: Http://www.globalize.org/lexicon/globalization.html

Lull, J. (1995). *Media, Communication, Culture: A Global Approach.* New York: Columbia University Press.

MacKenzie, D. (2000). Bioterrorism special report: Run, radish, run. *New Scientist, 164*(2217), 36–39.

Makary, M. A. (1998). The International Tobacco Strategy. *MS/Journal of the American Medical Association, 280,* 1194–1195.

Nadakavukaren, A. (1995). *Our Global Environment: A Health Perspective.* Prospect Heights, IL: Waveland [Online] Available: Http://www. oneworld.org/ips2/sep/biopriacy.html

Newton, S., & Kingsnorth, P. (1999). US fights rearguard action to protect "bipiracy". *The Ecologist, 29*(6), 368.

O'Reilly, E., & Alfred, D. (2000). *Making Career Sense of Labor Market Information.* British Columbia: Algonquin College [Available Online] Http:// workinfonet.bc.ca/lmisi/making

Repetto, R. (Ed.). (1985). *The Global Possible: Resources, Development, and the New Century.* New Haven: Yale University.

Sassen, S. (1998). *Globalization and Its Discontents.* New York: New Press.

Schiller, D. (1999). *Digital Capitalism.* Cambridge, MA: The MIT Press.

Taylor, R. (1996). Bioterrorism Special Report: All Fall Down. *New Scientist, 150*(2029).

Webb, A. C. (1995). Endangered Languages. *English Journal, 84*(5), 124.

WHO. (1998). *The World Health Report 1998 Executive Summary.* Geneva, Switzerland: World Health Organization [Online] Available: Http://www. who.int/whr/1998/exsum98e.htm

WHO. (1999a). *Tobacco Free Initiative.* Geneva, Switzerland: World Health Organization [Online] Available: Http://www.int/toh/worldnotobacco99/english/policies.htm

WHO. (1999b). *The World Health Report: Making a Difference.* Geneva, Switzerland: World Health Organization. Available: Http://www.who. org

World Bank Group. (2000a). *What Does the World Bank Do?* [Online] Available: Http://www. worldbank.org/html/extdr/about/role/htm

World Bank Group. (2000b). *Who Runs the World Bank?* [Online] Available: Http://www. worldbank.org/html/extdr/whoruns.htm

World Bank Group. (2000c). *Why Do We Need a World Bank?* [Online] Available: Http://www. worldbank.org/html/extdr/about/why.htm

World Trade Organization. (1999). *About the WTO* [Online] Available: Http://www.wto.org/ wto/inbrief/inbr00.htm

Yach, D., & Bettcher, D. (1998a). The globalization of public health, I: Threats and opportunities. *American Journal of Public Health, 88*(5), 735–37.

Yach, D., & Bettcher, D. (1998b). The globalization of public health, II: the convergence of self-interest and altruism. *American Journal of Public Health, 88*(5), 738–41.

3

Global Environmental Health

Edward A. Meister

One Earth, Three Worlds

As we begin the twenty-first century and look around the planet we see the people of Earth living in three very distinct worlds. The Technophiles are the post-industrial countries characterized by a society of technological immersion, with glitzy new advances in electronics, medical research, fiber optics, Internet shopping, electronic mail, and pharmaceuticals, as well as the dizzying computerization of all aspects of home and business life. The silicon chip, portable phones, virtual reality, smart homes and automobiles, cloning, DVD home movies, human genome mapping, surgical robotics, mass production of agricultural products, and remote sensing are all examples of the relentless pursuit of progress driven by the amalgamation of science and the digitalization of nature. As a consequence, the people of the Technophile world also experience a severely diminished connection to the natural environment.

The pre-Technophiles countries are propelling rapid social, industrial, and technological changes, driven by the ferocious desire to become the next Technophile giant of the planet. These countries have extensively relaxed (or completely suspended) environmental protection norms, and as a consequence will experience enormous belated health costs, as chronic and debilitating diseases eventually manifest in the population. The Poverty-Quagmire countries represent the third type of world. These countries have almost everything going wrong: overpopulation driven by high maternal and infant mortality rates, low literacy and education, military vandalism, capital flight, corrupt political leadership, deteriorating infrastructures, political instability and border wars, depleted agricultural soils, and the burden of inordinate infectious disease morbidity and mortality (Ayittey, 1999; *Lancet*, 1999).

Although these three worlds are caricatures, this typology will serve as a useful guide to understanding the complex nature of global environmental health problems. This chapter covers six main topical dimensions of global environmental health: (1) population change, (2) environmental change, (3) air pollution and health, (4) water resources issues, (5) infectious diseases, and (6) environmental health solutions. Although these topics are presented in separate sections, they are ultimately all interconnected and share a synergistic and dynamic relationship that is global.

An underlying tenet of this chapter is that many environmental health problems are transnational or global in origin, and thus their resolution necessitates global solutions. Secondly, the essence of environmental health is the science and politics of fostering and protecting the planetary ecosystem, a system in which all three worlds are ultimately immersed and upon which they are dependent.

Global Population Change

The impact that humans have upon the environment is a function of three interrelated dimensions: absolute population count, population density, and the level of industrial and technological organization of the society. Generally the greater the level of development the more adverse enviromental impacts extend beyond the local population and impact the global environmental (e.g. acid rains, ozone depletion, climatic warming). Humans have become the dominant species on the planet, and it is the quantitative advance in population numbers that will be assessed first.

Approximately 10,000 years ago Earth's human population was 5 million. In 1804 it hit 1 billion, in 1927 it reached 2 billion, in 1974 it was 4 billion, and it surpassed 6 billion in the fall of 1999. Currently, annual births are estimated at 78 million, with 97% occurring in the developing world. Just five countries—India, Peoples Republic of China, Pakistan, Indonesia, and Nigeria—will account for nearly 50% of the world's annual growth rate (United Nations, 1999). Every day in the world 400,000 births and 140,000 deaths occur, for a net gain of 260,000 people or 3 humans per second. To accomplish this level of global reproduction, humans average 200 million matings per day.

The positive news is that world population growth is currently slowing. This is due to a variety of factors including declining fertility rates (i.e., fewer children being born per woman), organized efforts by countries around the world to provide family-planning education and services, and increased mortality in developing countries due to infectious/chronic diseases such as HIV/AIDS and localized military conflicts such as those occurring in Rwanda, Burundi, Iraq, and Afghanistan. The United Nations Population Division is projecting 9 billion people by 2050; 7.8 billion in the developing countries and 1.2 in the developed (United Nations, 1999). The United States Bureau of Census projects a world population of 9.3 billion people. The population growth for an individual country is a function of four factors: births, deaths, immigration, and emigration (Gelbard, Haub, & Kent, 1999). The United States population, estimated at 275,000,000 in 2000, is projected to grow to 393,000,000 by the year 2050, representing a net increase of 118 million people (U.S. Bureau of Census, 2000). This is based on a gain of one person every 12 seconds. Each year in the United States there are approximately 4 million births, 2 million deaths, 1 million immigrants, and 200,000 emigrants. Since first-generation immigrants tend to have higher fertility rates, approximately 60% of the United States population gain in year 2050 will be due to immigration (Nowak, 1997).

Although a country may have less than replacement births (i.e., fewer than two children per family), its population continues to grow because of a phenomenon demographers term "population momentum." This continuing growth results from a country's having a large proportion of young people who are entering their reproductive years, hence the absolute number of people will continue to rise even if couples have fewer children per family. This population momentum phenomenon will be dramatically experienced in the Peoples Republic of China (PRC), where only one child per couple is permitted in the urban areas, yet over 30% of the population is under 15 years of age.

PRC has adopted specific family planning policies and penalties for violating such rules. The main content of PRC's current family planning policy is as follows: (1) To promote late marriage as well as later and fewer but healthier births and to avoid genetic and other birth defects; (2) To advocate "one couple, one child"; (3) To encourage rural couples who have practical difficulties and who wish for a second child to have proper spacing; and (4) To have the specific regulations and measures for minority nationalities to practice family planning decided by the governments of the relevant provinces and autonomous regions in accordance with local conditions (CFPC, 1999). These policies may seem controversial to those in Western cultures, where reproductive freedom is simply assumed. However, PRC has 22% of the entire Earth's population, and it is striving to advance the economic well-being of the entire country. To this end, restrictions on the number of births per family are seen as necessary.

Overall, the world population is increasing by an estimated 78 million persons per year after subtracting for deaths (see Table 3.1). By 2050, the world's more developed regions are expected to exhibit a population decline, while the less developed areas are projected to almost double, from 4.7 billion to 7.7 billion. Europe will have a population decline, while Asian countries will increase from 3.6 to 5.2 billion people (see Table 3.2). China and India will probably have the largest population by 2050, with over 1.5 billion each. Pakistan is projected to become the third largest country in the world, and the United States fourth (Haub, 1998).

Overall, worldwide fertility rates are declining from an average of six to three births per woman. In the Technophile countries, fertility has actually dropped below two children per woman, that is, less than replacement levels. Examples include the United States, Western European countries, Japan, and Australia. So why are the United Nations and other agencies still predicting a near doubling in world population by 2050? Even with the 50% decline in fertility, a woman birthing an average of three children produces a population increase with each surviving generation. In addition, overall mortality will continue to decline as life expectancies continue to increase with better standards of living, better ed-

TABLE 3.1   *World Vital Statistics Per Unit of Time: 1998*

Time Unit	Births	Deaths	Increase
Year	132,947,673	54,280,999	78,666,674
Month	11,078,973	4,523,417	6,555,556
Day	364,240	148,715	215,525
Hour	15,177	6,196	8,981
Minute	253	103	150
Second	4.2	1.7	2.5

Source: U.S. Bureau of Census Report WP198, World Population Profile: 1998, U.S. Government Printing Office.

TABLE 3.2   *World Population Projections to 2050*

World	8,909,000,000
Developed regions	1,155,000,000
Less developed	7,754,000,000
Africa	1,766,000,000
Asia	5,268,000,000
Europe	628,000,000
Latin America	809,000,000
North America	392,000,000
Oceania	46,000,000

Source: United Nations (1998).

ucation, better nutrition, and improved access to basic primary health care. Third, as previously discussed, many countries have plenty of population momentum— that is, a large mass of young people entering their reproductive years who will be generating more offspring, and hence increasing the world's population. Finally, reductions in country-specific fertility rates are reflecting the phenomena of pregnancy spacing and pregnancy delay.

Women in Technophile countries have been moving into extended career training involving higher education, attending graduate schools, and beginning productive professional careers. Collectively, this results in delayed marriage and postponement of births until later years after marriage and careers are established. These delays among the high-income countries have been termed "today's baby bust," and once these women begin reproducing, the fertility rates will rebound to the couples' desired level of two children per family (Bongaarts, 1998).

Pre-Technophile countries (e.g., China, India, and Southeast Asia) will continue to have enormous population growth due primarily to population momentum. Governmental family planning efforts have been achieving success in many developing countries, reducing fertility rates to 2.1 children per family or even lower. These levels of fertility reduction are evident in such countries as Barbados, Trinidad, Tobago, Seychelles, Mauritius, Cyprus, Sri Lanka, Azerbaijan, Kyrgyzstan, and Kazakhstan (Population Institute, 1998). For the Poverty-Quagmire countries, population projections reflect high increases, which will place greater burdens on existing natural resources. Examples include Liberia, Pakistan, Nigeria, Ethiopia, and Congo, where populations are projected to triple by 2050 (United Nations, 1999).

Much has been written about the "graying" of the baby boomers in the developed countries; however this is also occurring in many of the developing countries. This will result in increasing proportion of older and more dependent individuals. By 2050, 25% of the world's population will be over 65 years of age, and in the United States the number of people over 100 is estimated to increase from 37,000 to 4,000,000. These projections could be much higher if current research in life-extending drugs is successful (Schwartz, W. B., 1999).

Theories of Population Dynamics

In 1798 an English economist named Thomas Malthus expounded a theory that increases in agricultural production grow arithmetically, while human populations grow geometrically. He believed that sooner or later the human population would outgrow the ability of agricultural systems to provide an adequate food supply. In his own words:

> I think I may fairly make two postulates. First, that food is necessary to the existence of man. Secondly, that the passion between the sexes is necessary and will remain nearly in its present state. . . . Assuming then, my postulate as granted, I say, that the power of population is indefinitely greater than the power in the earth to produce subsistence for man. (Malthus, 1798)

Malthus is all too easily dismissed as shortsighted or too pessimistic, yet his *Essay* was undertaken because of his genuine concern for the well being and improvement of human societies. What Malthus could not have imagined from the late eighteenth century was the ability of technology to exponentially expand human economies and food production. For example, in 1900 one American farmer fed himself and six other people; today one farmer feeds 129 people. Nor could Malthus imagine the human ability to voluntarily control their reproductive numbers once they had reliable methods.

Recently, there has been a reexamination of Malthus's ideas that still have relevance, particularly the notion of "carrying capacity." In a strict ecological sense, carrying capacity is the maximum population that a particular environment or geographical area can maintain (Ricklefs, 1979). Food production technology (e.g., mechanized farm equipment, synthetic fertilizers, and pesticides) has allowed human populations to "overshoot" environmental carrying capacity (Catton, 1998; Rohe, 1997). Malthus contended that a negative-feedback process would reduce overpopulation by means of famine, disease, and mortality in a fairly rapid manner. However, this negative-feedback mechanism did not occur in human populations as rapidly as Malthus supposed (Catton, 1998). This is because humans experience a long period from birth to the time of their maximum resource consumption and because humans have exploited the fossil-fuel energy reserves of the planet. This results in a disjunction from the "normal" ecosystem constraints and feedback loops to which other species are vulnerable (i.e., bears and deer cannot turn up the air conditioner during very hot summers or the furnace in very cold winters).

Population ecologists use the concept of "carrying capacity" to argue that Earth's ecosystems do not have unlimited ability to maintain unlimited population growth, and at some level human population demands will result in a catastrophic population decline and collapse of environmental systems. This is of particular concern in view of the fact that the functioning of modern developed societies has become highly dependent on such nonrenewable resources as coal, natural gas, and crude oil. Carrying capacity also does not indicate the "quality of life" that would be available in all likelihood when populations near or exceed it. Some researchers take the extreme view of human population growth as the sole cause of all society ills: crime, ethnic conflict, joblessness, environmental degradation, overcrowding stresses, and greater commuting times (Grant, 1998).

Human population dynamics are more complex than natural animal examples, in which herbivore numbers go up and down with vegetative food supplies and predator numbers go up and down with the available prey. Humans reside in a multidimensional social matrix composed of political, economic, technological, philosophical, geographical, and historical factors—all of which impact population changes. Demographers are specialists in understanding human population changes, and they employ several theories or models to facilitate understanding and predicting these changes.

Demographic Transition (DT). DT, the oldest of population theories, was developed by Thompson in the 1930s and predicts that changes in fertility are based on the level of economic development within a society. According to DT, a society will progress through four distinct stages as a corollary to economic development. In Stage 1, a society has both high mortality rates and high birth rates, the former due to poor living conditions and diseases that shorten human life expectancies, and the latter as a necessary compensation to enable maintaining their population. In Stage 1, populations were vulnerable to the vagaries of the climate and encounters with new pestilence, which may explain the disappearance of many prehistoric peoples such as the Hohokam at Pueblo Grande in the Sonaran Desert of central and southern Arizona (Foster & Taylor, 1998). Stage 2 begins when societal conditions improve such that the mortality rate declines; however, the birth rate continues to remain high and may actually increase. The continuing high birth rate not only reflects the high value humans place on large families; it make take parents time to feel assured that they no longer need to have child "spares" to ensure survival of the children born (McFalls, 1998). In Stage 3 the birth rate gradually declines and begins to approximate mortality rate. At Stage 4, the birth rate and death rate oscillate in close proximity to each other. Developed countries in Western Europe, for example, are said to have completed their DT to Stage 4.

The DT model has been modified somewhat and is referred to as the Epidemiologic Transition (ET) (Bah, 1995; Gaylin & Kates, 1997; Omran, 1983), which correlates each stage of transition with the historical health status of Earth's population (see Figure 3.1) (Barrett et al., 1998). Stage 1 is characterized as the Age of Pestilence and Famine, a time of early death and high infant mortality, which predominates most of human history up until the nineteenth century. Stage 2 coincides with the period of the Industrial Revolution, and is termed the Age of Receding Pandemics. During this time, improving living conditions and public health practices begin to assert positive impact on human mortality. Stage 3, the Age of Degenerative and Man-Made Diseases, brings us to the latter twentieth century, and is characterized by the transition to low infant mortality rates primarily through the control of infectious and parasitic diseases. Stage 3 societies shift to chronic disease mortality as primary, most of which deaths are related to such behavioral and lifestyle factors as tobacco consumption and obesity. Stage 4 is called the Age of Delayed Degenerative Diseases, characterized by the adoption of health-promoting lifestyles such as the rational choice adjustments that extend and promote health. However, Stage 4 is also characterized by increasing incidence of late-life aliments such as rheumatoid and osteoarthritis, Alzheimer's disease, insulin-resistance syndrome, and obesity-related Type II diabetes mellitus. Clearly, the Technophile countries have moved into Stage 3 and to some extent also exhibit signs of Stage 4.

With either DT or the ET version, progression through each stage is not necessarily a preordained dynamic, nor is regression to a former stage impossible. There is some evidence that, since 1860, DTs are taking less time—for example, Taiwan, South Korea, and Kenya. This is primarily due to rapid decline in infant mortality rates in these developing countries (Guerrant, 1994).

With the collapse of the Soviet Union and the quasi-reorientation to a market-driven allocation of goods and services, Russia has undergone severe political, economic, and social upheavals. In Russia today, life expectancy for males has declined to 58 years of age, and birth rates have been below replacement levels, indicating a negative population growth throughout the 1990s (Ciment, 1999). In DT theory Russia currently represents almost an inverted Stage 2, with low birth rates and high adult mortality, in response to the series of social cataclysms. Demographers, however, caution that there are many factors contributing to the population changes in Russia. Russia since the 1950s has been undergoing a long-term shift in population composition such that by 2015 20% of the population will be over 60 years of age (Da Vanzo & Adamson, 1997). Secondly, the increase in adult male mortality is the result of violence, homicides, suicides, and an increase in chronic disease related to alcohol and tobacco consumption (e.g., heart disease, cancer, and chronic obstructive pulmonary disease). There has also been a resurgence of

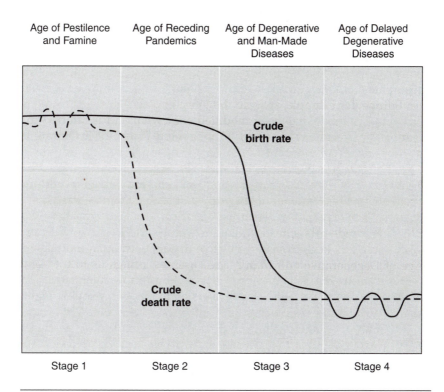

FIGURE 3.1 *Demographic and Epidemiologic Transitions*
Source: Barnett et al., 1998.

infectious diseases health problems caused by hepatitis A and B, diphtheria, and resistant strains of tuberculosis. All of these factors point to the real crisis in the public health care systems, which have severely eroded in the past ten years. Today the health care system is in a state of total turmoil since the government shifted from universal free medical care to a two-tiered system of deteriorating remnants of the old Soviet infrastructure and expensive private care that only a few can afford. Efforts are underway to address the many health care problems, and a first step has been to require compulsory health insurance that would be paid through taxes and approximate a managed care approach (Da Vanzo & Adamson, 1997). Reducing tobacco and alcohol use is critical for Russia, as well as for many other countries, and necessitates widespread public health interventions and revamping of social norms.

Theories of Couple Fecundity

There are several major theories that attempt to explain and predict the number of children each couple has. The Neoclassical Microeconomics Theory is a prominent population change theory from the field of economics (Schultz, 1973). This economic-based theory builds on three related premises regarding fertility decision making as follows: (1) The relative costs associated with reproducing a child when compared to other commodities, (2) the available family capital or income resources allocable to a child, and (3) a couple's desire for a child relative to other possible preference acquisitions. The Neoclassical Microeconomics Theory places its emphasis upon the decision making of the couple dyad, and offers little for assessing the macroeconomic influences within the larger society (e.g., inflation, high or low unemployment).

The Wealth Flows Theory (Caldwell, 1982) suggests that the decline in fertility is caused by "emotional nucleation" of the family, which results in the children becoming the net beneficiaries of family life rather than the parents. For example, in the agrarian period, when single-family farms predominated American rural life, each additional child added to the overall productivity of the farm (i.e., more acres could be brought under cultivation, more pounds of hoofed livestock could be raised and marketed). Hence, there was a net gain for the parents with each newly created child/farm hand. With the rise of the nuclear family, the emphasis of benefit shifts to the child—who seems to require two working parents who end up expending an enormous amount of physical and emotional capital for each child. Thus, emotional nucleation theory would predict that parents would want to have fewer children in order to restore higher levels of dyadic (couple) or self-investment happiness.

The Interactive Fertility Transition Model (IFT) is a more complex and multi-factorial model of fertility transition that has been elucidated by research demographer Mason (1997). In the IFT model, fertility is a function of the parental perceptions of child survival chances, the costs and benefits of having a child, and the actual postpartum costs—either emotional and/or financial—of raising a child. These parental percepts are impacted by preexisting societal mortality conditions, the degree of gender stratification (i.e., the relative degree of gender equality), and the availability of morally acceptable postpartum family reduction methods (e.g., adoption versus infanticide). Thus, in the IFT model, a couple's level of reproduction is a function of both personal self-interest calculations and child survival considerations.

All of these couple fecundity theories provide some insight and understanding into the phenomenon of population growth and change. The world community recognizes the importance of the issue of population growth, and of the need for taking action to bring down the Earth's expanding population. One of the foremost international efforts was the world summit held in Cairo, Egypt.

The Cairo Conference and Cairo +5

In 1994, over 180 nations and over 10,000 attendees met in Cairo from September 5th to the 13th to conduct the International Conference on Population and Development (ICPD). The conference attendees agreed on a set of principles to guide international programs and efforts to control population, encourage sustainable economic development, raise the level of primary care, and address the needs of gender equality.

The goals established by ICPD were as follows:

1. Stabilize Earth's population at 7.27 billion by 2050.
2. Provide women with education and access to economic and political power.
3. Provide family planning services.
4. Reduce infant mortality to <35/1,000.

Specifically for population control, ICPD agreed that the key issue is the empowerment of women, by means of equal access to education, economic resources, political power, and family planning services. Above all, education is the key to achieve sustainable development; it contributes to the reduction in both unwanted pregnancies and infant mortality. Education of women sparks the synergism of empowerment, leading to more control over their reproductive lives and their economic opportunities; and it provides role-modeling for young girls whereby they achieve a greater sense of self-responsibility leading to multigenerational progress.

On February 6th to the 12th, 1999, five years after the Cairo ICPD, representatives from world governments met in the Netherlands at The Hague Forum (Operational Review and Appraisal of the Implementation of the Program of Action of ICPD) to discuss and assess the accomplishments and further needs of the ICPD. The Hague Forum culminated in a special session of the United Nations General Assembly in the summer of 1999, and reiterated the importance of empowerment of women, gender equality, reproductive health and family planning, and access to the means of contraception.

Globally there is still enormous unmet need for contraceptive control. It is estimated that over 150,000,000 married women of reproductive age have unmet needs for contraception assistance (Rand, 1999). There are many impediments to contraception—relatively high expense (e.g., the contraceptive pill would be $100/year, an exorbitant amount in poor developing countries), limited availability of contraceptive means, and, more critically, the ability of a woman to exercise reproductive control or equality in reproductive decision making. Very often a woman, because of her societal conditioning or cultural history, is not able to assert her desires and wants regarding reproduction, often referred to as the "male domination" aspect of gender relations. The inability to space or prevent a pregnancy has important health consequences since there is increased risk of maternal mortality with unintended pregnancies. Since the Cairo ICPD tremendous progress has been made as evidenced by both governmental and international expenditures for family planning programs and the promising reductions in worldwide fertility. These programs have helped to accelerate the demographic transition, and their success is reflected in today's lower death and birth rates (Brown, 1999a).

TABLE 3.3   *World Internet Connections Box: World Population*

1. Interactive World Population Counter	Http://www.PopExpo.net
2. National Headquarters for Negative Population Growth Inc	Http://www.NPG.org
3. National Wildlife Fund International Population and Environment Site	Http://www.NWF.org/International/pop/
4. United States Bureau of Census	Http://www.Census.gov
5. Center for Overpopulation	Http://www.Overpopulation.com
6. World Population Council	Http://www.PopCouncil.org
7. Population Reference Bureau (USAID)	Http://www.Popnet.org
8. Population Index, Office of Population Research	Http://popindex.princeton.edu
9. Population Reference Bureau	Http://www.Prb.org

The Population and Environment Connection: Impact Models

Surprisingly there is considerable vexation and debate concerning the relationship between human health and the environment. The "environment" is the totality of all dimensions of Earth's environ—climate, topography, water, air, soils, flora, and fauna—all of which we often refer to as "nature." Humans have a history on Earth unique from other species in that we are not at all content with the slow process of genetic- and evolution-based adaptation to nature. Thus began the spiral of human ascendancy on the planet. First came control of fire, which increased the spectrum of available protein and carbohydrates from food sources, extended the hours of human activities (e.g., weaving or art after dark), provided for some defense against certain species that thought humans were sort of tasty treats, and allowed inchoative levels of altering the environment by burning areas of vegetation. Humans eked out a living as foragers or opportunistic hunters and gatherers. Survival was heavily dependent upon the resources of the immediate habitat.

Next came the control over food supplies for both humans and their domesticated animals, called agriculture. Approximately 12,000 years ago, in the upland areas of Mesopotamia in the Middle East, there appears the first evidence of human agricultural activity featuring wheat and barley (Bates, 1995). This advent was incredibly significant because we became the first species not only to cultivate (and hence control) our own food supply, but also to generate food surpluses. All of the subsequent specializations of human activities into trades and crafts, then sciences, and medicine are based on the ability of a society to move beyond individual family subsistence. Once a farmer could produce a surplus (i.e., more food than needed for individual family survival), then he could trade that surplus to others who in turn could make candles and tools, thus creating early forms of technology. Larger urban collectives arose, incorporating water and sanitation management practices and characterized by expanding centers of commerce.

In the eighteenth and nineteenth centuries, in the Industrial Revolution, machines were organized to mass-produce physical goods, which increased economies of scale such that large quantities were available and affordable. This industrial and economic expansion was concurrent with the modernization of agricultural production, which in turn led to reduced demand for children and thus slowed population growth (Schuh, 1995).

For example, cows have to be milked twice a day (morning and evening) and as such the size of the dairy herd is limited by the number of hands available for manual udder milking. The introduction of milking machines not only speeds up the process, and permits the farmer to have a larger dairy herd (and hence increased surplus production), but subtly reduces reproductive pressures to have a large family of "cheap" milking laborers. However, the mass production of agricultural products also lead to extraordinary environmental impacts from pesticide and synthetic fertilizer runoff into water systems, a dependency on fossil-fuel utilization for tractors and harvesting equipment, and concentration of animal wastes that can pollute ground water acquifers. Likewise the industrial production of goods has lead to enormous amounts of air, water, and soil contamination of the environment on a global level.

This is the crucial and defining uniqueness of human beings: Humans both utilize the environment and modify it to better achieve their needs for sustaining and expanding their population. By 40,000 years ago humans resided throughout Europe and Africa, north and south, and, with the Ice Ages between 25,000 and 11,000 years ago, three distinct waves of humans migrated across Beringia (the land bridge) from Siberia to the New World of the Americas (Powledge & Rose, 1996). Settlements of humans dispersed across North America down to the tip of South America. This worldwide migration was predicated on the ability of humans to exert sufficient skills in modifying the environment (e.g., to create clothing, fire, seed crops, and hunting tools).

Zooming forward in time, not only have human numbers vastly expanded from those early days but the impact—both intended and unintended—on the natural systems of the environment has attained a global scale of consequences: polar bears with DDT and PCBs in their body fat, thinning ozone layers in the troposphere, increasing atmospheric greenhouse gases, loss of fertile soils, pesticide contamination of ground water, species extinction, deforestation, climatic changes with rising temperatures, and acid rains. These global modifications are easily recited by any grade school student, as evidence of his or her awareness of these potential threats to the environment upon which human viability depends. Historically, this awareness was increased by means of the "environment movement" of the 1970s in the United States, and the "Green Movement" in Europe, and subsequent resulted in passage of a panoply of environmental laws.

What is often missing in this awareness is that humans, as individuals, are capable of rapid adjustments to adverse environmental changes (e.g., in response to thinning ozone, put on UV sun screen), while the rest of the flora and fauna of the Earth can only adapt by the relatively slow means of natural selection. Hence, the latter are much more vulnerable to alternation of environmental ecosystems. Early heroes of the United States environmental movement such as John Muir, Aldo Leapold, Henry David Thoreau, and Theodore Roosevelt often spoke of giving a voice to the many species that are unable to register their complaints over the human modifications of the environment that provide the conditions for their livelihood. Albeit that humans have a much greater vested interest in preserving and protecting their own species relative to nonhuman species, the modern science of ecology has thoroughly demonstrated the interconnectedness or interdependency among all species, plants and animals, and human life. It is crucial to keep in mind the certainty that all human life is still dependent on the process of photosynthesis within plants for the production of oxygen, and on the capturing of solar energy in the form of carbohydrates. The human ability to modify our relationship with the natural environment is both the essence of our immense success and, in the modern world, the source of potential collapse.

Recently the central environmental health issue was framed by the World Health Organization as follows:

> The interdependence of health, development, and environment is manifold and complex, but two aspects predominate: how well the environmental can sustain life and health, and how free the environment is of hazards to health. (WHO, 1997)

Notice the key term *sustain*. Just how many humans can Earth's environment sustain in an absolute numerical sense, at what level of quality of life can they live, and at what level of economic activity? These are the quandaries zealously debated among population ecologists, demographers, and world health authorities. There is also seemingly unending scientific uncertainty and disagreement regarding assessment of the relative harmfulness of human activity upon the Earth's ecosystems (e.g., global warming versus global cooling). Presumably this understanding of human interconnectedness and vulnerability with natural processes will engender an environmental ethic of enlightened self-interest, and better care will be undertaken to protect and avert irreparable harm to the environment.

This debate is often viewed as occurring between two camps: the optimists, who have unwavering faith in "human ingenuity" to solve all possible problems, versus the doomsday pessimists, who contend that the environmental systems are rapidly approaching their maximum threshold of endurance and will soon collapse. A second bifurcation to the debate is viewed as a demarcation between environmental resource managers and old-fashioned conservationists or preservationists (Livernash & Rodenburg, 1998). The former want to achieve the maximum ecosystem yield for human beings, and the latter want to minimize adverse human impacts on the environment and maintain the maximum amount of pristine and healthy habitat.

This fundamental question of the relationship between the environment and human population growth is addressed from more formal perspectives. Political economists argue that it is lack of development and unequal access to resources that cause environmental destruction and population growth. Hence the solutions reside in political changes that will result in more equitable distribution of wealth and resources. For ecologists, population growth is viewed as the crux of environmental degradation. Human populations simply exceed the natural carrying capacity, and with each new person more consumption of the finite resources will occur (Orians & Skumanich, 1997).

Paul Ehrlich, the famous University of Stanford population and butterfly biologist (Ehrlich & Ehrlich, 1991), first proposed a simple formula to assess the impact of human population growth on the environment. The formula is called IPAT and is expressed as follows:

$$I = P \times A \times T$$

where I = environmental impact, P = population, A = affluence, and T = technology. Environmental impact can be pollution (e.g., of air, water, soil), affluence can be expressed in mean gross domestic product per capita or consumption per capita, and technology refers to level of technology in use by that society (e.g., number of cars, amount of carbon monoxide produced). The IPAT model can be used to help understand the comparative impact of one country on the environment versus that of others. For example, if population tripled there would be triple the impact on the environment, or if technology in the form of air conditioners doubled, that would double the impact on the environment (in the form of electrical power generation, coal burning, or need for nuclear fuels). Ehrlich and Ehrlich give the example of the average American's using 280 gigajoules of energy per year, and the average person in Bangladesh using 2 gigajoules per year; hence the U.S. citizen has 140 times more impact on the environment. The obvious limitation of the IPAT model is that all of the factors could potentially interact with each other in more ways than demonstrated by simple multiplication. For example, the more wealth a society has the more its citizens insist on a quality environment and diminished pollution, and the more likely a society is to implement lower-polluting technology (e.g., electric cars, electric commuter trains). The more people in a society who are struggling for food in a growing population, the more they simultaneously degrade the environment by overtaxing reserves of soil nutrients, forest products for fuel, and water by contamination, all of which further worsen their survival efforts (Ehrlich, Ehrlich, & Daily, 1993). This is referred to as the population-environment-food trap. Inadequate nutrition results in premature deaths and the failure of each generation to achieve their full developmental potential.

Another popular model was developed by Park and elaborated by Catton (Catton, 1987) from the field of ecology and referred to as the POET (see Figure 3.2). The POET model contends that the interactions or relationships between human populations and the environment are impacted by the social organization and the technology used in the society. These impacts may be either destructive or ameliorative for the environment and for the human population. The POET model exhibits the importance of the dynamic and reciprocating relationship between humans and the environment, since humans both alter and are altered by the environment.

From these models one can distill three central themes. First, the effects of population on the environment's wellness and subsequent impacts on the health of the population are both corollaries of the quantity (i.e., the total size) of the population and the quality of the population's interactions with the natural environment (i.e., its level of social-technological sophistication, and its relative ability to harm and benefit natural systems). Second, population and environment are not simply interconnected; they are interrelated such that changes in one can manifest changes in the other. Third, the extent and locus of environmental impact and subsequent feedback consequences to the population vary with the relative state of economic and technological development (see Table 3.4).

China (PRC) is a perfect example of a pre-Technophile country that is undergoing rapid industrialization based on the use of high-sulfur coal for energy generation and home heating. The adverse environmental impact is both local and global—producing locally high sulfur dioxide and PM10 (small particulate pollution) levels and consequently generating 500,000 premature urban deaths by 2020 (McMichael & Smith, 1999; Wei et al., 1999). Carbon dioxide emissions contribute to global climatic warming by trapping solar heat within the Earth's atmosphere that would have otherwise dispersed into space. The United States contributes 4.8 billion metric tons of carbon dioxide that is released into the atmosphere annually, which primarily has an adverse global environmental impact (Livernash & Rodenburg, 1998). Public health researchers have also been concerned with both the within-country depositing of environmental wastes, and the export of such wastes

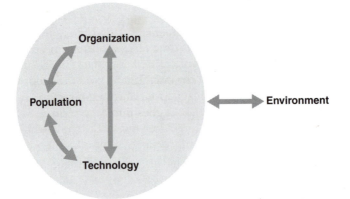

FIGURE 3.2   *POET Model*

Source: Catton (1987).

TABLE 3.4 *Potential for Adverse Environmental Impact by Society Type and Location of Impact*

The Three Worlds	Local Impact	Global Impact
Technophiles	Low	High
Pre-Technophiles	High	High
Poverty-Quagmires	High	Low

to developing countries. This topic of inequitable deposition of societal hazardous wastes among the lower socio-economic strata of the world is referred to as environmental equity (Hardening, 1993).

Time-Out for a Thought Experiment: The Tropical Island

Let's take a time-out and conduct a thought experiment regarding human needs and environmental effects. Suppose you and nine other humans were stranded on a tropical island of five acres (currently the amount of producing farmland for every ten Americans), what public health decision would your group of castaways have to make within the first few hours of arrival? Give up?

Where is everyone going to deposit his or her urine and feces? Random deposition would quickly create a multitude of problems. If you put it in the ocean, it can wash up on the beach; if you put it in a stream, it will contaminate your only source of fresh (unsalted) water. Beach burying may contaminate clam-digging sites, and so on. So just this simple biological need for coordinated disposing of human excreta must be carefully agreed upon by everyone, hence a public decision for the good of the whole. Without this agreement, both the environment and the group's health would quickly be in peril. Your second primary need will be locating and protecting a source of potable water, meaning that it is consumable without causing diseases. The human body can only last 48 hours without water, since you are losing it through excretion, respiration, and perspiration, and once the body water level drops below 45% a person goes into a state of dehydration and eventually coma and death. Third, it will not be long before the gastric system will make its needs known; that is, your stomach starts demanding food. Humans on average need about 2,500 kilocalories per day for normal patterns of activity and rest, along with the basic nutrients of protein, carbohydrates, and fats. Macro- and micronutrient needs are a more long-term concern, but without them certain diseases will be inevitable (e.g., vitamin C and scurvy, vitamin B-4 and pellagra, copper and mental functioning). Finally, some form of shelter (housing) will be needed from the elements of sun, wind, and rains. In the Technophile world, where one's needs are met with a flick of some switch, it is useful to think through exactly the essential human biological needs that must be met to ensure survival. Obviously this little group of ten will have many other organization needs to address regarding social functioning. To mention a few, there are differences in gender needs, workload assignments, emergency procedures, personal and public rights and privileges, and a means of adjudicating disputes and grievances. These social-functioning needs, however, are both necessary and secondary to the biological needs of humans who interact with the island environment.

Environmental Changes

Climatic Changes and Air Pollution

Perhaps no area of environmental impact by human activity is more contested than changes in global climate. Climatologists, who study long-term changes in the Earth's weather conditions, agree that there have been many cycles of climatic change on Earth over the eons of time—from tropics in North Dakota to Ice Ages in California. The extent to which climatic changes are the result of human activities is the Great Debate among scientists, centering mostly on global warming. The best data today from the NOAA (U.S. National Oceanic Atmospheric Administration) indicates that Earth's atmosphere has grown 1/10 of a degree Celsius warmer during the past twenty years. Most of this warming has occurred in the northern hemisphere, according to data from the NOAA satellites, which measure the Earth's temperature about one mile above the surface, called the National Environment Satellite Data and Information Service. The fastest warming area is Canada's Northwest Territories, which warmed up 1.6 degree C. (or 2.5 degrees F.). North America and Europe were all warmer, with Siberia, Mongolia, Northern China, Korea, and Japan (Nippon) warming up 1.4 degrees C. (or 2.5 degrees F.) (NOAA, 1999). Other evidence for global warming comes from University of Colorado at Boulder's National Snow and Ice Data Center (NSIDC) that monitors via satellite the ice shelves off the Antarctic Peninsula. The two main ice shelves, the Larsen B and the Wilkins, have been retreating landward for the past 50 years, with losses of 7,000 square miles. However, in 1998 the total ice loss was a staggering 3,000 square kilometers (NSIDC, 1999). The current size of the Larsen B ice shelf is at 7,000 square kilometers and the Wilkins ice shelf is about 14,000 square kilometers.

Therein lies the debate: Even if scientists agree that the Earth's atmosphere is heating up (and there is no firm consensus so far), there is considerable disagreement as to whether human activities are responsible. This is because global warming is a natural occurrence based on the "greenhouse" effect of trapping solar heat. In simple terms, solar energy hits Earth's surface and most of it should bounce back into space; however certain gases in the atmosphere collect the heat and prevent it from escaping into outer space. These collector gases include water, carbon dioxide, and methane. Hence, much like a greenhouse with all the windows shut and no exhaust vents, heat collects inside the Earth's atmosphere and temperatures increase. Since the planet is so huge and there are so many modifying variables that could impact global temperature, scientists use computer models in an attempt to simulate Earth's climate and make long-term temperature forecasts. Like any computer model, they operate on a great variety of assumptions, and scientists have reached no consensus on them.

Furthermore, the Earth's climate is constantly changing from tropical to glacial and back again, so just what is normal for the planet, given these immense changes? Scientists refer to climate change as some predominant alteration of the mean climate conditions, and climate variability indicates fluctuation around some average temperature (Rosenzweig & Hillel, 1998). Thus, one has to take into consideration the timeframe of the analysis, whether decades or thousands of years, to determine whether a true climatic change is occurring.

The main types of greenhouse gases, indicated in order of importance in their impact, are as follows: carbon dioxide, methane, nitrous oxide, and chloroflurocarbons (see Table 3.5). As can be seen, there are natural and human sources for most of the greenhouse gases; hence calculating the human or anthropogenic contribution is complex. Carbon dioxide is the major concern in terms of global warming, given that the atmospheric levels have increased in the last 150 years from 280 ppm (parts per million) to about 360 ppmv^3, an alarming 30% increase (IPEC, 1995). This jump is attributed to the Industrial Revolution, the burning of fossil fuels, and the extent of land use modification. Current measurements indicate a slight decrease in global carbon dioxide emissions from human sources of a half percentage to 6.32 billion metric tons per year (Sissell, 1999). International agreements, such as the Kyoto Protocol, call for the United States to reduce its carbon dioxide emissions 7% by 2010. U.S. transportation is the fastest growing contributor of atmospheric carbon (see Table 3.6). Regarding the other types of greenhouse gases, methane has jumped from 700 ppbv (parts per billion by volume) in the preindustrial period (end of the eighteenth century) to 1,720 ppbv, and nitrous oxide has increased from 275 ppbv to 310 ppbv, and CFCs were nonexistent prior to the Industrial Revolution (IPCC, 1995).

Antagonistic to the effects of greenhouse gases are sulfate aerosols formed by the interaction of sulfur dioxide, sulfur trioxide, and other atmospheric compounds. Sulfate aerosols are dispersed into the atmosphere from the combustion of fossil fuels and volcanic activity. In the atmosphere these particles reflect solar radiation away from the Earth (negative radiative forcing) and produce a cooling effect on Earth's temperature (Kaufman & Fraser, 1997). Hence, measuring or predicting climatic changes involves a complex analysis of many variables.

Consequences of Global Warming

If global warming is a real phenomenon, than what are the potential impacts that it would have? The first area of concern is worldwide agricultural production, which is highly dependent on stable climatic conditions (Bazzaz & Sombroek, 1996). Arid areas of the world that are currently marginal in their productivity due

TABLE 3.5   *Primary Greenhouse Gases and Their Sources*

Greenhouse Gas	*Natural Sources*	*Human Sources*
Carbon dioxide (CO_2)	Plants and oceans	Fossil fuels: coal, oil, cement production, and land use practices
Methane (CH_4)	Wetlands, termites, oceans, and freshwater lakes	Fossil fuels: cow gas, rice paddies, plant burning, human and animal sewage
Nitrous oxide (N_2O)	Oceans and soils	Fertilizers, burning plants
Chloroflurocarbons (CFCs)	None	Solvents, aerosol propellants

Source: IPCC (1995), IPCC (1997).

TABLE 3.6   *Carbon Dioxide Production by Source in the United States*

	Million Metric Tons per Year: 1997
Residential	286
Commercial	237
Industry	483
Transportation	473
Total	1,049

Source: NECI (1998).

to limited rainfall will be made worst. Second, temperature-sensitive crop insect pests could increase their geographical dispersion and extend over new ranges (Wittwer, 1995). This may also happen with weed plants that compete against agricultural crops. Third, sea levels will continue to rise (as the South Pole ice melts) creating severe disruption in some parts of the world that are already close to sea level (Eisma, 1995).

The impact of global warming on agriculture will not be all damaging. Some regions will experience a longer growing season (i.e., a reduction in the number of frost-free days) and be able to increase the quantity and types of growable crops. For example, the United States is considered a low-vulnerable region because only 10% of the cropland is irrigated compared to areas such as Egypt, which is virtually 100% irrigation dependent (Rosenzweig & Hillel, 1998). Some countries such as Canada may actually experience a gain in grain production as a result of an expanding growing season. Mexico, South Africa (Zimbabwe, Kenya, and Senegal), and Chile are high-vulnerable countries since they already have low national food security, and drier conditions would further reduce local food production and necessitate increased import dependency.

Impact of Global Warming on Health

Global warming may have its biggest impact on human health by enhancing the distribution of disease pathogens (agents) and disease vectors (transmitters). Researchers at NIH (National Institutes of Health) predict that rising global temperatures would increase the range of the Aedes aegypti mosquito, which transmits viral dengue hemorrhagic fever. The A. aegypti mosquito is restricted to the frost-free zones of the tropics and subtropical regions. Global warming would extend the range of the A. aegypti mosquito, increase the feeding needs of the mosquito (and thus increase dengue fever transmission rates), and decrease the dengue virus's incubation times within the mosquito (Peterson & Pettengill, 1998). Dengue is a dangerous killer disease with no vaccine or treatment drugs. Approximately ¼ of the world's population is currently at risk for dengue fever, and global warming will exacerbate the problem.

Another mosquito-distributed disease that would be accelerated by global warming is the world's second leading cause of human mortality: malaria. Malaria infects approximately 300 to 500 million people each year and results in over 1 million deaths. It is a disease of the topical regions—Africa, Southeast and Central Asia, and South America. The disease is caused by protozoa, called Plasmodium, and P. falciparum accounts for most of the cases that are the most deadly (Benenson, 1995). Global warming would increase the range of the Anopheline mosquitoes that transmit the malaria protozoa, by means of increased precipitation in and near endemic regions (creating stagnant water pockets in which the mosquito larva mature) and by extending the temperature-sensitive zones for mosquito reproduction. Children are particularly vulnerable, with 3,000 dying per day each year worldwide from malaria (WHO, 1999).

Global warming will also cause an increase in precipitation that will make floods more common in vulnerable areas. The secondary consequence of floods is contamination of sources of potable drinking water with disease-causing pathogens. One disease of particular concern is cryptosporidiosis, which causes gastrointestinal (GI) distress and emesis, and can be fatal in individuals with weakened immune systems (e.g., the elderly and HIV/AIDS patients). Cryptosporidiosis is caused by a protozoan parasite. The protozoa live in the GI track of farm animals and wildlife. As the oocytes (eggs) mature they are distributed into human sources of water by means of agricultural runoff and farming. Cryptosporidia are not destroyed by chlorination, and can be removed only by running water though very minute filters. Currently there is no curative treatment for cryptosporidiosis. Table 3.7 presents a summary of key vectorborne tropical disease, their current infection rates, and predicted probability of expanded impact on human health if global warming persists.

TABLE 3.7 *Major Vectorborne Tropical Diseases*

Disease	Worldwide Prevalence (in millions of cases)	Probability of Increase Due to Global Warming
Malaria	300 to 500	Extremely likely
Schistosomiasis	200	Very likely
Lymphatic filariasis	117	Likely
Leishmaniasis	12	Likely
Onchocerciasis	17.5	Very likely
American trypanosomiasis	18	Likely
Dengue fever	10–30 (new per year)	Very likely
Yellow fever	<.005 (new per year)	Very likely

Source: Monastersky (1996).

Finally, new research indicates that global warming may cause global warming! It turns out that when tundra regions have increased temperatures, the soils increase their release of carbon dioxide anywhere from 112% to 326% (Welker, Fahnestock, & Jones, 1999). Carbon dioxide is a significant cause of atmospheric heat trapping, as previously discussed. The arctic region covers approximately 1/5 of the planet's surface and contains 30% of the Earth's stored carbon in its soils. Researchers found that, even with increased snow cover (due to increased precipitation), carbon dioxide release was higher in warmed areas (Welker, Fahnestock, & Jones, 1999).

Much is made in the news regarding El Nino, the natural periodic warming of ocean water temperatures off the west coast of South America. El Nino's impact causes major weather changes with far-reaching effects—causing droughts in some regions and floods and excessive precipitation in others. New computer modeling research suggests that global warming may actually initiate El Nino into

TABLE 3.8 *World Wide Web Box: Climate Change and Global Warming*

1.	United States National Oceanic and Atmospheric Administration	Http://www.Ncdc.noaa.gov/ol/climate/globalwarming.html
2.	National Ozone Organization	Http://www.Ozone.org/page20.html
3.	United Nations Convention on Climate Change	Http://www.unfccc.de
4.	Climate Change and Human Health Web	Http://www.JHU.edu/~climate

a more or less permanently occurring weather phenomenon (Timmerman et al., 1999). This could occur because global warming would cause ocean surface temperatures to increase more in the eastern Pacific than in the west (because the western Pacific is already relatively warmer).

Air Pollution and Health

Humans probably first encountered air pollution when lightning struck and started a raging savanna fire, sending clouds of smoke in their faces. Fire or pyrolysis is a "dirty" process that manifests a variety of pollutants that can harm human health. Whether the exposure is outdoors or indoors, the combustion of fossil fuels or biomass (e.g., wood, and animal manure) releases a variety of harmful compounds. These are sulfur dioxide (SO_2), nitrogen oxides (NOx), carbon monoxide (CO), and ozone (O_3), along with small suspended particulate matter (SPM) (Schwela, 1996).

Beginning with the environmental movement in the United States in the 1970s, a variety of so-called "carrot and stick" environmental protection laws have been passed to reduce air pollution emissions from industrial and transportation sources. For example, coal power plants have been retrofitted with so-called "scrubber" technology to reduce SO_2 emissions, and automobiles are required to have catalytic converters to reduce CO and NO releases.

In the 1990s there was a shift of emphasis to indoor air pollution because of the advent of super-insulated home construction that permits fewer external air exchanges and hence tends to "trap" pollutants indoors. EPA studies identified alarming levels of radon gas in many homes in the United States. Radon is a naturally occurring radioactive gas emitted from rocks and soil and often seeps into homes through cracks in basement floors and walls. The EPA estimates a range of between 7,000 and 30,000 excess lung cancer deaths per year in the United States due to indoor radon exposure (Nadakavukaren, 1995). Indoor (or domestic) air conditions have also been implicated in the increasing incidence of asthma over the past three decades due to a variety of allergens (Jones, 1998). These "tighter" homes also trap more molds, dust mites, animal dander, and VOCs (volatile organic compounds) released from paints, carpets, and building materials.

In the developing world, most households must rely on the burning of unprocessed solid fuels such as wood, dried animal manure, and crop residues for cooking and heating. These sources of combustibles are very polluting and contribute to an estimated 2.5 million premature deaths worldwide (Rothman et al., 1999). Cleaner sources of fuel and safer technology are desperately needed throughout many of the Poverty-Quagmire countries.

Two new major air pollution problems that have been the focus of considerable research and evaluation are atmospheric ozone depletion and small-suspended particle matter. The ozone layer is a belt of O_3 gas that exists within the stratosphere ranging from 10 to 30 miles from the Earth's surface, and is most concentrated at 15 miles up. Ozone is produced naturally when energetic light from the sun strikes a molecule of oxygen (O_2) and splits it apart, creating O_1 atoms. The free-ranging O_1 atoms combine to produce ozone (O_3) gas. Ozone it-self is broken up by absorbing UV-B (ultraviolet B spectrum of light) radiation from the sun and protecting the planetary species below (see Figure 3.3). The threat to human health by ozone loss has to do with its blocking action of 99.8% of the sun's UV-B radiation (Lillyquist, 1985). Excess UV-B results in (a) in-creased risk of some skin cancers, (b) accelerated aging of the skin, (c) eye prob-lems such as cataracts and photokeratitis, and (d) reduced immunocompetency, which increases the risk of infectious diseases (Longstreth et al., 1998; Ma-dronich, 1998).

What causes ozone depletion? There are two main categories of threats: chlo-rine compounds and nitrogen oxides. Chlorine compounds remove the odd oxy-gen species of O_1 and O_3. These chlorine compounds are referred to as chloroflurocarbons (CFCs for short). Worldwide efforts have been undertaken to eliminate the use of CFCs in such aerosol products as hair sprays and shaving creams. Nitrogen oxides, produced by automobiles, commercial fertilizers, and commercial aircraft, react with ozone to produce nitrogen dioxide and oxygen (Lillyquist, 1985). The reaction is expressed as follows: $NO + O_3 \rightarrow NO_2 + O_2$. Ni-trogen dioxide then reacts with oxygen and the nitric oxide to further degrade ozone, expressed as follows: $NO_2 + O_1 \rightarrow NO + O_2$. Hence, nitrogen oxides can start a chain reaction of ozone depletion.

Much has been made in the media about the "ozone hole," which is actually a poor analogy. It is more like a thinning of the layer based on decreased concen-trations of the O_3 gas. Worldwide monitor efforts are ongoing to assess the chang-ing status of the ozone layer. Recently reported trend analysis by NOAA for the period 1992 to 1996 indicates that the levels of ozone-depleting chemicals in the

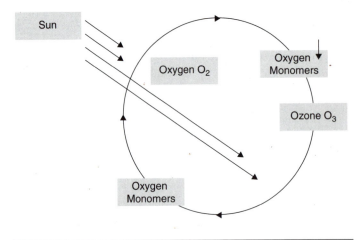

FIGURE 3.3 *The Ozone Cycle, Birth and Death*

atmosphere are declining. This decline is mostly due to reduction in the levels of methyl chloroform, a solvent that has been phased out of use worldwide. Other ozone-depleting chemicals such as CFC-12, used in refrigeration technology, continue to increase, while CFC-11, used in foam manufacturing, has decreased (Montzka et al., 1999, Fraser & Prather, 1999).

Small Particulate Matter (SPM)

SPM is very tiny particulate matter that remains suspended in air and can be readily ingested into the deep recesses of the lungs. The EPA estimates that there are 60,000 excess deaths per years in the United States due to exposure to SPM. The primary sources of SPM are diesel engine fumes, agricultural activities that generate dust, and certain industrial practices. The most dangerous and invisible SPMs are connoted as PM-10 (particle matter with a diameter less than 10 micrometers). The EPA has established two human exposure limits for SPM as follows: (1) Within 24 hours, not to exceed 158 micrograms per cubic meter of air (ug/m^3) more than three times per year, and (2) an annual mean exposure not to exceed 50 ug/m^3.

PM-10 and even smaller particles referred to as PM-2.5 cause deep inflationary response in the lungs, much like an allergic response by the immune system. This can often prove to be fatal for individuals with a preexisting respiratory condition such as emphysema or asthma. In Europe, a study found increased morbidity and mortality due to cardiopulmonary complications associated with elevated SPM levels (Monn & Becker, 1999). These lung injury deaths resulted from an imbalance of immune response inflammatory mediators (i.e., cytokines). A similar finding occurred in the United States (Schwartz, 1999). In California, a study found a strong association between mortality from nonmalignant respiratory diseases and PM-10 levels (Abbey et al., 1999). When PM-10 exceeds 100 ug/m^3 the relative risk for mortality was 1.18 among a 15-year cohort of nonsmokers, and relative risk was 2.38 for lung-cancer–related deaths (Abbey et al., 1999).

After the tent goes up, what do most campers do? What is considered the pinnacle of romance to cuddle next to? The answer is burning biomass! The campfire and the fireplace are seemingly harmless activities. Yet the World Health Organization estimates that 3 million preventable deaths and respiratory diseases per year worldwide are due to exposure to wood smoke (WHO, 1997). For example, fire from fireplaces and wood stoves is the single greatest source of PM-2.5 that enters people's homes in the United States. Just a few hours of wood burning by one family can cause all houses in the neighborhood to exceed SPM limits by a factor of 20. Governmental agencies in the United States are moving aggressively to monitor SPM levels and issue PM-10 alerts to the public. Diesel exhaust particles in particular are being investigated in connection with their role in global increases in allergic respiratory disease, such as allergic rhinitis ("hay fever"). Diesel exhaust contains a variety of chemicals called polyaromatic hydrocarbons. Once these chemicals are deposited in the lungs, they diffuse into the cell membranes— where they directly provoke an immune response that is typical of what allergy

TABLE 3.9 *World Wide Web Box: Air Pollution Resources*

1. United States EPA Office of Air and Radiation	Http://www.EPA.gov/airsdata
2. European Environmental Agency	Http://www.EEA.dk

suffers recognize (Peterson & Saxon, 1996). These studies have significant public policy implications as countries such as France and Germany begin to reevaluate and reverse their move to all-diesel vehicles, which began in the mid-1980s.

Water Resources

Water is second only to oxygen as a fundamental nutrient for human life. Anatomically, in humans water accounts for 40% to 60% of total body weight, and when this bodily constituent drops below 8% to 10% of total body weight, dehydration sets in, eventually leading to coma and death. Humans under "normal" conditions need to consume around 2,550 ml per day; however during strenuous exercise or high heat conditions humans can lose 3 liters of water per hour due to perspiration (McArdle et al., 1991).

Humans can live in societies that vary greatly in patterns of water usage, but all of them have certain minimal water needs. Biophysiological consumption need is around one gallon per day (losses occur from respiration, perspiration, and waste elimination), food preparation (cooking and cleaning of utensils), and sanitation, where water is used as a medium for disposal of human waste (e.g., in the United States, 3.4 gallons per toilet flush). Societies also need water for industrial practices, agricultural irrigation, and recreational and aesthetic purposes.

Freshwater Distribution

Water is a non-negotiable natural resource that is essential for human life; however, it is not equally distributed around the planet. Approximately 97% of the Earth's water is in saline form in the oceans. The majority of usable freshwater is locked up in glaciers, arctic ice caps, and deep ground water sites (Butts, 1997). The freshwater sources available for human usage are dependent upon the hydrologic cycle (HC), which is easy to understand. The sun causes warming of the oceans sufficient to create evaporation, whereby water changes from liquid to gaseous state. The gas rises and becomes the constituent of clouds. The switch from ocean water to water vapor lowers the salinity such that it is consumable for humans. Rain, or precipitation, is the conversion of water vapor back to liquid form (or snow) that falls into lakes, rivers, mountaintops, and on the soils, and then has the potential for human utilization (Berner & Berner, 1995).

Even groundwater was originally precipitation from clouds that fell on the soils and rocks and gradually seeped (percolated) down to form deep underlying reservoirs of water. Streams and rivers represent natural sources that return the ocean's precipitation back to the ocean, completing the HC. Hence, dams that humans construct are simply a means of telling the HC to "slow down . . . what is the big hurry?" Dams are a means by which humans can capture the kinetic energy of water to generate electrical power, but they are also the way to capture freshwater for human use. China, for example, is in the process of constructing the Three Gorges Dam on the Yangtze River. Spanning 1.2 miles in width and 607 feet in height, it will take 20 years to construct, requiring 40,000 workers who will create a reservoir 370 miles long (Childs-Johnson, Cohen, & Sullivan, 1996). The dam will generate hydroelectric power and permit shipping up the 1,500 miles of Yangtze River to markets in Chongqing.

The HC is a stable planetary process (albeit global warming may have long-term effects), and as a result the quantity of freshwater produced by HC is considered essentially finite. The distribution of freshwater varies great over the planet. As the Earth's population increases each person must extract minimum daily requirements of freshwater in order to survive and carry out life activities. Water is characterized by what economists term an inelastic demand (you have to have it), and this results in enormous freshwater-shortage problems. The Johns Hopkins Population Information Program projects that by 2025, 30% of the Earth's population will live in regions short of water (Hinrichen et al., 1998). Countries are classified as water-stressed if annual supplies are below 1,700 cubic meters per person per year, and water-scarce when supplies are below 1,000 cubic meters per person per year. In 1997 it was estimated that one third of the world's population is living under water-stressed conditions, and this could increase to 50% by the year 2025 (Roberts, 1999).

Water and Human Health

The central problem confronting growing populations, besides inadequate quantities of water, is poor quality of water. Public health uses the term *potable* to describe water that does not cause disease when consumed by humans (Last, 1997). Nonpotable water results in over 250 million cases of disease worldwide every year and 5 to 10 million premature deaths (Gleick, 1998). Potable water is directly connected to the level of human sanitary infrastructure. Humans need to treat their waste products such that excreta are rendered safe or disposed of at a distance from human habitation sufficient to prevent breeding and transmission of diseases. Proper sanitation requires a minimum of 20 to 40 liters of water per person on a daily basis. Further, potable water requires that water sources not be contaminated with pollutants from industrial or agricultural sources. For example, in Shanghai 15 million people dump 75% of their raw sewage directly into the Yangtze River, the Huangpu River, and Suzhou Creek. This amounts to 4.125 million cubic meters daily (Qide, 1998). With a projected water demand of 11 million tons per day by 2020, Shanghai is facing serious potable water needs (particularly because the city's main source of water is the Huangpu and Yangtze Rivers) (Qide, 1999). Even five-star hotels in Shanghai have embossed warning plates affixed to all faucet fixtures: Not Potable. Agricultural activity remains the overall largest source of water pollution in almost every country, which is due to runoff from fertilizers, pesticides, and animal wastes (Hinrichen et al., 1998).

The World Health Organization (WHO) classifies water-related diseases into four distinct groups: (1) waterborne diseases, resulting from excreta contamination that contains a pathogenic (disease-causing) bacteria or virus; (2) water-washed diseases, resulting from inadequate personal washing and hygiene; (3) water-based diseases, resulting from parasites residing in intermediate aquatic hosts; and (4) water-related diseases, resulting from vectors that use the water medium for part of their reproductive life cycle. The most significant cause of human morbidity (suffering) and mortality on an annual basis is referred to as diarrheal diseases—afflicting an estimated 1 billion people per year and causing the deaths of 3.3 million annually (WHO, 1999) (see Table 3.10).

The enteric diseases infect the human digestive tract and are caused by bacteria, parasites, and viruses. Common examples include cholera, giardia, and rotaviruses. Diarrheal diseases operate within a synergistic cascade of worsening host conditions. Infection occurs, then diarrhea, then because of inadequate absorption of nutrients (malabsortion) and dehydration the person's immune system becomes weakened, lowering resistance to diseases, resulting in greater morbidity and mortality (see Figure 3.4).

Progress has been made in combatting diarrhea disease with the introduction of ORT (oral rehydration therapy), yet often diarrheal diseases last for weeks and remain a major source of death and human suffering. What typically happens is that the microorganism must first stick (adhere) to a section of the intestinal mucosa lining. Once established, the microorganism can produce either a toxin (called endotoxin or exotoxin) such as cholera, or a cytotoxin (cell killer) such as Shiga, which causes a weakening of or disturbance to the mucosal stability (Guerrant, 1994). This loss of intestinal integrity begins the cycle of malabsorption of nutrients, malnutrition, and weakened host resistance (Nesheim, 1993).

As populations continue to grow, the demands for water will intensify, particularly in countries that are already water-stressed. In India, where the population growth will increase to over 1 billion in the near future, water usage rates are twice as much as aquifer recharge rates. This could cause acute water-stress problems for large numbers of people and force irrigation cutbacks that would reduce agricultural grain production (Brown, 1998). In Lagos, Nigeria, a city of 7 million, the daily demand for water is estimated at 250 million gallons, and with no ready water collection infrastructure millions must spend their days searching and collecting water from dug-out wells (Hinrichen et al., 1998). Globally 31 countries, with around 500 million people, face acute freshwater shortages, and this is projected to increase to 2.5 billion people (or 35% of the world's population) by 2025 (Brown, 1998).

Potable water is the preeminent structural component of any society's functional public health. Clean water cures diseases by eliminating the many waterborne

TABLE 3.10   *Infectious Diseases*

Diseases	Morbidity (episodes/year, or as stated)	Mortality (deaths/year)	Relationship of Disease to Water Supply and Sanitation
Diarrheal diseases	1,000,000,000	3,300,000	Strongly related to unsanitary excreta disposal, poor personal and domestic hygiene, unsafe drinking water
Infection with intestinal helminths	1,500,000,000	100,000	Strongly related to unsanitary excreta disposal, poor personal and domestic hygiene
Schistosomiasis	200,000,000	200,000	Strongly related to unsanitary excreta disposal and absence of nearby sources of safe water
Dracunculiasis	100,000	—	Strongly related to unsafe drinking water
Trachoma	150,000,000	—	Strongly related to lack of face washing, often due to absence of nearby sources of safe water
Malaria	400,000,000	1,500,000	Related to poor water management, water storage, operation of water points, and drainage
Dengue fever	1,750,000	20,000	Related to poor solid waste management, water storage, operation of water points, and drainage
Poliomyelitis	114,000	—	Related to unsanitary excreta disposal, poor personal and domestic hygiene, unsafe drinking water
Trypanosomiasis	275,000	130,000	Related to the absence of nearby sources of safe water
Bancroftian filariasis	72,800,000	—	Related to poor water management, water storage, water operations, drainage
Onchocerciasis	17,700,000	40,000	Related to poor water management in large-scale projects

Source: WHO (1997).

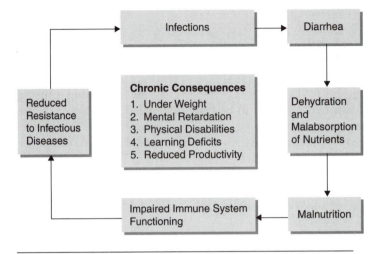

FIGURE 3.4   *The Diarrhea Disease Cycle*

TABLE 3.11   *World Wide Web Box: Water Resources*

1. National Institutes for Water Resources (NIWR)	˙Http://WRRI.NMSU.edu.NIWR
2. United States Environmental Protection Agency: Office of Water	Http://www.EPA.GOV/owow/index.htlm
3. Millennium Institute of Water	Http://www.IGC.apc.org/Millennium/ links/water.html

pathogens and allowing children to develop into healthy and productive adults. Water contributes to ending hunger by supporting agricultural production in order to sustain the population and undo the cycle of poverty that grips the Poverty-Quagmire countries.

Infectious Diseases

Herpes Virus

At the end of the twentieth century the topic of infectious diseases was supposed to be banished to old history books. Infectious diseases, formerly predicted to be controlled and eliminated, have formed brand new virulent pathogens (Binder et al., 1999). In the late 1970s, resurgent infectious agents appeared in the form of an odd little genital rash. A virus was identified as the etiological agent, and modest efforts were begun toward pharmaceutical remedies. The disease that sent anxious tremors throughout the sexually active community was herpes simplex II virus (HSV-2). Today the U.S. prevalence is estimated at 45 million, with an annual incidence rate of 500,000 new cases (CDC, 1998). There is no vaccine and no cure for this nonfatal disease; however, such new drugs as Valtrex (Valaciclovir-Hcl) and Famvir (Famciclovir) appear to better manage the episodic dermatological outbreaks.

Today, the forms of human herpes virus are expanding, causing new pathologic diseases that have yet to be fully delineated and nomenclatured (see Table 3.12). These human herpes viruses are ubiquitous in human populations, being transmitted by infant exposures to infectious saliva (airborne) and body fluids (HHV-1, HHV-3, HHV-4, HHV-5, HHV-6, HHV-7), whereas others appear to be mostly transmitted by sexual contact (HHV-2 and HHV-8) (Drago & Rebora, 1999). HHV-8 has been the focus of considerable recent research, since it appears to be the cause of a fatal form of skin cancer that primarily occurs in AIDS patients (i.e., Kaposi's sarcoma).

TABLE 3.12 *New Human Herpes Viruses*

Herpes Identification Name	Type of Disease	Pathology Descriptions
Herpes virus 1 (simplex 1)	Dermatological lesions	Typically oral cavity sores
Herpes virus 2 (simplex 2)	Dermatological lesions	Typically genital cavity sores
Herpes virus 3 (varicella-zoster)	Dermatological lesions	Whole-body dermal sores, known as chicken pox
Herpes virus 4 (Epstein-Barr)	Mononucleosis	Fever, sore throat, splenomegaly, and lymphocytosis
Herpes virus 5 (cytomegalovirus)	Systemic multi-organ infection	Malaise; hepatitis; infection of kidneys, pharynx; lymphoadenopathy
Herpes virus 6	Inflammatory disorders and malignant diseases; CNS diseases	Liver inflammation, auto-immune diseases, skin rashes, lymphomas, leukemia, infantile febrile illnesses
Herpes virus 7	Inflammatory disorders	Pityriasis rosea, exanthema subitum, chronic fatigue syndrome, infantile febrile illnesses
Herpes virus 8	Inflammatory disorders and malignant diseases	Kaposi's sarcoma, lymphoma, Castlemans disease, myaloma

Source: Adapted from Drago & Rebora (1999); Benenson (1995).

HIV and AIDS

If it were not for an obscure publication in the CDC's *Morbidity and Mortality Weekly Report,* June 5, 1981 and the subsequent AIDS (Acquired Immunodeficiency Syndrome) epidemic, herpes would have continued to dominate the world stage of infectious disease for many decades. The introduction of HIV/AIDS in the United States began with five cases of young homosexual males reported to the CDC as having died from a type of pneumonia (Pneumocystis carinii, that almost always infects the elderly) following the virtual collapse of their functioning immune system. It took several years before researchers Robert Gallo, of the United States, and Luc Montagnier, of France, actually identified the HIV virus that caused this collapsing immune system disease syndrome, the latter eventually receiving sole discovery credit (Alcamo, 1993).

Today, HIV/AIDS is a worldwide pandemic that continues to expand its range (Satcher, 1999). Some 34 million persons are currently infected with the HIV virus, with close to 6 million new cases occurring each year (UNAIDS, 1999). Deaths for 1999 stood at 2.6 million, with a total mortality count of 16.3 million since the epidemic began (UNAIDS, 1999). The WHO reported that over 95% of the worldwide HIV infected population reside in the developing regions of the world, and this is also where 95% of the mortality occurs. Sub-Saharan Africa is the region hardest hit by the HIV/AIDS pandemic, with an estimated 60% of the cases, and particularly devastating are the high infection rates among young women and children. For example, in Botswana, 25% of the adult population is infected, which adversely impacts the productivity of the society and transfers child rearing to the grandparents as young couples die off. Zimbabwe is projected to have 2,400 people dying per week of AIDS, leading to a 45% level of orphaned children (WHO, 1998). Swaziland now has the third-highest rate of HIV infection in the world, and the problem is exacerbated by limited government funding of educational prevention and the funding of AZT drug therapy only for those who have contracted the disease by means of needle contact or contaminated blood. Throughout Sub-Saharan Africa the primary means of HIV transmission is through heterosexual contact.

HIV/AIDS has been very "successful" from a pathogen's perspective, because it kills its host relatively slowly (an average of 11 years) and is spread by the two most fundamental drives humans possess—sexual activity and breast feeding. HIV also interacts with other STDs (sexually transmitted diseases), such as HSV-2, by taking advantage of STDs infectious sites that permit easier entry of the HIV into the bloodstream. HIV/AIDS is also particularly devious and devastating because it attacks and kills the cells of the human immune system (CD4 and CD8), the very system that provides protection from invading pathogens. Finally, HIV would never have become the global pandemic it represents if not for the fact that the virus was able to gain access to male semen. Semen is the critical linkage in the spread of HIV/AIDS—hence it is essentially a males-as-vector-based disease. Its origins have been established as a natural and inevitable transmission from the reservoir animals in equatorial West Africa; the HIV-1 type came from chimpanzees (pan troglodytes troglodytes) and the HIV-2 type from the Sooty Mangabey monkeys (Ceroccocebus atys) (Feng et al., 1999; Simon, 1999).

Currently there is no cure available, only drug combinations that slow the pace and postpone symptoms of declining immune function. The key may be developing clinical therapies that rebuild the immune system. Testing of vaccines (termed clinical trials) is underway, but it has been a particularly difficult task because the HIV virus is able to mutate very rapidly, which is termed viral polymorphism. In addition, this mutability leads inevitably to ineffectiveness of the combination drug treatments, known as drug resistance. The HIV replications can produce 10 billion viral particles daily in a person, thus eventually triumphing over the goal of drug therapy of eliminating the HIV infection (Erbelding, 1999). In time the complex virology of HIV will be controlled, but for the immediate future, behavior changes (i.e., "safer sex") that reduce the transmission of the virus are the most crucial means of preventive intervention. The young people alive today are the first generation to grow up always knowing about AIDS. Unlike syphilis, which ravaged and killed millions of people all of the world for 500 years, the AIDS pandemic will run its historical course and probably soon go the way of smallpox (i.e., will no longer be a threat to human health).

Newly Emerging and Reemerging Diseases

There are many new infectious threats to human health worldwide, along with the revival of infectious diseases that were once confined to minor epidemic levels. Some of these diseases are completely new; others are old ones that have been repackaged into new forms; still others are old diseases that, due to societal and environmental changes, have recently reemerged worldwide (see Table 3.13). For example, cholera, which is typically thought of as a killer disease of nineteenth-century England spread by fecal contamination of human drinking water, recently emerged in a new strain in Madras India designated 0139 (Balakrish et al, 1994). This new form of cholera attacks adults more often than children. New food-borne transmission concerns are being raised because survival of the cholera pathogen is actually enhanced by refrigeration and freezing, which may have contributed to rapid spread of the 0139 version (Albert, Neira, Motargemi, 1997).

Whether we like it or not, all humans are a delightful place in which to live, reproduce, and raise offspring for the millions of organisms inside us. Most of these masses of organisms reside in a more or less harmless manner, and some actually provide important nutrient-capturing services in the intestinal tract. Further, host and parasite relationships have evolved into a relationship of symbiosis in which one is benefited and the other is unaffected, termed commensualism (Tortora et al., 1997). These relationships take time to evolve, and there is a distinct survival advantage to organisms that are "nice" to their hosts, since promoting the death of one's host is not a very good way for a species to survive (Lappe, 1992). Disease pathogens such as the Ebola virus, which immobilizes and destroys its host in a manner of days, probably will not become very "successful" in terms of

TABLE 3.13 *Newly Emerging Infectious Diseases*

Disease	Year
Lasa fever	1969
Human toxoplasmosis	1970
Lyme disease	1975
Ebola fever	1976
Legionnaires' disease	1976
Cryptosporidiosis	1976
Rift Valley fever	1977
Hepatitis D	1980
Eschericia coli 0157:H7	1981
Human herpes virus-6	1986
Human ehrlichiosis	1986
Salmonella enteritis PT-4	1988
Hepatitis C	1989
Human herpes virus-7 and 8	1990
Vibrio cholera 0139	1992
Hantavirus pulmonary syndrome	1993
Hendra virus (Previously the morbillivirus)	1994
Human monkeypox	1996
H5N1 Avian influenza	1998
Nipah virus	1999

Sources: Karlen (1995); Pimentel et al. (1998).

worldwide distribution. Many of the newly emerging pathogenic agents are thus harmful to us because, in terms of evolutionary time, our meetings have been exceedingly quick.

A great variety of critical interconnected factors contributing to the emergence of new disease pathogens have been discussed throughout this chapter—population growth, malnutrition, pollution of air and water resources, and global warming. Other factors that epidemiologists contend are instrumental in the emergence of new disease pathogens include rapid international travel and trade, ecological disruptions of native environments, breakdown of essential public health systems due to regional military conflicts or inadequate governmental funding, development of antimicrobial resistance, microbial adaptation and change, and changing human social behaviors (Gubler, 1998; MacDonald & Osterholm, 1995).

The Globalization of the Human Immune System

Human population growth, international immigration, and the movement of peoples into urban centers contribute to the spread of infectious disease by simple crowding and rapid levels of interpersonal transmission. This is particularly relevant for airborne pathogens such as TB (tuberculosis) and influenza, which can race through concentrated populations. The twentieth century has also given rise to the prodigious expansion in international travel for both tourism and business. This can result in the direct importation of pathogens on persons, within foods, or in unrelated cargo. For example, approximately 70% of the fruits and vegetables eaten in the United States are grown in developing countries (MacDonald & Osterholm, 1995). A nurse treating Ebola patients in Kikwik, Zaire, gets on an international flight, lands at Orly Airport in Paris, switches to a second international flight, and, within a few hours, is landing at Toronto International Airport. This demonstrates with shocking reality how pathogenic exposure potentials have radically changed—what health experts refer to as "porous borders" (Shalala, 1998). Epidemiologists once used a concept called "herd immunity," which defines the minimum number of population-level immune systems needed to enable fending off a particular pathogen. The underlying presumption of the herd immunity concept is that adequate numbers of immune systems not resistant to a particular pathogen are sufficiently isolated so as not to transmit the disease further. What is fundamentally changing is the globalization of the human immune system (HIS). The HIS no longer operates in isolated population clusters (e.g., Santa Fe, Shanghai, or Budapest) surrounded by resistant protectors, but is more and more connected to the planetary pathogenic load. For example, TB bacterial strains that no longer respond to antibiotics (resistant strains) are incubated in Russian prisons and migrate westward across Europe and worldwide. Bacterial-resistant strains appear in some U.S. hospitals, and within months are identified in hospitals in Southeast Asia. The urban concentration of populations coupled with the international movement of people and products are the key changes that are leading to the globalization of the human immune system.

Ecological Disruption of Natural Environments

Many emerging infections result from pathogens that are ubiquitous in the environment and are essentially held at a status quo level by the natural functional limits of the indigenous ecosystems. These pathogens may can gain a selective advantage and infect new host populations following human disruption of the environment (Epstein, 1995; Morse, 1999). Deforestation and reforestation can dramatically alter the local ecosystem, resulting in the emergence of new diseases (CDC, 1994; Walsh et al., 1993). Removing forests not only puts humans into contact with new heretofore isolated microbial populations, but causes disruption of the soils that can potentially release new forms of E. coli, helminthes, and other microbes (Pimentel et al., 1998). Reforestation of the New England areas of the United States concurrent with intrusive urbanization brought humans in close proximity with the deer ticks that are the principle vectors of Lyme disease. Lyme disease is a devastating arthritis-type disease caused by a spirochete (Borrelia burgdorferi) that is transmitted by different forms of the Ixodes tick. The reservoirs for the spirochete are deer, mice, and migratory ducks. As the forested and brush areas of New England expanded, so did the the range of the deer and mice populations. As people bought or built houses in these semiforested tract subdivisions (e.g., Lyme, Connecticut), the transmission of Lyme disease to humans began.

Agricultural practices such as concentrated rice paddy farming in China are largely responsible for the emergence of the Hantann virus (named after the Hantann River in Korea) which causes Korean hemorrhagic fever. The Hantavirus lives harmlessly within a field mouse (Apodemus agrarius) that thrives in rice fields, and is transmitted to humans during annual harvesting times. The Hantavirus was brought to the United States by soldiers returning from the Korean conflict and has now established itself primarily in the Southwest United States (Ksiazek et al., 1995).

Japanese encephalitis (JE) is caused by a flavivirus that is spread by the Culex (tritaeniorhynchus) mosquito, which breeds primarily in rural pig-farming and rice-farming areas of Asia (Hennessy, 1996). JE results in 7,000 deaths per year in Asian countries (Morse, 1999). JE is a vaccine-preventable disease that occurs from India to Japan, as well as in China (Steinhoff, 1996). Of those infected with JE virus usually only 20 per 1,000 actually go on to develop the full-blown brain infection. In actual cases of JE, 40% recover completely, 30% recover with permanent neuralgic damage (e.g., paralysis), and 30% die. The incubation period of contact to illness is 6 to 8 days, and JE usually begins like the flu, with fever, chills, body ache, nausea, and vomiting. The symptoms can also be accompanied with mental confusion and agitation. China has undertaken a massive JE immunization program that has inoculated over 100 million children (Hennessy et al., 1996).

In early 1999, the CDC confirmed a new encephalitis virus, among patients of the Perak (Malaysia) outbreak of JE, that is a member of the Paramyxovirus family of viruses. The outbreak, involving 251 cases and 95 fatalities, was originally believed to be caused by JE. This new virus is 80% genetically similar to the Hendra viruses (which first appeared in Brisbane, Australia) and is now being designated as the Nipah virus. The reservoir for the Nipah virus is hogs, with around 5% infected; thus the Malaysian health authorities have recently put to death over 800,000 pigs in an attempt to end the epidemic (Enserink, 1999a).

Everywhere humans go they alter, change, or disrupt the ecology of a region's microbial inhabitants, which can also impact the population of microbial vectors (Gratz, 1999). Each spring at the CDC influenza tracking section has to determine which new strains of influenza A and B will emerge on the world stage and need to be immunized against the coming fall. The fact that virtually every year a new variant of influenza spreads across the world and predictably appears in the U.S. population is attributable to farming practices in rural China. Pigs and ducks are reservoirs for the influenza virus, and because they are raised in close proximity, the virus is able to leap back and forth and form new protein spikes on its outer shell sufficiently strong that the human immune system must prepare a whole new set of antibodies to attack it. The annual "flu shot" against these influenza strains is not an effort to combat a minor health threat. Historically the swine flu influenza of 1918 and 1919 (originating either in Iowa at a swine breeder county fair or possibly from a burning pile of hog manure at Fort Riley, Kansas) resulted in some 20 million deaths worldwide and still worries influenza specialists since it is never known when the next influenza virus will emerge. In 1997, the influenza A(H5N1) created a serious outbreak in Hong Kong, yet fortunately did not spread very far. Then, in 1998, another new influenza strain designated A(H9N2) emerged in Hong Kong that was genetically distinct from the GI/97(N9N2) virus. Fortunately, this new influenza produces only mild symptoms, no medical complications, and no fatalities. Continuing surveillance is essential to enable mounting a coordinated response should the next new influenza prove to be the catastrophic one that could threaten millions of lives.

Mosquitoes around the world are the primary transport (vector) of human death and disease through spreading malaria, Japanese encephalitis, Cache Valley fever, eastern equine encephalomyelitis, yellow fever, and many others. This is why the CDC is closely monitoring the spread into some 25 U.S. states of the "Asian tiger mosquito," Aedes albopictus (Moore & Mitchell, 1997). Albopictus arrived in the United States in shipments of used tires from northern Asia, demonstrating the ease with which potentially new disease vectors become transmitted globally.

Development of Antimicrobial Resistance

There is a certain irony that the race for earthly supremacy is between humans and microbes invisible to the human eye. At the beginning of the twenty-first century human influence has certainly predominated over the planet, yet we are seemingly only a few steps ahead of the microbial world. The societal threat from infectious disease is not just from novel microbes, but from microbes that are able to alter themselves to evade our best pharmaceutical weapons: the antibiotics. Antibiotic drugs, or, better, antimicrobials, have been around for the second half of the twentieth century, and have alleviated countless cases of infectious diseases, extending the life of hundreds of millions of people. Penicillin was discovered in 1928, when Dr. Alexander Fleming returned from vacation to St. Mary's Hospital in London and found that a Staphylococcus aureus culture had been killed out by a common soil mold (fungi) called Penicillium that had grown on the dish. By the early 1950s, antibiotics such as penicillin and sulfa drugs were in use worldwide.

There is no question that humanity has vastly benefited by the mass manufacture of antimicrobials. The diseases syphilis, tuberculosis, pneumonia, cholera, and plague terrified humans for centuries. The subduing of these microbial diseases was one of the greatest triumphs of human ingenuity. However, they have been subdued but not vanquished. They have been taking a tremendous beating, but they have not been dying passively. To understand how microbes in general developed the ability to evade our best antimicrobial drugs, we must first gain some understanding of the working mechanisms of antibiotics.

Antibiotics work by complementing the immune system's response to a pathogen by either bacteriostatic action, stopping the reproduction of the germ, or bactericidal action, which actually destroys the organism. Antimicrobials have essentially five mechanisms of action against a pathogen: (1) blocking microbial protein synthesis, (2) interfering with microbial cell wall synthesis, (3) changing microbial cell wall permeability such that germ waste products cannot escape, (4) blocking the microbial synthesis of DNA or RNA (stopping microbial reproduction), and (5) inhibiting microbial metabolism (Lambright-Ecker & Stimmel-Fair, 1996). Antimicrobials accomplish these actions as a result of their chemical structure, the beta-lactam ring.

Recent research indicates that antimicrobials work indirectly against the pathogen by causing it to kill itself. Researchers at Saint Jude Children's' Research Hospital in Memphis have found that the antibiotic penicillin causes the bacterium to release an enzyme called autolysin, which actually dissolves the bacteria's cell wall. Since bacteria are likely to live together in colonies, they will even sacrifice themselves for the "good" of the colony when conditions are unfavorable to the survival of the whole. Thus, the autolysin mechanism serves the purpose of allowing individual bacteria to commit suicide (Travis, 2000). Researchers hope to better exploit this suicide-signaling pathway by having drugs trigger the gene for the sensor proteins (Novak et al., 2000).

The microbial underworld has, over time, responded to the introduction of antimicrobial drugs into "their" host environment by a variety of very intriguing and at times ingenious adaptations. Their first challenge is to outwit the human immune system's army of attacking cytotoxic T-cells, antibody-producing B-cells (mature plasma cells), and the sophisticated system of "nasty" (depends on your perspective) attacking proteins called complement. Microbes do this by sometimes changing their outer capsule layer such that complement (C3b) can no longer "ripen" them up for attack (opsonize them), rendering the complement system inoperative. At other times they modify their fatty (lipopolysaccharide) complement binding sites on their surface. Still others evade phagocytosis, immune cell engulfing, by escaping before complete digestion can occur (the bug actually escapes the phagosome before it merges with the cell's lysomome). Another approach is for the microbe to alter the surface binding sites that antibodies use, such they are rendered ineffective. Finally, some microbes will coat their surface with human proteins, such as fibronectin, so that the immune system mistakes the microbe as being part of the human host and does not attack it.

When it comes to antimicrobial pharmaceuticals the microbes are equally smart. Their first line of circumventing antimicrobials is to simply change themselves sufficiently that the antimicrobial drug binds poorly and thus has a reduced effectiveness. Secondly, the microbe can produce an enzyme called beta-lactamase, which attacks the beta-lactam ring, rendering it useless. Microbes are also developing extended-spectrum beta-lactamase (ESBL) resistance (in their plasmids), meaning that they are able to produce mutant enzymes that confer variable levels of resistance (Sirot, 1995; Lautenbach, 1999). These enzymes are able to hydrolyze the beta-lactam antibiotics, rendering them inactive (Kohler et al, 1999). In addition, microbes are able to gain resistance over the so-called broad-spectrum beta-lactam antibiotics (BSBL), such as the third-generation cephalosporin, used to combat multiple microbes at the same time.

Microbes may also engage in what is termed "active efflux," in which the drugs are disengaged from the binding sites on the microbe's surface. They may reduce a drug's access to a given microbe by impairing the drug's ability to penetrate it. All of these mechanisms lead to what is termed "resistance," the ability of the microbe to resist or defeat an antimicrobial drug. Finally, the DNA of the microbe can simply and spontaneously change, called a mutation, whereby it now has the ability to fend off the antibiotic.

The most alarming phenomenon involving microbial resistance involves plasmids—little packets of genetic material outside a cell's nucleus in the cytoplasm. Microbes can pick up genes that are resistant to an antibiotic and store them in their plasmids. From there the antibiotic-resistant genes can be passed on to other microbes of the same species, and even to other microbial species! There are several means by which plasmid genes are transferred, the most interesting of which is referred to as conjugation (Burton, 1992). With conjugation, bacteria attach to each other by means of a tentacle-like structure called a pilus; they then engage in a sort of "sexual act" and pass along genes that code for resisting the antibiotic. These plasmids can also pass along genes that code resistance not just for one but for many different antibiotics, termed multiple drug resistance (MDR).

Why Is Antibiotic Resistance Happening Now?

Antibiotic resistance is not a new phenomenon, and resistant microbes developed soon after the introduction of antibiotics into population-based usage in 1942. Today, however, we are dealing with an accelerated pace of antibiotic resistance that threatens to overwhelm most of the tried and true antibiotic drugs in the medical arsenal. The key anthropogenic factors in this global problem can be summarized as follows: (1) the overprescribing of antibiotics, (2) the inappropriate prescribing of antibiotics for illnesses that are not treatable by antibiotics, (3) overuse of antibiotics as a feed supplement for livestock production, (4) rapid worldwide dispersing of antibiotic-resistant strains, and (5) the failure of the patient to properly use the prescribed antibiotic (Farmer, 1996; Huemer & Challem 1997).

Antibiotic prescriptions exceed 100 million per year in the United States (Wu, 1999), and as a result the microbes have ample opportunity to undergo adaptive changes in order to survive. This phenomenal rise in antibiotic prescription use results in part because people want quick fixes to illnesses, and when a child is sick the parents can be very insistent in obtaining a prescription. This leads to inappropriate prescribing of antibiotics for diseases that they were never intended to treat (e.g., bronchitis or sinuus when caused by a virus). Another major contributor to antibiotic resistance as mentioned, is the patients not completing the entire prescription. The patient feels better in a few days and does not take the entire course of the antibiotics. This is a particular concern with TB, and results in many surviving bacteria that are now resistant to the particular antibiotic used. Other problems include excessive presurgical administration of antibiotics (even among dentists) because of the rise of nosocomial infections—those that patients get just by going to a hospital or clinic. In the United States, there are over 2.5 million of these infections each year and some 88,000 deaths (Weinstein, 1998), and approximately 15% of these deaths are due to antibiotic resistance cases. Hospitals are major breeding grounds for microbes, staff pass them from patient to patient, and there are many antibiotic prescriptions to combat them, all of which contributes to further antibiotic resistance and more antibiotic-resistant deaths. The most dangerous place in the hospital for nosocomial infections is the ICU (intensive care unit), where the acquisition rates are 5 to 10 times greater than in other parts of the hospital (Weber et al., 1999). There are even reports of community-acquired antibiotic resistance, particularly in large urban centers (Herold et al., 1998).

The extensive use of antibiotics as a growth promoter among livestock may also be contributing to antibiotic resistance. Cows, chickens, and pigs are all given antibiotic supplements, such as chlortetracycline, on an ongoing basis, to promote rapid growth and weight gain (Huemer & Challem, 1997). The antibiotics are given at subtherapeutic levels, which provides an opportunity for bacteria to become resistant. Subsequently, antibiotic-resistant bacteria such as E. coli and Salmonella can make their way into the human population.

A recent study by the Minnesota Department of Health regarding fluoroquinolone resistance found that Minnesotans returning from foreign travel had antibiotic-resistant Campylobacter jujuni. These travelers apparently acquired the resistance bacteria as a result of consuming foreign meats, such as beef and chicken.

Key Microbes Gaining Resistance

Which are the key microbes that are gaining resistance? The first microbe that gained resistance to penicillin was Staphylococcus aureus, a bacteria that is usually a benign occupant in the human host but can turn hostile and produce pneumonia (see Table 3.14). Streptococcal pneumococcus can cause purulent meningitis, bacteremia, community-obtained pneumonia, and acute otitis media, and has reached levels of penicillin resistance of 40% in North America (Butler & Cetton, 1999). Campylobacter jejuni causes over 2 million cases of gastrointestinal dysentery each year in the United States, with 1/1000 developing GBS (Guillain-Barre syndrome), which causes 20% of the cases to have varying levels of permanent neuromuscular paralysis (Altekruse et al., 1999).

Bacteria are not the only microbes gaining resistance. The protozoa Plasmodium falciparum, which causes most of the 300 million annual malaria cases, has developed resistance to chloroquine, one of the commonly employed prophylaxis drugs (Lobel & Kozarsky, 1997). The fungus Candida albicans, which causes havoc for AIDS and cancer patients, appears to be gaining resistance. The human immunodeficiency virus is also developing resistance to the antiviral drugs currently employed in treatment (Hirsch et al., 1998).

TABLE 3.14 *Bacteria Resistant to Antibiotics and Their Diseases*

Pathogen	Diseases
Entrobacteria	Pneumonia, urinary tract infections, bacteremia
Haemophilus influenza	Ear infections, pneumonia, and meningitis
Mycobacteria	Tuberculosis
Neisseria gonorrhea	Sexually transmitted disease, dermal lesions
Shigella dysteria	Dysentery (bloody diarrhea)
Pseudomonas aeruginosa	Pneumonia, urinary tract infections, bacteremia
Staphylococcus aureus	Bacteremia, pneumonia
Camplylobacter jejuni	Dysentery, Guillain-Barre syndrome
Staphylococcus pneumoniae	Purulent meningitis, bacteremia, pneumonia, and otitis media
Bacteriodes	Septicemia, pneumonitis
Acinetobacter	Nosocomial infections, pneumonia
Klebsiella	Pneumonia, meningitis
Escherichia coli	Gastro-intestinal diarrheal diseases
Enterococci	Bacteremia, meningitis, sepsis

Source: Adapted from Butler (1998); Huemer & Challem (1997); Wisner et al. (1999).

Antibiotic Resistance: Individual and Global Solutions

At the individual level, people need to practice as many safeguarding measures as possible so that antibiotics will be effective when they are really necessary. First, they should be used only when appropriate, realizing that they are not effective against viral infections (e.g., the "common cold"). Second, an individual who gets a prescription should take the entire regimen and at the indicated time intervals. Third, people should never use leftover prescriptions—their own or, particularly, those of others—since self-administration of antibiotics may be for an incorrect infection and have diminished or lapsed potency. Finally, the public's attitude toward antibiotic must change. Antibiotics are not "medical candy," but powerful drugs that should be prescribed when needed. They should not be the result of pressure on the physician to calm one's undue fears.

Globally, medical practice needs to use antibiotics with much greater restraint and prudence. Prescribing an antibiotic for viral bronchitis is the best example of inappropriate and excessive usage. Results of laboratory tests must be more rapid so the patient does not have to wait several days to find out if an antibiotic really is needed. Second, nosocomial infection stands at 2,000,000 per year in the United States, and is mostly due to inadequate professional hygiene practices between patient contacts. Hospital and clinic staff need to improve noso-comial control by simple measures such as equipment sterilization and hand washing. Third, cross-border movement of antibiotics and self-medication is another problem, particularly across the American southwest where U.S. citizens cross into Mexico and purchase over-the-counter antibiotics (i.e., not prescription based). The practice is illegal in the United States, but when one is returning from Mexico, pharmaceuticals do not need to be declared to U.S. Customs. Finally, at the global level, undertrained pharmacists in developing countries often do not know the proper use of antibiotics. Uneducated parents whose child has a chronic condition (e.g., asthma, MS, or MD) end up switching doctors and treatments, hoping to find the "magic cure," all to no avail (Schwartz & Casillas-Miranda, 1998). All of this inappropriate use and misuse of antibiotics contributes to the international issue of antibiotic resistance. We also need better worldwide hospital and clinic-based surveillance systems that can monitor and report resistance events, to enable better orchestrated responses.

Mad Cow Disease

The new pathogens, which are sometimes old ones in new packages, just keep coming. "Mad cow disease," also known as bovine spongiform encephalopathy (BSE), is caused by a totally new pathogenic agent—a rogue protein called a prion (proteinaceous infectious particles). The primary outbreak was among British cows, beginning in 1996, but the disease has spread to cows in Ireland, France, Portugal, Switzerland, and Italy. Thus far, no U.S. cows have developed BSE. The human corollary of BSE is called transmissible spongiform encephalopy (TSE), because of the spongy degeneration of brain and because it can be transmitted to lab animals (WHO, 1999). Creutzfeldt-Jakob disease (CJD), the most common form of TSE, attacks the human brain much like runaway dementia, leading to loss of bodily functioning and death. The etiology of TSE transmission is still not fully understood, with 85% of cases occurring sporadically, 10% inherited, and 5% iatrogenic (a result of a medical procedure) (WHO, 1999). There is an epidemiological association with eating bovine meats and exposure to bone meal. Iatrogenic cases have occurred after blood transfusion, corneal transplantation, and neurological surgery (Alter, 2000; Collins et al., 1999). CJD is also changing in that there have been 24 reported cases in the United Kingdom of a new variant form that is more closely linked to BSE (Will, 1999).

E. Coli on the Attack

In 1982, a new strain of E. coli, designated as 0157:H7, emerged. The initial outbreak in the United States occurred in Portland, Oregon, and was traced to exposures to undercooked bovine meats. E. coli 0157:H7 causes severe gastrointestinal distress such as acute hemorrhagic colitis and diarrhea (Tarr, 1995). The organism lives harmlessly in the guts of cows and is the source of subsequent meat contamination; unlike its older cousin, it requires only a few microbes to result in infection (Huemer & Challem, 1997). In 1994, another new strain of E. coli erupted in Montana. It was traced to contaminated bovine milk and is designated 0104:21. It, too, causes rapid onset of diarrhea, emesis, and fever. In 1996, Nippon had an outbreak of 0157:H7 that resulted in over 9,000 cases and several deaths. The exposure was to undercooked beef. New vehicles of transmission for 0157:H7 include unpasteurized apple cider, lettuce, and salami.

Flesh-Eating Bacteria

A common bacteria found in the human throat and on the skin is called Group A Streptococcus pyogenes (GAS), and it has recently turned into a killer dubbed by the media as "flesh-eating bacteria." GAS also causes the deadly toxic shock syndrome (Benenson, 1995). GAS is the common microbe that causes "strep throat," and is thus easily spread by ordinary human-to-human contact. When infectious microbes attack and kill human muscle and adipose tissue, the disease is termed necrotizing fascitis (NF) (Kotrappa et al., 1996). NF begins when a person's normal defenses of the integument (skin barrier) are weakened and/or a person's immune system is diminished. There have even been reports of NF as a result of toothpick injuries (Gilad et al., 1998). In Nippon there have been cases of NF caused by eating raw seafoods, and subsequent liver disease caused by vibrio vulnificus (Fujisawa et al., 1998). In the United States, the Centers for Disease Control and Prevention report some 10,000 cases of GAS per year, with 800 involving NF. Treatment involves the very aggressive administration of antibiotics, since multiple organ system failure can rapidly overwhelm the victim.

Infectious Diseases: Future Solutions

Worldwide infectious diseases remain the single greatest cause of an estimated 17 million deaths per year. New antimicrobial pharmaceuticals are in development that will move away from the "broad sprectrum" approach—that wipes out the "bad guys" along with bacteria that are beneficial for humans—and attack the microbe with much greater specificity. However, in the most promising new line of research, vaccines will be developed that actually "switch off" the microbe genes that cause a given disease (Enserink, 1999b). Many pathogens have the gene that produces the protein DNA adenine methylase (DAM). When the DAM is knocked out, the bacteria are then incapable of producing disease (Heithoff et al., 1999). Thus, one vaccine that inactivates the DAM gene would work against a whole host of diseases, including cholera, plague, yellow fever, dysentery, influenza, meningitis, and syphilis, and it may have applications to combat HIV/AIDS and cancer. Switching off the microbe genes that cause the disease may hold great promise in the near future. Another line of important research, genetic engineering, involves improving the functioning of human immune system cells. In a recent breakthrough, researchers were able to improve the receptor site on T-cells so that they would better bind to and attack a pathogen. This would be most beneficial in combating diseases such as AIDS and cancer that develop from a failure of the immune

TABLE 3.15 *World Wide Web Box: Infectious Diseases*

1. National Center for Infectious Diseases	Http://www.cdc.gov/ncidod/
2. Journal of Emerging and Infectious Diseases	Http://www.cdc.gov/ncidod/eid/index.htm
3. World Health Organization: Communicable Disease Surveillance and Response Center	Http://www.who.int/emc
4. National Center for HIV, STD & TB Prevention	Http://www.CDC.gov/nchstp/od/nchstp.html
5. Emerging Infectious Information Network	Http://info.med.yale.edu/EIINET/welcome.html
6. AGIS: Sisters of St. Elizabeth of Hungary	Http://www.aegis.com
7. Infectious Disease Links	Http://Pages.prodigy.net/pdeziel
8. Outbreak News	Http://www.Outbreak.org/cgi-unreg/dynaserve.exe/index.html
9. Johns Hopkins HIV Service	Http://www.hopkins-aids.edu
10. Joint United Nations Program on HIV/AIDS	Http://www.us.unaids.org

system to mount a successful antibody response. In addition, this biogenetic engineering opens the door to blocking the immune system in treating such inappropriate autoimmune diseases as rheumatoid arthritis and multiple sclerosis. Other new research involves blocking the ability of microbes to move bodily cells around with them, referred to as "cellular hijacking." The body's cells move by means of a signaling proteins, called actin. A microbe, like Listeria, is able to gain control of the actin, enabling it to dash about the body creating disease (Prehoda et al., 1999). These fantastic new developments at the molecular and gene level have led some researchers to once again raise the possibility of a disease-free future (Schwartz, 1998; Schwartz, 1999).

Global Environmental Health Solutions

Throughout this chapter the topics related to global environmental health have been presented in a linear manner to better enable the reader to digest the diverse information. However, the functioning world ecosystem is just that—a dynamic, holistic manifold of interconnected and interacting biological, hydrological, geophysical processes, all driven by our extraterrestrial sun. Humans have been one of the most successful species on the planet, and they have attained that status not by the passive process of evolution among countless ancestors. They have advanced by emerging in the Pleistocene with their complex brains to constantly strive to proactively adapt the environment to comply with their needs and desires. We need water for our crops, so we build irrigation dams or dig wells. In order to move into severe winter climates, we harness heat sources such as oil, gas, and coal, and we build insulated homes. When paleontologists first uncovered the so-called "ice man" that was remarkably preserved over a thousand years, what most impressed them was the fact he was wearing what would have passed for shoes. We do not wait for Darwinian selection to grow fur on the bottoms of our feet so we can move into cold climates; we invent tools that permit our rapid adaptation to new environmental conditions. By projecting symbolic communications both verbally and in written form, humans are able to dominate all other species. We can organize ourselves to carry out mutually beneficial activities, such as procuring food and shelter, and forming common defense strategies. Zoologists accurately refer to humans as the "big brained apes" because of our unparalleled capacity to learn, store, process, and apply symbolic knowledge. No other species has evidenced such ability.

Collectively, these interrelated components are the very core of our human nature and are what has propelled our enormous success as a species. However, it is this ability to bend the environment to meet our adaptive needs that now poses severe challenges to our survival. Population size is a critical dimension in all the global environmental health concerns that have been presented here. It contributes to ecosystem degradation as it causes air, water, and soil pollution, as well as the release and dissemination of newly emerging infectious agents.

However, population per se is only part of the dynamics of the problem. How humans individually and collectively constitute their society's utilization of the natural world is preeminently critical. With only 20% of the population, people in the developed world utilize the majority of Earth's resources (Davis & Meyer, 1999). The world's ecosystem would be taxed to the maximum and could not sufficiently absorb the abuse that would occur if, for example, everyone in China and India drove gas-hog sport utility vehicles. However, if we used nonpolluting hydrogen-based automobiles, this would produce much less environmental degradation that current vehicle types cause.

Knowledge Export and the Poverty-Quagmire Countries

The poor countries of the world are different in many ways from the developed world, but what is most striking is the enormous disparity in knowledge levels. The Poverty-Quagmire countries have vastly diminished means for knowledge transfer to their populace. Generating knowledge and transferring it to people are costly tasks that are often beyond the resources of a developing country.

Poor countries often undertake large-scale industrial projects or massive purchasing of armaments which result in huge external debt. To repay these loans they have to sell off their limited natural resources (e.g., hardwoods, petroleum), and/or undergo debt "restructuring," which results in (a) further depletion of local ecosystem and (b) reduction in funding of knowledge-generating and knowledge-transferring institutions (i.e., education) (Davis & Meyer, 1999). The solution resides in two basic kinds of knowledge importation (IBRD, 1999). Knowledge about technology is simple know-how of things—for example, maternal and child developmental nutrition, computer software usage, immunization, and maintaining of potable water sources. Knowledge about attributes is knowledge that enables a person to assess the quality of goods and services offered in the marketplace. For example, consumers need to be able to assess the quality of goods and services so that producers of low- or poor-quality goods and services do not gain an unfair competitive advantage over those producers with good- and high-quality products. A society also needs to have the legal and institutional structures to make attribute assessments such that consumers can have a functioning level of trust and utility in the products they acquire. The developed world has extensive means of training, credentializing, and licensing individuals who perform various technical functions in the society (e.g., medical doctors, nurses, CPA accountants, health education specialists, etc.). It also has the legal means to enforce contracts for goods and services, along with legal disincentives for failures to fulfill these contracts (e.g., punitive lawsuits and criminal incarceration).

In simple terms, for a person to survive and progress he or she has to know a lot of stuff. Yet developing countries do not have to reinvent computers, vaccines, tractors, irrigation pumps, or solar-based photovoltaic roof shingles for generating electricity. They do need sufficient and focused educational training to enable technology utilization and knowledge transfers. Education has an important impact on all aspects of a society, particularly regarding the public health. A study that examined a total of 45 developing countries found a dramatic decrease in infant mortality as education levels increased among women (see Table 3.16)

The link between parental knowledge and family health and productivity can be illustrated with many examples. Household maintenance of potable water reduces diarrhea-causing diseases, and when infections occur the employment of

TABLE 3.16   *Infant Deaths and Education Levels of Mothers*

Education Level	*Infant Deaths per 1,000 births*
No formal education	144
Primary education	106
Some secondary education	68

Source: International Bank for Reconstruction and Development (1999).

ORT (oral rehydration therapy) can be lifesaving. Respiratory infections kill some 4,000,000 infants annually, and many of these deaths are related to lack of knowledge regarding harmful smoke exposure within the household. Greater knowledge results in greater family productivity, increasing standards of living, and reduced parental fertility. The linkage is simple to understand: When parents have greater security in the survivability of their children, they are more likely to (a) reduce the number of compensatory births, and (b) exhibit greater psychological investment in any particular child that is born. This latter change results in greater willingness to expend household resource investment for a child's education, health maintenance, and overall advancement.

The Poverty-Quagmire countries need sustained and increased assistance from the Technophile countries. The Technophiles could partner with these struggling countries as "mentors" to further their sustainable development. Many of these Poverty-Quagmire countries are experiencing "demographic fatigue"—a sort of societal demoralization, under the crushing struggle to educate their children, create new employment opportunities, and manage massive environmental degradation problems (Brown, Gardner, & Halwell, 1999). On top of this, the Poverty-Quagmire countries are experiencing what WHO calls the "double burden" of endemic infectious disease morbidity and mortality and escalating chronic disease (e.g., lung cancer, heart disease) caused by older populations and high rates of tobacco consumption (WHO, 1999). Hence, they need a system of educational transfer that includes health promotion to enable curtailing the adoption of the unhealthy lifestyle aspects of the developed countries. It would be ironic and tragic indeed if the developing countries simply traded in the burden of infectious diseases for the chronic diseases related to high fat/low fiber diets (with inferior nutrient density) and the excesses of alcohol and tobacco consumption.

Population and Environment Linkage

Ecologists conceptualize organisms and environments as inseparable, interactive, and dynamic systems. Through time these plant/habitat/animal interactions have evolved into more or less balanced ecosystems. Plants capture solar energy, stored as carbohydrates, and nutrients from the soils; these nutrients flow through predator/prey hierarchy and eventually are returned to the habitat. Humans transcend their ecosystems by means of technology and knowledge that is always pursuing greater control over resource-converting systems. This is both our great strength and vulnerability as a species and now threatens the global ecosystems by which we as functioning mammals are still intimately sustained and on which we are dependent.

The environment has two basic sources of hazards for human life—hazards of human origin such as pesticides, fertilizers, industrial chemicals, and hazards that occur naturally such as infectious pathogens. Addressing both of these sources poses different strategic needs; however, both require international, hence global, cooperation. For less developed countries the linkage between population, poverty, and the environment manifests hazards that result in the depressive cycle of habitat degradation, high birth rates, and lack of social-economic opportunities. This negative linkage cycle is particularly acute when the society: (a) is subsistence based with a high dependence on natural resources, (b) has a scarcity of potable water, (c) has costly levels of soil rehabilitation, (d) has low educational development, particularly for women, (e) has low social equity for women, and (f) has inequitable access to natural resources (UNFPA, 1998). Breaking this cycle necessitates empowerment of women; basic food, water, and medical security; habitat restoration; land tenure security; effective cooperative management of resources; and investment credits to spur economic opportunities.

This chapter elucidated the many potential consequences and harms to the global environment that are associated with population growth. Some population researchers even contend that uncontrolled population growth per se is the principle cause of worsening environmental destruction. Yet most of the potential global-level environment harm is caused by the Technophile and pre-Technophile countries that have declining population growth or are at least moving toward population stability. The developing countries and Poverty-Quagmire countries have tremendous environmental degradation problems, with the consequences typically contained at the local level. What is changing is the globalization of environmental disruptions and the degradation to human social-economic systems. The primary global threats are long-term climatic changes (such as global warming), because any efforts at correction will take decades if not longer time spans to bring into effect.

Second, there are the acute health threats posed by antibiotic resistance and newly emerging infectious diseases. For example, when the Marburg virus suddenly jumps from horses to humans in Australia, when new influenza virus strains emerge from pig/duck flocks in rural China, when antibiotics no longer work at a hospital in Bagley, Minnesota, and when resistant virulent strains of TB are encountered in Russian prisons, the consequences are all too real and threatening for everyone on the planet. This is sometimes referred to as the "death of distance" (Brown, 1999b), or the beginning of nonlocality. Like it or not, each person's immune system is becoming immersed in a global world, and human damage and disruptions to the environment have harmful consequences for the entire human species.

Summary

This past century exhibited unparalleled epidemiology transitions as societies moved from high infant mortality rates and high birth rates to low infant mortality rates and slowing birth rates. World fertility rates are declining, yet the Earth's population is still increasing, due mostly to population momentum (i.e., a larger number of young females entering their reproductive years). As the burden of infectious diseases declines in developing countries, problems are rapidly shifting to noncommunicable chronic diseases. Today these noncommunicable diseases account for 39% of the lost years of potential life in the low- to moderate-income countries, and 81% in the high-income countries (WHO, 1999).

The developed world cannot retreat from providing the necessary knowledge transfer to those countries struggling to sustain their populations. We cannot expect poor countries to contribute to solving environmental problems until they are able to meet their basic food, water, sanitation, education, and health care needs, nor can they develop environmentally sound economies that support the health and well-being of its citizens (Brown, 1999b). Ultimately we need a moral commitment to contribute to the sustainability of basic human needs. This commitment will entail a fundamental shift from the values of excess consumption to an ethic of meaningful aesthetics. These values will come from the globalization of our awareness. We all know the disruption that one sick family member can create in a household, and it is this fundamental realization that everyone is part of the human household that will foster in the dawn of universal compassion and preserve this marvelous blue- and green-colored planetary orb called Earth for future generations to come.

Discussion Questions

1. Why would a country's population continue to grow when fertility rates are below two children per woman?

2. What are some of the societal consequences of an increasing DR (dependency ratio)?

3. What are the societal factors that Malthus did not foresee that have allowed world population to increase so dramatically?

4. Discuss the potential for adverse environmental effects based on a society's level of technological development.

5. What are the possible adverse health effects of global warming?

6. Why is thinning of the atmospheric ozone layer alarming to public health officials?

7. Discuss the four main types of water-related diseases that have been identified by WHO.

8. Discuss the factors that have contributed to the reemergence of infectious diseases.

9. What does "globalization of the human immune system" mean?

10. What is antibiotic resistance and what factors contribute to it?

11. Summarize how global environmental problems can be addressed.

12. How do the quantitative and qualitative dimensions of population growth impact the sustainability of ecosystems, and how do these aspects of population growth impact the quality of life in any given society?

References

Abbey, D. E., et al. (1999). Long-term inhalation particles and other air pollutants related to mortality in nonsmokers. *American Journal of Respiratory and Critical Care Medicine, 159*(2), 373–382.

Albert, M. J., Neira, M., & Motargemi, Y. (1997). The role of food in the epidemiology of cholera. *World Health Statistics Quarterly, 50*(1–2), 111–118.

Alter, M. (2000). How is Creutzfeldt-Jakob disease acquired? *Neuroepidemiology, 19*(2), 55–61.

Alcamo, E. I. (1993). *AIDS: The Biological Basis.* Dubuque, IA: William C. Brown Communications, Inc.

Altekruse, S. F., Stern, N. J., Fields, P. I., & Swoedlow, D. L. (1999). Campylobacter jejuni: An emerging foodborne pathogen. *Emerging Infectious Diseases, 5*(1), 28–35.

Armstrong, G. L., Conn, L. A., & Pinner, R. W. (1999). Trends in infectious disease mortality in the United States during the 20th century. *Journal of the American Medical Association, 281*(1), 61–66.

Ayittey, G. (1999). *Africa in Chaos.* New York: St. Martins Griffin.

Bah, S. M. (1995). Quantitative approaches to detect the fourth stage of the epidemiologic transition. *Social Biology, 42*(1–2): 143–148.

Balakrish et al. (1994). Spread of Vibrio choleraw 0139 Bengal in India. *Journal of Infectious Disease, 169*(5), 1029–1041.

Barrett, R., Kuzawa, C. W., McDate, T., & Armelagos, G. J. (1998). Emerging and re-emerging infectious diseases: The third epidemiologic transition. *Annual Review of Anthropology, 27,* 247–271.

Bates, D. G. (1995). *Cultural Anthropology.* Needham, Mass: Allyn and Bacon, Inc.

Bazzaz, F., & Sombroek, W. (1996). *Global Climate and Agricultural Production.* New York: Food and Agriculture Organization, United Nations.

Benenson, A. S. (Ed.). (1995). *Control of Communicable Diseases Manual* (16th Ed.). Washington, DC: American Public Health Association.

Berner, E. K., & Berner, R. A. (1995). *Global Environment: Water, Air, and Geochemical Cycles.* Upper Saddle River, New Jersey: Prentice Hall.

Binder, S., Levitt, A. M., Sacks, J. J., & Hughes, J. M. (1999). Emerging infectious diseases: Public health issues for the 21st century. *Science, 284*(5418), 1311–1313.

Bongaarts, J. (1998). Demographic consequences of declining fertility. *Science, 282*(5399), 419–420.

Brown, L. (1998). Food scarcity: An environmental wakeup call. *The Futurist, 32*(1), 34–38.

Brown, L. R. (1999a). *Beyond Malthus: Nineteen Dimensions of the Population Challenge.* Scranton, PA: W. W. Norton & Company.

Brown, L. R. (Ed.). (1999b). *State of the World.* New York: W. W. Norton & Company.

Brown, L. R., Gardner, G., & Halwell, B. (1999). Sixteen impacts of growth. *The Futurist, 33*(2), 36–41.

Burton, G. R. W. (1992). *Microbiology for the Health Sciences.* Philadelphia: J. B. Lippincott Company.

Butler, J. C., & Cetron, M. S. (1999). Pneumococcal drug resistance: the new "special enemy of old age." *Clinical Infectious Disease 28*(4): 730–735.

Butts, K. H. (1997). The strategic importance of water. *Parameters, 37*(1), 65–83.

Caldwell, J. C. (1982). *Theory of Fertility Decline.* London: Academic Press.

Catton, W. R. (1987). The world's most polymorphic species: Carrying capacity transgressed two ways. *BioScience, 37*(6), 413–419.

Catton, W. R. (1998). *Malthus: More Relevant Than Ever.* Negative Population Growth Forum Series [Online] Available Http://www.npg.org/forums/catton_malthus.htm.

CDC. (1987). Staphylococcus aureus with reduced susceptibility to vancomycin: United States 1977. *Morbidity and Mortality Weekly Report, 46*(33), 765–766. Atlanta: U.S. Public Health Service.

CDC. (1994). Addressing emerging infectious disease threats: A prevention strategy for the United States. *Morbidity and Mortality Weekly Report, 43*(RR-5), 1–18. Atlanta: U.S. Public Health Service.

CDC, Division of STD Prevention. (1998). *Sexually Transmitted Disease Surveillance, 1997.* U.S. Dept. of Health and Human Services. Public Health Service. Atlanta: Centers for Disease Control and Prevention.

CFPC. (1999). Basic Views and Policies Regarding Population and Development. Beijing, Peoples Republic of China: China's State Family Planning Commission [Online] Available Http://www.sfpc.gov.cn

Childs-Johnson, E., Cohen, J. L., & Sullivan, L. R. (1996). Race against time: Chinese scholars scramble to save sites threatened by the world's biggest dam. *Archaeology, 49*(6), 30–45.

Ciment, J. (1999). Life expectancy of Russian men falls to 58. *British Medical Journal, 319*(7208), 468.

Collins, S., Law, M. G., Fletcher, A., Boyd, A., Kaldor, J., & Masters, C. L. (1999). Surgical treatment and risk of Creutzfeldt-Jakob disease: A case-control study. *Lancet, 353*(9154), 693–697.

Da Vanzo, J., & Adamson, D. (1997). *Russia's Demographic "Crisis": How Real Is It?* Santa Monica, CA: RAND. Center For Russian and Eurasian Studies: Labor and Population Program. RAND Issue papers. Website Address: Http://www.RAND.org/publications/IP/IP/62

Davis, S. M., & Meyer, C. (1999). *Blur: The Speed of Change in the Connected Economy.* Boston, MA: Little Brown & Company.

Drago, F., & Rebora, A. (1999). The new herpesviruses: Emerging pathogens of dermatological interest. *Archives of Dermatology, 135,* 71–75.

Ehrlich, A. H., & Ehrlich, P. R. (1991). Why isn't everyone as afraid as we are? *Focus, 1*(1), 15–18.

Ehrlich, P. R., Ehrlich, A. H., & Daily, G. C. (1993). Food security, population, and environment. *Population and Development Review, 19*(1), 1–32.

Eisma, D. (Ed.). (1995). *Climate Change: Impact on Coastal Habitation.* Boca Raton, FL: Lewis Publishers.

Enserink, M. (1999a). New virus fingered in Malaysian epidemic. *Science, 284,* 407–410.

Enserink, M. (1999b). Gene may promise new route to potent vaccines. *Science, 284,* 883.

Epstein, P. R. (1995). Emerging diseases and ecosystem instability: New threats to public health. *American Journal of Public Health, 85*(2), 168–172.

Erbelding, E. J. (1999). *Resistance Testing: A Primer for Clinicians.* The Hopkins HIV Report. Maryland: Johns Hopkins Hospital.

Farmer, P. (1996). Social inequalities and emerging infectious diseases. *Emerging Infectious Diseases, 2*(4), 259–269.

Feng, G., et al. (1999). Origin of HIV-1 in the chimpanzee pan troglodytes troglodytes. *Nature, 397,* 436–441.

Foster, M. S., & T. Taylor (1998). A doomed people: The collapse of the Hohokam at Pueblo Grande. *Archaeology, 51*(5), 44–46.

Fraser, P. J., and Prather, M. J. (1999). Uncertain road to ozone recovery. *Nature, 398,* 663–664.

Fujisawa, N., Yamada, H., Kobda, H., Tadano, J., & Hayashi, S. (1998). Necrotizing fasciitis caused by vibrio vulnificus differs from that caused by streptococcal infection. *Journal of Infection, 35*(3), 313–316.

Gaylin, D. S., & Kates, J. (1997). Refocusing the lens: Epidemiologic transition theory, mortality differentials, and the AIDS pandemic. *Social Science and Medicine, 44*(5):

Gelbard, A., Haub, C., & Kent, M. M. (1999). *World Population Beyond Six Billion,* Washington, DC: Population Reference Bureau. Website Address: http://www.prb.org/pubs/bulletin/bu54-1.htm

Gilad, J., Borer, A., Weksler, N., Risenberg, K., & Schlaeffer, F. (1998). Fatal necrotizing fasciitis caused by a toothpick injury. *Scandinavian Journal of Diseases, 30*(2), 189–190.

Gleick, P. H. (1998). *The World's Water 1998–99: The Biennial Report on Fresh Water Resources.* Washington, DC: Island Press.

Grant, L. (1998). *Juggernaut: Growth on a Finite Planet.* Santa Ana, CA: Seven Locks Press.

Gratz, N. G. (1999). Emerging and resurging vector-borne diseases. *Annual Reviews of Entomology, 44,* 51–75.

Gubler, D. J. (1998). Resurgent vector-borne diseases as a global health problem. *Emerging Infectious Diseases, 4*(3), 442–450.

Guerrant, R. L. (1994). Twelve messages from enteric infections for science and society. *American Journal of Tropical Medicine and Hygiene, 51*(1), 26–35.

Harding, A., & Holdren, G. (1993). Environmental equity and the environmental professional. *Environmental Science & Technology, 27*(10), 1990–1993.

Haub, C. (1998). UN projections assume fertility decline, mortality increase. *Population Today, 26*(12), 1–2.

Heithoff, D. M., Sinsheimer, R. L., Low, D. A., & Mahan, M. J. (1999). An essential role for DNA adenine methylation in bacterial virulence. *Science, 284,* 967–970.

Hennessy, S., Liu, Z., Tsai, T. F., Strom, B. L., Wan, C. M., Liu, H. L., Wu, T. X., Yu, H. J., Liu, Q. M., Karabatsos, N., Bilker, W. B., & Halstead, S. B. (1996). Effectivensss of live-attenuated Japanese encephalitis vaccine (SA14-14-2): A case-control study. *Lancet, 347*(9015), 1583–1586.

Herold, B. C., et al. (1998). Community acquired methicillin-resistant staphylococcus aureus in children with no identified predisposing risk.

Journal of the American Medical Association, 279, 593–598.

Hinrichen, D., Robey, B., & Upadhyay, U. D. (1998). *Solutions for a Water-Short World.* Population Reports, Series M, No. 14. Baltimore: Johns Hopkins University, School of Public Health, Population Information Program.

Hirsch, M. S., et al. (1998). Anti-retroviral drug resistance testing in adults with HIV infection. *Journal of the American Medical Association, 279,* 1984–1991.

Huemer, R. P., & Challem, J. (1997). *The Natural Guide to Beating the Supergerms.* New York: Pocket Books.

IBRD (1999). *The World Bank Annual Report 1999.* Washington, DC: The International Bank for Reconstruction and Development.

IPCC (1995). *Second Assessment Report: Climate Change.* New York: United Nations, Intergovernmental Panel on Climate Change.

IPCC (1997). *Stabilization of Atmospheric Greenhouse Gases: Physical, Biological, and Socio-Economic Implications.* New York: United Nations, Intergovernmental Panel on Climate Change.

Jones, A. P. (1998). Asthma and domestic air quality. *Social Science Medicine, 47*(6), 755–764.

Karlen, A. (1995). *Man and Microbes: Disease and Plagues in History and Modern Times.* New York: A Jeremy P. Tarcher/Putnam Book.

Kaufman, Y. J., & Fraser, R. S. (1997). The effect of smoke particles on clouds and climate forcing. *Science, 277*(5332), 1636–1639.

Kohler, J., et al. (1999). In vitro activities of potent, broad-spectrum carbapenem MK-0826 (L-749, 345) against broad-spectrum beta-lactamase- and extended-spectrum beta-lactamase-producing Klebsiella pneumonia and Escherichia coli clinical isolates. *Journal of Antimicrobial Chemotherapy, 43*(5), 1170–1176.

Kotrappa, K. S., Bansal, R. S., & Amin, N. M. (1997). Necrotizing fascitis. *American Family Physician, 53*(5), 1691–1697.

Ksiazek, G. T., et al. (1995). Identification of a new north american hantavirus that causes acute pulmonary insufficiency. *American Journal of Tropical Medicine and Hygiene, 52*(2), 117–123.

Lambright Eckler, J. A., & Stimmel Fair, J. M. (1996). *Pharmacology Essentials.* Saint Louis, Missouri: W. B. Saunders Company.

Lancet. (1999). An African Solution. *The Lancet, 355*(9153), 603.

Lappe, M. (1992). *Evolutionary Medicine: Rethinking the Origins of Disease.* San Francisco: Sierra Club Books.

Last, J. M. (1997). *Public Health and Human Ecology* (2nd ed.). Stamford, CT: Appleton & Lange.

Lautenbach, E. (1999). Control of outbreaks due to organisms producing extended-spectrum Beta-lactamases. *Journal of the American Medical Association, 281,* 1080.

Lillyquist, M. J. (1985). *Sunlight and Health: The Positive and Negative Effects of the Sun on You.* New York: Dodd, Mead, & Company.

Livernash, R., & Rodenburg, E. (1998). Population change, resources, and the environment. *Population Bulletin, 53*(1), 2–44.

Lobel, H. O., & Kozarsky, P. E. (1997). Update on prevention of malaria for travelers. *Journal of the American Medical Association, 278*(21): 1767–1771.

Longstreth, et al. (1998). Health risks. *Journal of Photochemistry and Photobiology, 46*(1–3), 20–39.

MacDonald, K. L., & Osterholm, M. T. (1995). Emerging infectious diseases: Controversies, causes, and control. *Minnesota Medicine, 78,* 41–44.

MacFarquhar, N. (1996). With Iran population boom, vasectomy receives blessing. *New York Times, 1,* 1:1, Sept. 8.

Madronich, S., et al. (1998). Changes in biologically active ultraviolet radiation reaching the earth's surface. *Journal of Photochemical and Photobiological Biology, 46*(1–3), 5–19.

McMichael, A. J., & Smith, K. R. (1999). Seeking a global perspective on air pollution and health. *Epidemiology, 10*(1), 1–4.

Malthus, T. R. (1798). An essay on the principle of population. pages, 15–130. In Appleman (Ed.), *An Essay on the Principle of Population: Text Sources and Background Criticism* (pp. 15–130). New York: W. W. Norton and Company, 1976.

Mason, K. O. (1997). Explaining fertility transitions. *Demography, 34*(4), 443–454.

McArdle, W. D, Katch, F. I., & Katch, V. L. (1991). *Exercise Physiology* (3rd ed.). Melvern, PA: Lea & Febiger Pubishers.

McFalls, J. A. (1998). Lively Demographics. *Population Bulletin, 53*(3), 3–48.

Monastersky, R. (1996). Health in the hot zone: How would global warming affect humans? *Science News, 149,* 218–219.

Monn, C., & Becker, S. (1999). Cytotoxicity and induction of proinflammatory cytokines from human monocytes exposed to fine ($PM_{2.5}$) and coarse particles ($PM_{10-2.5}$) in outdoor and indoor air. *Toxicology and Applied Pharmacology, 155*(3), 245–252.

Montzka, S. A., Butler, J. H., Elkins, J. W., Thompson, T. M., Clarke, A. D., & Lock, L. T. (1999). Present and future trends in the atmospheric burden of ozone-depleting halogens. *Nature, 398*(6729), 690–694.

Moore C. G., & Mitchell, C. J. (1997). Aedes albopictus in the United States: Ten-year presence and public health implications. *Emerging Infectious Diseases, 3*(3), 329–324.

Morse, S. S. (1999). *Factors in the Emergence of Infectious Diseases.* New York: Rockefeller University [Online] Available Http://www.cdc.gov/ncidod/EID/vol1no1/morse.htm.

Nadakavukaren, A. (1995). *Our Global Environment: A Health Perspective* (4th ed.). Prospect Heights, IL: Waveland Press Inc.

NEIC (1998). *Emissions of Greenhouse Gases in the United States, 1997.* Washington, DC: National Energy Information Center.

Nesheim, M. C. (1993). Human nutrition needs and parasitic infections. *Parasitology, 107,* S7–S18.

Novak, R., Charpentier, E., Braun, J., Tuomanen, E., (2000). Signal transduction by a death signal peptide: Uncovering the mechanism of bacterial killing by penicillin. *Molecular Cell, 5,* 49–57.

NOAA. (1999). *Global Warming.* Washington, DC: National Oceanic and Atmospheric Administration. [Online website]: Http://www.ncdc.noaa.gov/ol/climate/globalwarming.html

Nowak, M. W. (1997). *Immigration and U.S. Population Growth: An Environmental Perspective.* Arlington, VA: Negative Population Growth Organization. Website Address: http://www.npg.org/imm&cuspopgrowth.htm

NSIDC. (1999). *Antarctic Ice Shelves Breaking Up Due to Decades of Higher Temperatures.* University of Colorado at Boulder, National Snow and Ice Data Center [Online] Available: Http://www NSIDC.colorado.edu/NSIDC/ICESHELVES

Omran, A. R. (1993). The epidemiologic transition theory: A preliminary update. *Journal of Tropical Pediatrics, 29*(6), 305–316.

Orians, C. E., & Skumanich, M. (1997). *The Population-Environment Connection: What Does It Mean for Environmental Policy?* Seattle: Battelle Seattle Research Center. [Online] Available: http://www.battelle.org/

Peterson, J., & Pettengill, L. (1998). *Global Warming Would Foster Spread of Dengue Fever into Some Temperate Regions.* Bethesda, MD: National Institutes of Health. [Online website] Http://www.niehs.nih.gov/oc/news/global.htm

Peterson, B., & Saxon, A. (1996). Global increases in allergic respiratory disease: The possible role of diesel exhaust particles. *Annals of Allergy, Asthma and Immunology, 77,* 263–270.

Pimentel, D., Tort, M., D'Anna, L., & Krawic, A. (1998). Ecology of increasing disease. *Bioscience, 48*(10), 817–826.

Population Institute (1998). *21 Century Monograph Series.* Washington, DC: Population Institute.

Powledge, T. M., & Rose, M. (1996). Colonizing the Americans. *Archaeology, 49*(6), 58–60.

Prehoda, K. E., Do J. Lee, D. J., & Lim, W. A. (1999). Structure of the enabled/VASP homology 1 domain-peptide complex: A key component in the spatial control of actin assembly. *Cell, 97*(4), 471–480.

Qide, C. (1998). Clean-up drive aims to bring fish back to local rivers. *Shanghai Today, 1*(4), 24–25.

Qide, C. (1999). City Needs Clean Water. *Shanghai Star,* 08(0580), 1. Tuesday, March 30.

RAND. (1999). *International Family Planning: Labor and Population.* Santa Monica, CA: RAND Corp. Research Brief [Online] Available: http://www.RAND.org/publications/RB/RB5022

Ricklefs, R. E. (1979). *Ecology* (2nd ed.). New York: Chiron Press.

Roberts, R. D. (1999). Global Water Review, Issue 1. Global Water Project [Online] Available: Http://www.cciw.ca/gems/global-water-reviw-1.99.html

Rohe, J. F. (1997). *A Bicentennial Malthusian Essay: Conservation, Population and the Indifference to Limits.* Traverse City, MI: Rhodes and Easton.

Rosenzweig, C., & Hillel, D. (1998). *Climate Change and the Global Harvest: Potential Impacts of the Greenhouse Effect on Agriculture.* Cary, NC: Oxford University Press.

Rothman, K. J., et al. (1999). Seeking a global perspective on air pollution and health. *Epidemiology, 10*(1), 1–4.

Rubin, R. J. (1999). The economic impact of staphylococcus aureus infection in New York City hospitals. *Emerging Infectious Diseases, 5*(1), 9–17.

Satcher, D. (1999). The global HIV/AIDS epidemic. *Journal of the American Medical Association, 281*(16), 1479.

Schuh, G. E. (1995). The world food production and population growth. *Proceedings of the American Philosophical Society, 139*(3), 240–246.

Willis, R. J. (1973). A new approach to the economic theory of fertility behavior. *Journal of Political Economy, 81*(2), 514–564.

Schwartz, J. (1999). Air pollution and hospital admissions for heart disease in eight U.S. counties. *Epidemiology, 10*(1), 17–22.

Schwartz, W. B. (1998). *Life Without Disease.* Berkeley, CA: University of California Press.

Schwartz, W. B. (1999). The conquest of disease: It's almost within sight. *The Futurist, 33*(1), 51–55.

Schwartz, N. A., & Casillas-Miranda, R. (1998). Antibiotic prescribing and respiratory tract infections. *Journal of American Medical Association, 279*(4): 271–273.

Schwela, D. (1996). Exposure to environmental chemicals relevant for respiratory hypersensitivity: Global aspects. *Toxicology Letters, 86,* 131–142.

Sellers, R., (1998). Nine global trends in religion. *The Futurist,* 20–25.

Shalala, D. E. (1998). Collaboration in the fight against infectious diseases. *Emerging Infectious Diseases, 4*(3), 354–357.

Simon, F., Robertson, D., & Ayouba. A., et al. (1999). The characterizations of four novel SIV strains from Cameroon: Implications for primate lentivirus diversity. *6th Conference on Retroviruses and Opportunistic Infections,* Chicago, Ill.

Sirot, D. (1995). Extended-spectrum plasmid-mediated beta-lactamases. *Journal of Antimicrobial Chemotherapy, 36*(Supplement), A19–A34.

Sissell, K. (1999). World CO2 emissions dip. *Chemical Week, 161*(30), 41.

Smith, T. L., et al. (1999). Emergence of vancomycin resistance in staphylococcus aureus. *New England Journal of Medicine, 340*(7), 493–501.

Steinhoff, M. C. (1996). Japanese encephalitis: A Chinese solution? *Lancet, 347,* 1570–1571.

Stevens, D. L. (1999). The flesh-eating bacterium: What's next? *Journal of Infectious Diseases, 179*(Supplement No. 2), S366–S274.

Tarr, P. L. (1995). Escherichia coli O157:H7: Clinical, diagnostic, and epidemiological aspects of human infection. *Clinical Infectious Disease, 20*(1): 1–8.

Timmerman et al. (1999). Increased El Nino frequency in a climate model forced by future greenhouse warming. *Nature, 398,* 694–695.

Tortora, G. J., Funke, B. R., & Case, C. L. (1997). *Microbiology: An Introduction,* 6th edition. San Francisco, CA: Benjamin and Cummings Science.

Travis, J. (2000). Drugs order bacteria to commit suicide. *Science News, 157,* 100–101.

UNAIDS. (1999). *AIDS Epidemic Update: December, 1999.* Geneva, Switzerland: World Health Organization.

UNFPA. (1998). Report of the International Workshop on Population-Poverty-Environment Linkages: Key Results and Policy Actions. NY, New York: United Nations Population Fund. (1999). *Press Release: POP/711.* New York: Commission on Population and Development.

United Nations. (1999). *World Population Prospects: The 1998 Revision.* New York: United Nations Population Division.

United States Bureau of the Census. (2000). *Current Population Projections.* Washington, DC: Department of Commerce [Online] Available: Http://www.census.gov/population/www

U.S. Bureau of the Census, Report WP/98, *World Population Profile: 1998.* Washington, DC: U.S. Government Printing Office, 1999.

Waldvogel, F. A. (1999). New resistance in staphylococcus aureus. *New England Journal of Medicine, 340*(7), 556–557.

Walsh, J. F., Molyneux, D. H., and Birley, M. H. (1993). Deforestation: Effects on vector-borne disease. *Parasitology, 106,* S55–S75.

Weber, D. J., Raasch, R., & Rutala, W. A. (1999). Nosocomial infections in the ICU: The growing importance of antibiotic resistant pathogens. *Chest, 115*(3-S), 34S–41S.

Wei, F., Teng, E., Wu, G., Hu, W., et al. (1999). Ambient concentrations and elemental compositions of PM10 and PM2.5 in four Chinese cities. *Environmental Science and Technology, 33*(23), 4188–4193.

Weinstein, R. A. (1998). Nosocomial infection update. *Emerging Infectious Diseases, 4*(3), 416–420.

Welker, J. M., Fahnestock, J. T., & Jones, M. H. (1999). Annual CO2 flux in dry and moist Arctic tundra: Field responses to increases in summer temperature and winter snow depth. *Climatic Change, 44*(5), 139–150.

WHO. (1997). *Health and Environment in Sustainable Development: Five Years after the Earth Summit.* Geneva, Switzerland: World Health Organization.

WHO. (1999). *The World Health Report 1999.* Geneva, Switzerland: World Health Organization.

Will, R. (1999). New variant Creutzfeldt-Jakob disease. *Biomedical Pharmacotherapy, 53*(1), 9–13.

Wittwer, S. H. (1995). *Food, Climate, and Carbon Dioxide: The Global Environment and World Food Production.* Boca Raton, Fl: CRC Press, Inc.

Wu, C. (1999). Beyond vancomycin: Understanding an antibiotic of last resort may lead to new weapons against deadly bacteria. *Science News, 155*(17), 268–269.

4

The Challenge of Global Malnutrition

Robert W. Buckingham, Theresa H. Hollingsworth, and Heather L. Smith

Forms of Malnutrition in the World

On a global basis, hunger and malnutrition remain among the most devastating and debilitating problems facing the world's economically disadvantaged population. The tragic consequences of malnutrition have continuously dominated the health of the poorest nations. Indeed, nearly 30% of the world's population suffers from one or more of the travesties of malnutrition (WHO, 1999). Sadly, nearly 49% of the 10 million deaths among children under age five in the developing world are due to complications of malnutrition. It is a disease that is responsible for nearly half of all children's and infants' deaths worldwide, and has taken more lives than the entire Black Death that ravaged Europe in the Middle Ages. This disease steals away a child's natural curiosity, dulls intellectual capacity, and often causes its victim to develop lifetime learning disabilities. The immune system becomes chronically incapacitated, leaving the child vulnerable to illness. A vicious cycle occurs because illness is frequently a consequence of malnutrition, and conversely, malnutrition is often a result of illness. At the same time, an epidemic of global proportions is happening, especially in industrialized and developed countries—the epidemic of obesity that is emerging in children, adolescents, and adults. More than half the adult population is affected in many developed countries, which leaves them more susceptible to increasing death rates from heart disease, hypertension, stroke, and diabetes. In addition, the diets of many people in developed nations leave them at an increased rate for different forms of cancer, especially colon cancer.

Malnourishment can take on many forms. Appropriate nourishment is not, as many presume, a simple matter of eating until one's appetite is satiated. Just because a child can get enough to eat to satisfy his or her immediate hunger does not mean that the child is not malnourished. Indeed, three quarters of the children who die worldwide due to causes related to malnutrition show no outward signs of malnutrition or other problems to a casual observer (U.S. Committee for UNICEF, 1998). Malnutrition is not simply a lack of nutritious food—it is often compounded by a lack of essential vitamins and minerals, which leads to increased problems associated with deficiencies of various sorts. Iron deficiency, which manifests itself as anemia, is thought to afflict more than two billion people on a worldwide basis (U.S. Committee for UNICEF, 1998), and the World Health Organization estimates that 51% of children in developing countries are anemic (WHO, 1998). Protein-energy malnutrition (PEM) is one of the major nutritional crises in developing countries, yet it often goes unnoticed. A lack of sufficient amounts of iodine, taken for granted in the diets of most westernized nations, causes severe problems.

Therefore, malnutrition is not only a real and persistent problem, it is a silent worldwide crisis. Hunger and malnutrition can ravage entire families and societies, and will therefore have a crippling impact on the future of these societies. Children who are persistently hungry and malnourished have diminished futures and face the possibility of reduced cognitive functioning. They become adults with decreased productivity and decreased intellectual abilities, and they often suffer higher levels of chronic diseases. As previously stated, a vicious cycle occurs because illness is frequently a consequence of malnutrition, and conversely, malnutrition is often a result of illness. For example, in parts of Africa, malaria causes about a third of the cases of childhood malnutrition, and leaves pregnant women more susceptible to it as well. As countries struggle to improve their educational systems, the fact remains that they cannot overcome the consequences of years of undernourishment in their children. In 1990 it was estimated that the worldwide loss of social productivity caused by malnutrition amounted to 46 million years of productive, disability-free life (U.S. Committee for UNICEF, 1998).

Malnutrition is not necessarily confined to developing nations. Each night, millions of children in the United States go to bed hungry. Researchers estimate that 13 million children under the age of 12 cannot get enough to eat, and over 20% of U.S. children live in poverty (U.S. Committee for UNICEF, 1998). Widening gaps in income, reductions in social support systems, and lack of education all contribute to this insidious problem. Even more disheartening is the fact that nutrient deficiencies are occurring more frequently in families that are considered fairly well off—in the United States, a recent study found that 6% of children aged 1 to 5 were lacking in dietary folate, vitamin C, and food energy (U.S. Committee for UNICEF, 1998).

On the other side of the malnutrition spectrum lies the problem of overnutrition. For example, in the United States and other industrialized nations, fresh fruits and vegetables are available all year round; meats and other canned goods line the aisles of grocery stores; and a huge assortment of grains, cereals, breads, and other processed foods awaits the expectant consumer. Food is heavily abundant in most industrialized countries. With such ready food supplies, it seems that malnutrition would not be a problem in developed countries. On the contrary, a ready and convenient food supply does not necessarily bring about good nutrition and balanced diets. Indeed, obesity is one of the major nutrition-related problems in the United States. Between 1976 and 1994, obesity in the Unites States increased from 14.5% to 22.5%. Obesity carries with it increased risk of cardiovascular disease, certain cancers, hypertension, and noninsulin-dependent type diabetes. In industrialized countries, nutrition-related chronic diseases are among the major causes of morbidity and mortality (U.S. Committee for UNICEF, 1998).

Food Issues in Developing Nations

As stated previously, it is important to note that there is not one kind of malnutrition. It often takes on a variety of forms that result from deficiencies of certain nutrients, especially the micronutrients. The extent of malnutrition involves a complex interplay between the physical environment (household money, family size, safe drinking water, and safe sanitation) and our bodies' own internal environment. The most basic level of malnutrition is caused by inadequate dietary intake and the presence of disease. However, social, political, cultural, and economic elements play a large role in malnutrition. In many areas of the world, a lack of education and of access to good health care also contribute to malnutrition. Though there are many deficiencies that cause malnutrition, throughout the world it seems that a few particular deficiencies target developing nations the most.

The five biggest nutrition problems in developing nations are protein-energy malnutrition (PEM), micronutrient deficiencies (vitamins A, B, C, and D), iodine deficiencies, iron deficiency, and nutrition-related chronic diseases. Though these nutrition problems can often exist simultaneously to some extent in populations, some groups will exhibit one or more of the problems more seriously.

Protein-Energy Malnutrition (PEM) Diseases

Protein-energy malnutrition (PEM) is the world's most widespread form of malnutrition today, affecting over 500 million children (Torfin & Chew, 1994). Overall progress in reducing the incidence of PEM among infants and young children has been exceedingly slow, and nowhere near the goal of reducing global malnutrition by 50% by the year 2000 (WHO, 1999). However, this is an improvement from 1980; at that point, there were 175.7 million children in the world suffering from PEM. Today, there are 149.6 million children who suffer from it. Though it mainly strikes young children, older children and adults can also fall victim to PEM. The term *protein-energy malnutrition* fails to take into account that it is often micronutrient deficiencies, such as iron, zinc, and vitamin A, that bring about the condition of PEM itself. In addition, nondietary factors, such as infections and improper child care, can also lead to PEM in an indirect manner. The term *PEM* can also refer to a series of other conditions that manifest as protein deficiencies, such as marasmus and kwashiorkor. However, generally PEM refers to the etiology of undernutrition in young children. Signs of PEM include insufficient height gain relative to age; generally, when this occurs, there has been long-term malnutrition and poor health. Wasting, which occurs when there has been recent acute malnutrition, is an insufficient weight gain relative to height. Children who are afflicted with PEM during early childhood appear to be at an increased risk for abdominal fat, obesity later in life, hypertension, and increased mortality from cardiovascular disease. The effect of childhood malnutrition gives easier access to disease, thus increasing the chances of childhood mortality.

PEM due to undernutrition is prevalent in Africa, Central America, South America, the Near East, and the Far East, as well as for those living in poverty within developed countries (Sizer & Whitney, 1994). Two hundred-thirty million children in developing countries have low height for their age, and 50 million children have low weight for their age, reflecting severe undernutrition and disease (WHO, 1999). Adult PEM can also be seen in hospitalized persons with infections such as AIDS, cancers, tuberculosis, and eating disorders such as anorexia nervosa.

PEM is similar to other nutrient-related diseases in that it can be cured by obtaining adequate intake of essential nutrients. The prevention of this disorder begins in the home with appropriate nutritional management during and after illness, exclusive breast feeding for six months, good hygiene practices, and giving appropriate food at the right age. Also, psychosocial care, such as attention, affection, and encouragement, also plays vital roles in good nutrition and growth (WHO, 1997). Obviously, in many economically stricken countries, there are simply not enough family resources to provide such care. It is then that the public health system must bridge the gap.

Marasmus.   Marasmus is a term for the physical process of starvation. Often, it is accompanied by protein-energy malnutrition (PEM), and is common in children whose mothers have recently had another child and have weaned the first child off of breast milk. The first child often is forced to go from a diet high in nutrients (breast milk) to a thinned-cereal substance, such as rice or barley water. This child then begins to waste away. Without extra stores of fat, carbohydrate, or protein, the muscles begin to break down and become used by the body to fulfill energy requirements. The heart becomes increasingly weaker, and the face begins to look old. The child cannot keep warm and fails to grow. The body begins to systematically shut down nonessential functions, including the ability to cry. The immune system weakens, and the child becomes vulnerable to infection; often these secondary infections lead to the death of the child.

As with PEM, the only prevention for marasmus is adequate nutrition. Sufficient amounts of micronutrients are crucial, and exclusive breast feeding in the first six months of life gives an infant an increased chance of maintaining a good nutritional status. Obviously, one cannot ignore the fact that many women who are infected with HIV can pass the virus into their milk and then to their children.

However, a 1995 study in Kenya found that vitamin A–deficient mothers were five times as likely as non-vitamin A–deficient women to shed the virus in their breast milk.

Kwashiorkor. The symptoms of this disease are very similar to those of marasmus, and again, when this disease is involved, severe protein deficiency occurs, which can subsequently lead to death. Among the most common symptoms are failure to grow, edema, hair and skin disorders, and liver enlargement. To compound the problem, diarrhea and anemia occur, leaving the child even more nutritionally devastated. Those with kwashiorkor often have swollen bellies due to hypoalbuminemia, as well as skin depigmentation and other dermatoses. The child may intake energy or have a source of nutrition, but because of severe protein deficiency in the diet, repair, replacement, and growth of tissues become compromised. Interestingly, kwashiorkor occurs most often in children who have a severe lack of protein, but whose dietary intake of carbohydrates is dangerously high. For example, in regions where cereal grains cannot be grown, people often rely on starchy vegetables to supply most of their calories. While these crops often have high yields, their primary disadvantage is their very low protein content (Whitney & Rolfes, 1999).

Kwashiorkor leads to protein deficiency because the body often begins to metabolize its own protein sources. Logically, this disease is most common in children who live in underdeveloped countries. Inadequate intake of micronutrients, such as zinc, iodine, and vitamin A, often helps accelerate the disease by leading to a diminished immune system. As with marasmus, this disease leaves the victim open to infections that he or she could previously fight off.

Replacing nutrients that are lacking in the diet·is the most successful treatment. In many countries, the iodization of table salt and increases in zinc supplementation in common foods (such as breads) has led to an overall reduction in severe protein malnourishment.

Micronutrient/Vitamin Deficiency Diseases

The consequences of deficiencies are so dire, and the effects of restoring the needed vitamins so dramatic, that people spend billions of dollars every year on vitamin pills to cure a host of ailments, as well as to prevent them. In actuality, a vitamin can cure only the disease caused by a deficiency of that vitamin (Rolfes & Whitney, 1993). However, in countries where diets are severely lacking in both micronutrients and macronutrients, often a vitamin supplement will help provide security against other diseases of malnutrition.

Vitamin A Deficiency. Vitamin A deficiency is one of the major nutrition problems reported on a global basis. More than 100 million children worldwide have some degree of vitamin A deficiency, making them vulnerable to infectious disease (Humphrey, West, & Sommer, 1992). Deficiency of this vitamin causes a disorder known as *night blindness*, which can progress into permanent blindness (xerophthalmia). Though it was not known until recently in which of the many ways vitamin A deficiency increases childhood mortality, results of many field studies conducted in Brazil, Ghana, and India indicate that supplementing the diets with vitamin A can reduce deaths from diarrhea (U.S. Committee for UNICEF, 1998). In Bangladesh, the babies of breast-fed mothers who were given a single high dose supplement of vitamin A shortly after childbirth showed significantly fewer days of illness due to respiratory and diarrheal illnesses during the first six months of life than did breast-fed infants of unsupplemented mothers. There is also emerging research that suggests that vitamin A supplementation could reduce the transmission of HIV from the mother to her unborn child, as well as decrease maternal mortality. However, it is important to emphasize that these data are only preliminary.

A major goal of the World Health Organization (WHO) and the United Nations International Children's Emergency Fund (UNICEF) has been to seek child survival throughout the world by the control of vitamin A deficiency, and to eradicate the problem by the year 2000. Though this goal has not been completely met, many improvements have been made. For example, in Niger, with better irrigation methods and improved fertilizers and seeds, staple crop yields tripled, and new vitamin A–rich foods, such as amaranth and baobab leaves, were being produced. Women began incorporating these vitamin A–rich foods into their usual meals, and soon began noticing that night blindness was decreasing among their children. Word of mouth between villages prompted other women to do this as well, and the result has been a huge decrease in vitamin A–deficiency night blindness (U.S. Committee for UNICEF, 1998).

Other ways of improving vitamin A deficiencies are through fortification of basic foods, and supplementing children's diets with just two capsules of vitamin A per year; this would have a tremendous impact on the devastating problems caused by vitamin A deficiency (U.S. Committee for UNICEF, 1998). Educating developing nations on proper crop and fertilizer management, as well as in simple ways to maintain vitamin A in the diet, would be effective as well.

Iodine Deficiency Diseases (IDD).   Though very small amounts of iodine are needed by the body, a minimal amount is crucial to maintain human health. An inadequate level of iodine can cause ill health at any age, but it is most serious in pregnant women and children. Iodine deficiency is one of the world's most common preventable causes of mental retardation (DeLong, 1993). In pregnancy, iodine deficiency may result in fetal death; if the fetus survives, it will usually suffer from severe physical and mental retardation, a disease known as cretinism. In childhood, it may result in speech and hearing defects, delayed motor development, and impaired growth. Adult iodine deficiency results in goiter, which is a swelling of the thyroid gland.

Iodine deficiencies can be reversed if iodine is replaced in the diet before the damage becomes so severe that cretinism develops. In adults who have goiters due to iodine deficiency, adequate intake of the micronutrient will make milder forms completely disappear. Development of older children who are mildly affected can also be improved, though severe forms, such as cretinism, can be prevented only by adequate intake of iodine during pregnancy (U.S. Committee for UNICEF, 1998).

Iodine deficiency disorders are a public health problem in 18 countries; there are over 1 billion people living in environments deficient in this mineral, with approximately 70 million sufferers per year (WHO, 1999). In many parts of the world, the soil has very low levels of iodine; therefore any crops grown in the soil are iodine deficient (U.S. Committee for UNICEF, 1998). Though few countries had large-scale iodization programs as of 1990, it is estimated that 60% of all edible salt in the world is now iodized.

Iron Deficiency Diseases.   Iron deficiency manifests itself most commonly as anemia; it mostly results from inadequate dietary intakes of iron. Anemia occurs most often in women of childbearing age and young children. Women who are pregnant can easily become iron deficient; the increased nutritional demands placed on the mother's body by the fetus often leave the mother lacking in iron. Among pregnant women, 56% are anemic in developing countries, while only 18% are anemic in developed nations (U.S. Committee for UNICEF, 1998). A similar prevalence is thought to occur with preschool-aged children in these countries.

If left uncorrected, iron deficiency leads to severe anemia, diminished learning capacity in children, increased susceptibility to infections, and greater risk of death associated with pregnancy and childbirth. In addition, it retards fetal growth, causing low birth weights and increased infant mortality. Iron deficiency is also wholly blamed for at least 20% of maternal deaths in developing countries (U.S. Committee for UNICEF, 1998).

Increasing the intake of iron-rich foods, and those foods that enhance iron absorption, is the easiest preventative measure. Fortifying the commonly used foods in poor countries, or supplying those countries with low-cost iron tablets, is another alternative in treating this problem.

Vitamin D Deficiency.   Although vitamin D has been known to be important for decades, diseases caused by its deficiency still occur in large numbers of children worldwide. Vitamin D, essential for strong bone production and growth, is produced by the body through the effects of sunlight on the skin. Vitamin D deficiency occurs where people live in areas with long winters, or where people are covered up or remain indoors for most of the time (as happens often with disabled children).

In vitamin D deficiency, production of calcium-binding protein slows; even when calcium in the diet is adequate, it passes through unabsorbed, leaving the bones lacking in calcium. The bones then cannot calcify properly, leading to the most obvious sign of vitamin D deficiency—bone and skeletal abnormalities. Infants born to mothers with vitamin D deficiency may develop bone deformities as well. For example, young children who are deficient in this vitamin will develop rickets. The damage done by this deficiency can be overcome by exposing the face and arms to sunlight for 10 minutes a day.

Vitamin C Deficiency.   When vitamin C is deficient in the diet, the gums bleed easily, and the person feels weak and fatigued and has severe aches in the bones, muscles, and joints. Normal immune system functioning becomes compromised, and infections become frequent. In severe cases, sudden death is likely, caused by severe atherosclerosis or by massive bleeding into the joints and body cavities (Rolfes & Whitney, 1993).

Scurvy was responsible for most of the deaths among the pilgrims in the Massachusetts Bay Colony during their first hard winter (Anderson, 1982). The cause was a dietary lack of ascorbic acid (vitamin C). On long ocean voyages, fresh fruits and vegetables were used up early, and for the rest of the trip, foods that preserved better were eaten. However, these foods often lacked vitamin C, as well as other micronutrients.

Vitamin B Deficiency.   Beriberi is a vitamin-deficiency disease caused by a lack of thiamin, one of the B-complex vitamins. Beriberi has great cultural and historical significance—especially among the Chinese, due to the high consumption of polished rice. When the brownish coat on rice is removed, so is the thiamin content. Lack of thiamin can lead to symptoms such as an enlarged heart, heart failure, and edema. The nervous system eventually begins to degenerate, which can lead to paralysis.

Nutrition-Related Chronic Diseases and Their Impact on Human Health

Overnutrition is defined as an excess of energy or nutrients, a condition that generally leads to one of the most dangerous high-risk factors for chronic diseases, obesity (Whitney & Rolfes, 1999). A person who becomes obese is much more vulnerable to diseases associated with overnutrition, such as heart disease, cancer, and diabetes (Whitney & Rolfes, 1999). This section will discuss some of these diseases, nutritional high-risk factors, and possible methods for avoiding such problems.

Of all the industrialized countries, the United States probably has some of the unhealthiest eating habits, as well as the largest overall lack of regular exercise. Americans, on the whole, consume more calories than they expend in exercise (Whitney & Rolfes, 1999). Though this may not seem that significant, the increased calories, compounded with a lack of exercise, can cause significant weight gains over a period of time. Recent studies indicate that it is not actual body weight that counts so much as the weight (over-fat). In other words, what's more important to weight are health indicators such as blood pressure and cholesterol, and healthful lifestyle habits, such as plenty of regular exercise and low-fat diets (Whitney & Rolfes, 1999). People who are overweight are much more likely to succumb to cardiovascular disease (CVD) than are their underweight counterparts. Similarly, people with high sodium intakes are at higher risks for hypertension than are those who have normal sodium intake. Following is a description of the diseases most often caused by overnutrition.

Cardiovascular Disease.   Arterial lesions and lipid accumulation in humans were identified and described at least as early as the seventeenth century. Dietary fats and blood cholesterol, however, were not seriously implicated until coronary heart disease (CHD) reached epidemic levels in the United States around 1950 (National Research Council, 1989). The association of blood cholesterol concentrations with atherosclerosis and myocardial infarction was widely recognized by middle of the century (Dock, 1946).

Cholesterol has become a dreaded word, especially among American society. Although it has an unmistakable role in heart disease, it is a necessary component in our bodies for proper metabolism. Cholesterol performs vital functions in activities such as growth and reproduction, and is also a component of many hormones and cell membranes. The human body actually produces its own supply of cholesterol within the liver and intestines, and it is here that the problem often lies. If people are already producing adequate supplies of cholesterol and are, in addition, consuming high levels of it, there is an elevated level of risk for heart disease.

Atherosclerosis is the process by which fatty streaks and fibrous plaques are deposited in the inner layers of the arteries. Atherosclerosis often begins in childhood and develops over the years. The arteries are already 60% to 70% blocked when symptoms are first recognized. High amounts of cholesterol in the bloodstream initiate the fatty deposits, which in turn initiate the process of atherosclerosis.

There are two types of dietary cholesterol—high-density lipoprotein cholesterol (HDL) and low-density lipoprotein cholesterol (LDL). HDL has been called "good" cholesterol and LDL has been called "bad" cholesterol. Men with high levels of the HDL form of cholesterol were found to have a lower incidence of coronary heart disease than those with low levels. HDL can be thought of as a "street sweeper" that cleans up arterial cholesterol and takes it to the liver, where it can be cleared from the body in the form of bile, which is lost in the feces (Loomis, 1978).

"Bad" cholesterol, or low-density lipoprotein cholesterol, contributes to the production of atherosclerosis and increases the risk of cardiovascular disease. Low-density lipoproteins deliver cholesterol in a form that can irritate an area on the interior surface of an artery. This triggers a bump on the arterial wall that protrudes into the bloodstream. Particles accumulate and begin to choke the blood flow. The sticky substance that accumulates is called plaque. As this process continues, so does atherosclerosis, which may then lead to cardiovascular disease.

How do we influence HDL and LDL cholesterol to reduce the risk of heart disease? Examining the prevalence rates of coronary heart disease and atherosclerosis of various peoples around the world points to diet as our primary means of control. Certain cultures show almost nonexistent rates of coronary heart disease.

Dietary cholesterol is found only in animal-derived foods. Products high in cholesterol are meat, poultry, egg yolks, dairy products, and organ meats such as kidney and liver. There is no cholesterol in plant foods; all fruits, vegetables, seeds, and nuts are cholesterol-free. Only dietary cholesterol and saturated fatty acids have the ability to raise blood cholesterol.

Hypertension.   Several epidemiological studies over the course of the years have repeatedly identified a positive relationship between dietary intake of sodium and blood pressure levels. Randomized control trials have also demonstrated that a reduced sodium intake leads to an overall reduction in blood pressure (ADA, 2000). Given these facts, it seem obvious that reducing dietary intake of sodium is one of the easiest ways of controlling blood pressure and cardiovascular diseases, since long durations of hypertension highly increase the risk of heart attacks and stroke.

Hypertension is the most common cardiovascular disorder, affecting 8% to 18% of adults worldwide (World Health Report, 1995). Abnormally high blood pressure is a major contributor to heart disease, stroke, kidney failure, and other health problems (World Health Report, 1995). Arterioles—tiny blood vessels—are thought to be in a state of constriction, and it becomes harder for blood to flow through them, causing a backup of pressure inside the blood vessels. This forces the heart to push harder, causing unrelenting stress on the walls of the blood vessels.

When both hypertension and atherosclerosis are present, they act as antagonists of each other. The kidneys operate on a filtering system based on pressure, and when there is inappropriate blood pressure, the kidneys are forced to work harder. This causes a hormonal response to the heart to further increase blood pressure. High blood pressure then increases the hardening of the arteries because cholesterol is spread on the arterial walls at an increased rate. This process is wearing to the heart and the blood vessels. Researchers have found a strong correlation between obesity and hypertension in most epidemiological studies of blood pressure throughout the world. Some have even attempted to show possible causation (Rocchini, 1994).

Obesity.   Obesity is defined as an excessively high body fat in proportion to lean body tissue. It is considered a major public health problem today, and the prevalence appears to be increasing—especially among highly developed nations. Excess body fat accumulates when people take in more food energy than they can expend. Obesity places numerous hardships on the body, many of which place the person at higher risk for more diseases, such as cancer.

Perhaps the most important indicator of healthy body weight is the body-mass index (BMI). This is calculated by dividing a person's weight in kilograms by the square of his or her height in meters. Studies show that adults with a BMI between 20 and 30 are in relatively good health, and those with BMIs below 20 and above 30 tend to have health problems and thus lower longevity (Whitney & Rolfes, 1999). The desirable body mass index for women is 21 to 23, and for men it is 22 to 24. People who are obese generally have a BMI at 28.5 to 33, where serious obesity begins. In the United States, the growing trend is toward a higher BMI, whereas in developing countries, the trend is often toward BMIs lower than 18.

Fat cells grow in number during childhood and level off once adulthood is reached. In adulthood, fat cells can increase in size, but do not increase in number. Obese children increase fat cell numbers more rapidly, and therefore monitoring is critical. This is one key to preventing obesity in later years. Obesity due to an increase in the *number* of fat cells is called hyperplastic obesity. Obesity due to an increase in the *size* of fat cells is referred to as hypertrophic obesity.

Sedentary lifestyle is a major factor in the occurrence of obesity. Fewer than half of all adults in the United States exercise regularly; underactivity is probably the most important single contributor to obesity problems in the United States. Television watching may contribute most to physical inactivity (Gortmaker, Dietz, & Cheung, 1990). Watching television takes very little energy and often encourages snacking, especially of the high-fat foods that are advertised. Researchers have found that children who watch the most television have the highest prevalence rates of obesity (Dietz & Gortmaker, 1985).

Eating Disorders.   Diet, as described thus far, has referred to any food or drink consumed. Dieting, as defined in society, refers to the behavior adopted for the purpose of losing body weight. It is astounding to note that for a society with a general overabundance of food and large rates of obesity, the body ideals fall in the other extreme. Of the developed nations, the United States has one of the highest rates of dieting practices in the world. American obesity has become such a problem that weight-loss schemes are rampant. Fad diets and exaggerated claims are easier to promote than valid research findings and often dictate public knowledge.

This behavior often can become obsessive and unhealthy; excess dieting often carries with it its own ramifications. Many who try to become "healthy" by dieting often end up compromising their health. An estimated 2 million people in the United States suffer from eating disorders (Rolfes & Whitney, 1993). Many more have not been diagnosed, but have "dieted" to the point of harming their health. *Anorexia nervosa* is a disease that causes extreme dieting behavior, including self-starvation. Throughout the last 20 years, several high-profile celebrities in the United States have perished due to this disease's overtaking their lives. *Bulimia* is another dieting disease that is characterized by an intense fear of becoming fat, and involves binge-purging behavior. Proper nutrition often becomes vital in reestablishing compromised health due to these behaviors. Nutrition counseling is often needed, but psychological counseling is the key to successful treatment.

Cancer.   According to the American Cancer Society, diet plays a significant causal role in nine forms of cancer, which account for approximately 73% of cancer deaths:

lung, colorectal, breast, prostate, pancreas, stomach, ovary, bladder, and liver. Just as bad diet can play a causal role, good diet can help protect against the progression and incidence of these cancers.

In 2000, it is estimated that cancer will kill 552,200 Americans, and 1.2 million cases will be diagnosed (CDC, 2000). Although heart attacks are often deadly and tremendously feared, if one survives the initial attack, with lifestyle change, the patient can live healthily thereafter. On the other hand, cancer victims often must undergo severe, disfiguring, dehumanizing, and painful treatment. Cancer is most commonly fought by attempting to destroy "bad" cells while protecting healthy cells through techniques known as chemotherapy and radiotherapy. This involves either radiation or high concentrations of powerful drugs—or both—that target cell proliferation.

While nothing can guarantee prevention of human cancer, diet can influence the risk of cancer. Epidemiological studies have found evidence associating dietary factors with cancer at specific sites. Internationally, strong correlations have been observed in esophageal, stomach, colorectal, liver, pancreatic, lung, breast, endometrial, ovarian, bladder, and prostate cancers. In general, dietary fats can act as promoters of cancer, while vegetables and legumes act as antipromoters.

The following is a direct response from the American Cancer Society to help combat cancer risk with nutrition:

a. *Maintain a desirable body weight.* A study conducted by the American Cancer Society over a twelve-year period established that obese people are at increased risk of dying from certain cancers. This study found an association between increased deaths from cancers of the uterus, gallbladder, kidney, stomach, colon, and breast and varying degrees of overweight. Obese women, 40% above desirable weight, had up to a 55% greater mortality, and similarly obese men had up to a 33% greater mortality from cancer than did those with normal prevalence for certain cancer. For people who are obese, weight reduction is a good way to lower cancer risk. Weight maintenance can be accomplished by reducing intake of total calories and by maintaining a physically active lifestyle. Exercise and increased physical activity assist in weight maintenance.

b. *Eat a varied diet that is high in fruits, vegetables, and fiber.* The dietary advice in this report can be epitomized in two words, variety and moderation. Numerous human population studies have shown that daily consumption of vegetables and fruits is associated with a decreased risk of lung, prostate, bladder, esophageal, and stomach cancers. Vegetables and fruits contain varying amounts of vitamins, minerals, fiber, and non-nutritive constituents—alone or together—may be responsible for reducing cancer risk. It is desirable to vary the selection of vegetables and fruits.

Dietary fiber is a term used to cover many food components that are not digested in the human intestinal tract. These substances, abundant in whole grains, fruits, and vegetables, consist largely of complex carbohydrates of diverse chemical composition. A large body of epidemiologic evidence indicates that colon cancer is low in populations on other continents that live on a diet of largely unrefined food high in dietary fiber. It is not clear, however, that these data are applicable to the general population of the United States. Even if specific types of fiber may not ultimately prove to have a direct protective effect against cancer, high fiber—containing vegetables, fruits, and cereals can be recommended as wholesome low-calorie substitutes for high-calorie fatty foods.

    c. Cut down on total fat intake. The American Cancer Society recommends reducing total fat consumption from the current average of about 40% to 30% or less of total calorie intake. Substantial evidence from both human population and laboratory studies suggests that excessive fat intake increases the risk of developing cancers of the breast, colon, and prostate. Numerous experimental studies have also shown that high-fat diets increase the incidence of chemically induced breast and colon cancers in experimental animals. However, fat-restricted diets are not recommended for infants and very young children (2 years of age or less).

Stroke.   Excluding heart disease and cancer, stroke is the leading cause of death in the United States. Worldwide, stroke killed about 4 million people in 1996 (CDC, 2000). As blockage in a cardiac artery causes a heart attack, blockage of a brain artery causes stroke. Clots form around deposits protruding from arterial walls. Sometimes a blood clot (embolus) that is traveling through the bloodstream becomes wedged in one of the brain's arteries, which leads to a stroke. The bursting of a brain artery can also lead to a stroke by causing cerebral hemmorhage. An aneurysm, a blood-filled pouch that balloons out from a weak spot in the wall of an artery, may also cause hemorrhaging in the brain if it bursts.

Diabetes Mellitus.   Diabetes mellitus is a metabolic disorder characterized by an abnormally elevated level of blood glucose. The use of carbohydrate (which becomes glucose) is ineffective due to an absolute or relative lack of insulin. In other words, even though there is enough glucose to fuel the body, the cells actually starve because the glucose cannot enter the cells due to the lack of insulin. There are two types of diabetes mellitus; together, they are the seventh leading cause of death in the United States (CDC, 1996).

    Type I insulin-dependent diabetes mellitus (IDDM) is usually the result of the destruction of the insulin-secreting cells and may have genetic links. Approximately 5% to 10% of diabetics have IDDM, which is also called juvenile-onset diabetes. Noninsulin-dependent diabetes (NIDDM, Type II) is often not seen until adulthood; indeed, the likelihood of having NIDDM appears to double with each decade of life and with every 20% of excess body weight (Bland, 1981).

    NIDDM is much more common and is associated with aging, adiposity, and unknown genetic factors. Among countries of the world, incidence rates are correlated to the level of socioeconomic development. Rates in Central America and Southeast Asian countries are generally lower than those in western countries (National Research Counsel, 1989). The World Health Organization estimated that 100 million people would suffer from diabetes by the end of the twentieth century, with around 90% having NIDDM (World Health Report, 1995).

    Hispanics, blacks, Asian Americans, and Native Americans are especially at high risk. In several migrant populations, the prevalence of diabetes has increased along with westernized diet; these include Japanese who moved to Hawaii and

California and Yemenites who migrated to Israel (West, 1978). The only factor that has been consistently related to the prevalence of diabetes mellitus is relative body weight. Regular table sugar has not been shown to influence the risk of diabetes, but rather diets with high fat intakes have had an effect. The American Diabetes Association (2000) recommends carbohydrates from fruits and vegetables as a substitution for fats in the diabetic diet. The primary dietary recommendation for NIDDM is to achieve ideal body weight. Diet and exercise are usually the methods of controlling noninsulin-dependent diabetes mellitus.

Food Patterns in Different Nations

The World Health Organization has divided the world into six regions according to similar patterns of health development and concerns. Trends, goals, and food patterns will be discussed according to individual countries and the six regions: Africa, the Americas, Eastern Mediterranean, Europe, and Southeast Asia and the Western Pacific. People of all areas of the world rely on food not only for life sustenance but for a variety of other reasons; cultural, economic, social, and psychological factors play major roles in food choices. It is difficult to generalize food patterns in areas of the world due to the tremendous influence of modern communication and transportation methods. Nevertheless, most areas of the world have traditional diets unique to their own history. Table 4.1 illustrates the amount of food energy deficit in the world according to region (WHO, 1999).

Africa

Africa has 29 of the world's 47 least developed countries. Health care availability is poor and health care expenditure is very low. Maternal mortality rates are astoundingly high, and 50 million preschool children suffer from protein-energy malnutrition. Recently, natural disasters and those caused by humans have forced 16 million Africans to become refugees. One million of those suffered severe mal-

TABLE 4.1   *The Current Spectrum of Malnutrition Around the World*

Intrauterine growth retardation	30 million births/year
Protein energy malnutrition	149.6 million children < 5 years
Iodine deficiency disorders	740 million
Vitamin A deficiencies (blindness)	2.8 million children < 5 years
Iron deficiency anemia	1.5 million women, children, and men
Obesity	203 million adults, 21.9 million children
Cancer (due to diet)	Of 10.3 million cases every year, 3–4 million preventable with diet/exercise

Source: WHO, 1999

nutrition. Many strategies for improvement have been accepted, but action is more difficult. Africa's disease environment is largely determined by its poverty (World Health Report, 1995).

Ethiopians are at high risk for malnutrition, diarrhea, and vitamin A and B deficiencies, including night blindness (Geissler, 1994). Greater attention to water safety, sanitation, maternal and child health, and nutrition is essential for all of Africa.

Boiled peanuts, okra, and black-eyed peas are of African origin (Rolfes & Whitney, 1993). When slaves were brought to America, so came agricultural techniques and foods as well. Many southern dishes are made rich in fat and salts. The trick to choosing health-promoting rural southern food is to prepare vegetables without salt and without overcooking them, to eat plenty of beans, rice, and corn-bread (easy on the butter), and to use fatty meats, biscuits, and gravy sparingly (Rolfes & Whitney, 1993).

The Americas

There is great diversity among the populations of the Americas. All stages of development can be seen in country comparisons. In Latin America and the Caribbean, 46% of the population live in poverty (World Health Report, 1995). Health promotion is one of the priorities that the World Health Organization put into action for the years 1995–1998, and it has focused on public policies, living conditions, lifestyles, and food and nutrition.

The Mexican traditional diet is known for its complete vegetable protein: rice and beans. Chili pepper is also sacred to Mexicans, who are supposed to be blessed in health if they use it plentifully. Many dishes are wrapped in a corn or flour tortilla and referred to with different names, depending on the interior filling. Many of these fillings include cheese, onions, shredded lettuce, avocados, tomatoes, sauces, and sometimes meat. Mexican food can be lower in fat if lard, sour cream, and frying techniques are monitored.

In the United States, a large number of people of all different national origins and ethnic backgrounds provide many urban areas with a great variety of cuisine. Food patterns in the United States may be looked at regionally as the South, the Southwest, the Far West, the Midwest, the East Coast and New England, metropolitan areas, and isolated communities. Perhaps the food practice that unites the United States is its highly developed food technology. Foods take a variety of forms, and many can be available during all seasons.

Eastern Mediterranean

In terms of language, ethnicity, religion, social values, and customs, this region shares many commonalties. Life expectancy at birth gained 7 years in the past decade due to decreases in infant and childhood deaths (World Health Report, 1995). In Morocco, taking the foods that are being served is preferred more than reaching for foods, and fasting is often practiced by healthy adults (Geissler, 1994).

Muslim beliefs predominate in this area, which includes other countries such as Egypt, Iran, Lebanon, Pakistan, and Tunisia.

Europe

Many changes have occurred with the dissolution of the USSR and Yugoslavia. Infectious diseases are on the rise, and assistance has been targeted to this area by WHO, including support in setting up nutrition and health surveillance (World Health Report, 1995). Other areas of Europe, such as Sweden, are actively involved in health promotion and enjoy one of the world's highest standards of living.

Southeast Asia and the Western Pacific

Recently, cardiovascular diseases, cancer, and other noncommunicable diseases have begun to rank as major causes of death in this region's countries with the highest life expectancies, such as the Democratic People's Republic of Korea, Sri Lanka, and Thailand. Substantial progress in health education has been reported by WHO (World Health Report, 1995).

In India, Bangladesh, and Nepal, there is a serious problem of malnutrition and hunger; less than 90% of the average daily energy requirements are met (Kiple, 1993). The Indian Council of Medical Research found that about 35% of children have protein-calorie malnutrition and goiter with both having high regional prevalence.

Hypertension, diabetes, and cancer are the leading causes of death in China (Geissler, 1994). Of all fatal cancers in China, 60% are associated with the upper alimentary tract, and particular attention has been given to the role of diet and food hygiene (Kiple, 1993). Fluorine poisoning is reported to affect 21 million Chinese, according to epidemiological surveys. Further surveys suggest that about 35,000,000 suffered from endemic goiter and another 250,000 from endemic cretinism before salt was iodized in 1985 (Kiple, 1993). Both of these were caused by insufficient iodine. The promotion of health is important in Chinese society. Chinese culture has a rich, long history and a diet that has supported its people for thousands of years. With over a billion people, the traditional Chinese diet is land-efficient, and most of it comes from plant sources. On the whole, Chinese people eating traditional foods consume three times the fiber of people eating the American way, take in about half the fat, and have blood cholesterol values about half of what they are in the United States (UNICEF, 1998). Rice, vegetables, eggs, soups, small amounts of meat, and fruits are prepared with a wide array of seasonings and sauces. Although high in sodium, the traditional Chinese diet is low in fats and alcohol.

Japan has one of the lowest infant mortality rates in the industrialized world (Geissler, 1994). Japanese cuisine is, overall, a boon to those on low-fat diets (AHA, 1992). The Japanese often make a whole meal out of noodles with broth, pickled vegetables, cold rice, or snacks of sushi. Presentation is important in Japanese dishes. Even the simplest one-dish meal is attractively served, and an elaborate party meal, served in 10 or 12 separate and colorful dishes of different shapes, is truly a work of art (Anderson, 1982).

Summary

This chapter has emphasized the importance of good nutrition and the positive effects it has on overall well-being and health. At the same time, it has pointed out the ramifications of malnutrition and poor eating habits, and the different effects that cultural influences can have on the nutritional status of a country.

In developing countries, the issue of hunger is more extreme than in the United States, but the main cause is still the same, poverty. In general, people do not realize the intensity of this problem, though one fifth of the world's 6 billion people own no land or possessions at all (Whitney & Rolfes, 1999). Most of these people are illiterate, lack safe drinking water, and live on less than one dollar a day. The leading causes for this world hunger are extreme issues in themselves— food shortages, chronic malnutrition, and diminishing food supply (Whitney & Rolfes, 1999). When we think of food shortages, we imagine famines caused by drought, floods, and pest problems, but this is usually not the case. The problem is often related to increases in food prices along with a sudden drop in workers' incomes. Although famine may be always associated somewhat with world hunger, the number of people affected by famine is actually small compared to those affected with malnutrition.

Until the year 1988, the world's index of the sufficiency of the world food supply increased almost yearly. However this changed during the 1990s; the world's food production rate cannot keep up with the growth rate of nearly 90 million people yearly. In the past decade, the world's supply of the three primary grains—wheat, rice, and corn—has slowed or reached a plateau in production. Other factors that add to the problem are decreases in food production, environmental degradation, and drought in agricultural areas (Whitney & Rolfes, 1999).

Deficiency diseases and disease trends are susceptible to many factors influenced by the diet. Many factors are involved in people's preferences in the types of food they consume, how they consume them, and when and why they consume them. In general, people continue to eat the foods they grew up eating, and every region in the world has its own typical foods and ways of combining foods to make meals. These preferences reflect not only the people and the region they live in, but also the availability of the foods. Another important factor is the economic and political events of the current time and situation. Food choices may reflect people's concerns regarding the environment as well as their political views. Some of the strongest influences on food choices are cultural and religious beliefs. Politics could play a role in that a person may not eat a specific fruit due to a boycott for some type of exploitation or abuse. Another example is how some people buy only foods that are packaged in recycled containers. The last but sometimes the strongest factor that may be present is that of basic economics—a person may not be able to afford to purchase certain types of foods. Rice and beans may be more inexpensive than fresh fruits and vegetables, but these may not give the best nutritional outcome over a large period of time.

Heart disease, stroke, and cancer have become leading causes of death among technologically advanced countries. This directly correlates with the type of diet found in these countries. As our society has become more fast-paced, our demands for quick, easy foods have increased. This has led to a decrease in the amount of healthy foods that are consumed.

In underdeveloped countries, the lack of enough food to fulfill the daily needs of all people is often the biggest problem they have to face on a day-to-day basis. Starvation, nutrient-deficiency diseases, and poorly balanced diets often lead to a decrease in the overall health status of the country.

Though different countries have different eating patterns, the basic nutritional requirements for all humans remain the same. A diet high in fiber, fruits, and vegetables with moderate amounts of carbohydrates, proteins, and fats is the ideal for everyone, regardless of residence. Each country has its own version of diet staples, but on a worldwide basis we all need the same nutrition.

Discussion Questions

1. What does dietary intake have to do with the incidence of cardiovascular disease?

2. List the energy nutrients and their basic functions within the body.

3. Compare and contrast the different nutrient diseases in overnourished countries and in undernourished countries.

4. Describe the steps a person can take to lower the risk of cancer.

5. In primary health care, what role does nutrition play, and how?

6. Describe malnutrition and hunger; whom does it affect?

7. Why is maternal/infant nutrition such a large problem in underdeveloped nations?

References

American Cancer Society. (1991). *Diet: Nutrition and Cancer.*

American Heart Association. (1992). *Dining Out: A Guide to Dining Out.*

Anderson et al. (1982). *Nutrition in Health and Disease* (17th ed.). Philadelphia: J. B. Lipincott Company.

ADA (American Dietetic Assoc.), 2000. "Facts about Sodium and Healthy Blood Pressure." Available online: http://www.eatright.org

Amercian Diabetes Association (2000) "Diabetes Y2K." Avail. Online: http://www.diabetes.org/nutrition

Barr, D. P., Russ, E. M., & Eder, H. A. (1951). Protein-Lipid Relationships in Human Plasma. *American Journal of Medicine,* 11.

Berkson, D. M., & Staniler, J. (1981). Epidemiology of the Killer Chronic Diseases. In M. Winick (ed.). *Nutrition and the Killer Diseases.* New York: Wiley.

Bland, J. (1981). *Your Health Under Siege: Using Nutrition to Fight Back.*

Brandt, R., Blankenhom, D., Crawford, D., & Brooks, S. H. (1977). Regression and Progression of Early Femoral Atherosclerosis in Treated Hyperlipoproteinemic Patients. *Annals of Internal Medicine, 86.*

CDC. (2000) Report of Vital Statistics. Available online: http://www.cdc/gov/cancer

DeLong, G. R. (1993). Effects of Nutrition on Brain Development in Humans. *American Journal of Clinical Nutrition, 57.*

Dietz, W. H., & Gortmaker, S. L. (1985). "Do We Fatten Our Children at the Television Set?" Obesity and Television Viewing in Children and Adolescents. *Pediatrics, 75.*

Dock, W. (1946). The Predilection of Atherosclerosis for the Coronary Arteries. *Journal of the American Medical Association, 131.*

Dreon, D. M. (1988). Dietary Fat: Carbohydrate Ratio and Obesity in Middle-Aged Men. *American Journal of Clinical Nutrition, 47.*

Gebo, S. (1992) *What's Left to Eat?* New York: McGraw-Hill.

Geissler, E. (1994). *Pocket Guide to Cultural Assessment.* New York: Mosby Publishing.

Gortmaker, S. L., Dietz, W. H. Jr., & Cheung L. W. Y. (1990). Inactivity, Diet, and the Fattening of America. *Journal of the American Dietetic Association, 90.*

Hjennann, I., Byre, K. V., Holme, & Leren, P. (1981). Effect of Diet and Smoking Intervention on the Incidence of Coronary Heart Disease. *Lancet 2:* 1303–1310.

Hultman, E., Thomson, J. A., & Harris, R. C. (1988). *Work and Exercise, in Modern Nutrition in Health and Disease* (Ed.) M. D. Shils and V. R. Young. Philadelphia: Lea and Febiger.

Humphrey, J. H., West, K. P., & Sommer, A. (1992). Vitamin A Deficiency and Attributable Mortality among Under-5-year-olds, *Bulletin of the World Health Organization, 70.*

Kiple, K. (1993). *The Cambridge World History of Human Disease* (p. 473). New York: Cambridge University Press.

Loomis, H. (1978). Preferential Utilization of Free Cholesterol from High-density Lipoproteins for Biliary Cholesterol Secretion in Man. *Science,* April 7.

National Institute on Alcohol Abuse and Alcoholism. (July 1995). *Alcohol Alert Newsletter,* No. 29.

National Research Council. (1989). *Diet and Health.* Washington, DC: National Academy Press.

Olson, R. E. (1978, June), Clinical Nutrition: An interface between Human Ecology and Internal Medicine, *Nutrition Reviews, 36,* 13–24.

Pickett, G., & Hanlon, J. J. (1990). *Public Health: Administration and Practice.* St. Louis: Times Mirror/Mosby College Publishing.

Roberts, L. (1988). Diet and Health in China, *Science, 240, 27.*

Rocchini, A. P. (1994). American Institute of Nutrition Symposium Proceedings. Adapted from *Journal of Nutrition, 125* (6S).

Rolfes, S. R., & Whitney, E. N. (1993), *Understanding Nutrition.* St. Paul: West Publishing Company.

Shils, J. A., Olson, R., & Shike, M. (19**XX**). *Modern Nutrition in Health and Disease.*

Sizer, F., & Whitney, E. (1994). *Nutrition Concepts and Controversies.* St. Paul: West Publishing Company.

The Surgeon General's Report on Nutrition and Health: Summary and Recommendations. (1988). DHHS (PHS) publication no. 88-5021-1. Washington DC: U. S. Government Printing Office.

Symposium: Insulin Resistance, Obesity, and Hypertension. (1994). AIN Symposium Proceedings.

Torfin, B., & Chew, F. (1994). *Protein-Energy Malnutrition in ME.* Philadelphia: Lea & Febiger.

U.S. Committee for UNICEF. *Nutrition/World Hunger.* (1993). 331 East 38th Street, New York, NY.

U.S. Committee for UNICEF. *The State of the World's Children.* (1998). 331 East 38th Street, New York, NY.

West, K. N. (1978). *Epidemiology of Diabetes and Its Vascular Lesions.* New York: Elsevier/North-Holland.

Whitney, E. N., & Rolfes, S. R. (1999). *Understanding Nutrition.* Belmont, CA: Wadsworth.

Work Study Group on Diet, Nutrition, and Cancer. American Cancer Society, 1992.

World Health Report. (1995). *Bridging the Gaps.* Report of the Director-General, World Health Organization, Geneva, Switzerland.

World Health Report. (1999). "Making a Difference" *Report of the Director General,* World Health Organization, Geneva, Switzerland

World Health Report (1998). "Life in the 21st century: A Vision for All." *Report of the Director General,* World Health Organization, Geneva, Switzerland.

World Health Organization. (1997). *Fact Sheet 129.* Available online: http://www.who.int/

World Health Statistics Annual. (1986). Geneva, Switzerland: World Health Organization.

5

Primary Health Care: The Global Response

Robert W. Buckingham and Tracy Brannock

Primary Health Care

Primary health care (PHC) is both a goal for the world community and an organizational structure for the provisioning of clinical medical services. PHC is historically associated with the World Health Organization, which sponsored the famous health care conference in Alma-Ata (renamed Almaty), Kazakhstan, in 1978. The attendees from countries around the world agreed on a statement of the makeup of PHC, and the formal declaration contained key principles.

PHC is essential health care made universally accessible to individuals and families in the community by means acceptable to them, through their full participation and at a cost that the community and country can afford (WHO, 1978). It forms an integral part both of the country's health system, of which it is the nucleus, and of the overall social and economic development of the community (WHO, 1978; WHO, 1981). PHC is a basic level of health care that includes programs directed at the promotion of health, early diagnosis of disease or disability, and prevention of disease. PHC is provided in an ambulatory facility to limited numbers of people, often those living in a particular geographic location. Primary health care includes continual access to health care, regardless of a person's stage of development or level of income, and recognizes people's desire for improvement in their state of health. It provides greater access to a wide range of health-related services and allows people to enjoy the benefits of scientific and technological advances that will assist in those aims (Elling, 1984). The Alma-Ata Declaration goes beyond what one typically thinks of as primary care, because it includes public health measures such as sanitation and potable water needs for populations (Donaldson et al., 1996).

This chapter will provide an overview of PHC origins, practices, and future goals. PHC has been adopted by the international community and provides a basic structural goal for all countries to work toward and achieve.

Primary Health Care Services

Primary health care is not dedicated to one typical health service. The services vary depending on the location of the health care facility. The main focus of PHC is defined as essential health care based on practical, scientifically sound, and socially acceptable methods and technology made to maintain or improve health at every stage of development in a spirit of self-reliance and self-determination. It is the first level of contact with individuals, the family, and the community, bringing health care as close as possible to where people live and work; and it constitutes the first element of a continuing health care process. The basic services of PHC can be broken down into six components. The basic idea for each PHC program is focused around these components because these are the main turning points to improving health, and have been found to be the greatest concerns in developing countries that lack health care.

Primary Health Care Core Components

The core components of PHC, as promulgated by WHO, involve the promotion of adequate food supply and proper nutrition, an adequate supply of safe water and basic sanitation, maternal and child health care (including family planning), immunization against vaccine-preventable disease (such as measles, diptheria, tetanus, pertussis, and polio), and the prevention and control of locally endemic diseases by means of timely diagnosis, treatment, and vector control.

The health status of people is the foundation of national development. Due to the erroneous health policies of the past, basic health services remained unavailable to the most needy people, those of remote and backward areas. This is the main reason that the majority of the population still remains in very poor health. PHC is designed to make these services available to low socioeconomic families to help decrease the rate of poverty.

An estimated 1.3 billion people live in conditions of abject poverty—existing on less than a dollar per day (UN, 1998). Billions of people lack basic sanitation and drinkable water, have no minimal health care access, and lack adequate dietary calories and protein (Haines, 2000).

Primary Health Care Support

The success of every human endeavor depends on support, and PHC requires promotional, developmental, and functional types of support from the health care system. Several major assists are needed to effectively organize the health care system support for PHC. These include accessibility to service, selection of proper health techniques, control of the cost of services, and public and professional support.

In order for the PHC system to be accessible, it has to address both geographical and social components. In developing countries, the progression of even minimal health care has been slow due to lack of attention to these components. Thus, health care services have been inaccessible for many people. They can be geographically and socially burdened for a number of reasons. Geographically, facilities may not be within reach of all individuals, thus limiting their access to service. This may be due to factors related to climate, transportation, travel distances, and time. Socially, individuals may not have the proper knowledge of the services that are available to them, which in turn limits their access as well.

To properly select the technique used to educate and provide service, an evaluation of the major health concerns for each selected region is necessary. Each region may have different health barriers that isolate them from the rest of the world. The socioeconomic makeup of the community must be known. Certain diseases are more likely to occur in certain socioeconomic neighborhoods than in others (Buttery, 1991). Thus, to properly improve the health status, a thorough analysis is crucial. Several factors that should be evaluated include keeping epidemiology up to date with social trends in health status of the studied region, implementing and acting on new health procedures that are available, and keeping these services and education within reasonable cost, depending on the economy. The cost of keeping even a small number of hospitals up to date can have a drastic impact on the economy.

The increased cost of health care services has caused heightened concern in both developing and industrialized countries. It is due to a variety of factors, including the use of expensive techniques, the cost of training the staff, and other problems related to the organization and financing of health services. Increasing cost of services is most detrimental to developing countries because they lack the most services, yet their economies cannot afford to provide more.

Public and professional support is necessary to make any system work. The health care system must be unanimously accepted by the public as characterized by measures that the majority of citizens believe will help increase their health. The support of leaders and decision makers at each level is always required to keep the services funded and properly maintained. The personnel who are to be working and providing these services should also support these policies to ensure that proper procedures are carried out. The support will assist the PHC programs in continuing the services that are needed to increase health status. No sector involved in socioeconomic development can function properly in isolation. Activities in one impinge on the goals of another; hence constant consultation between major social and economic sectors is essential to ensure development and to promote health as part of it. Primary health care, too, requires the support of other sectors, which can also serve as entry points for the development and implementation of primary health care.

Primary Health Care Needs and Problems

One of the major issues that affect the health of the people is their access to health care. Access to health care includes more than having health care resources available and the economic means for obtaining them (Paulanka & Purnell, 1998). Geographic barriers can exist as well. The main challenge is reaching all the people who need these services, and it can be viewed through individual concerns or societal concerns.

Individuals and Poverty

Individuals may have difficulty in attaining services to benefit their health due to poverty, lack of transportation, or lack of education. These factors have an impact on health, but can be changed or provided for. Poverty is a lack of material wealth needed to maintain existence. Without material wealth, access to health care may be very difficult. Health care is very costly. With the investment in primary care made by federal programs has come significant progress in improving access to primary care for the poor and other disadvantaged groups (Miller, 1983). Detailed studies of the nature and extent of poverty in particular countries show that the problem is of truly gigantic proportions (Seligson & Smith, 1998). The global poverty picture as we begin the twenty-first century is one of stalled progress and of rising numbers of poor people everywhere. The number of people living below a dollar a day was estimated at 1.2 billion in 1998 (WB, 2000). A total of 33 countries have seen a decline in life expectancy since 1990. They are mostly countries hit hard by AIDS, and other countries grappling with negative economic growth, such as Russia (WB, 2000). The United States poverty rate continued to decline from a high of 39,000,000 in 1990 to 34,000,000 in 1998 (DC, 1999).

PHC tries to develop services necessary for each individual country at a cost that it can afford. Primary health care aims at providing the whole population with essential health care. Population coverage has often been expressed in terms of a numerical ratio between services for providing health care and the population to be served—for example, the number of hospital beds per unit of population, the number of doctors and nurses per unit of population, or the number of people for whom a health center has been established. Such ratios are often misleading. It is necessary to relate the specific components of health care being provided to those who require them—for example, to relate the provision of child care to the total number of children in the community, female as well as male, in order to make sure that such care is in fact available to all children. Even then, such ratios express the mere existence or availability of services and in no way show to what extent they have been used, let alone correctly used. To be used they have to be properly accessible. Providing services that are accessible to a greater percentage of the population is one step toward resolution of lack of services. However, health care is still dependent on means of transportation and is hampered by lack of education.

What makes the current situation so unacceptable is that the tragedy of mass exclusion from education is avoidable. With international cooperation, universal primary education could be achieved, even in the poorest countries, and illiteracy could be eradicated within one generation (Oxfam, 1999). Universal primary education is very costly, but eliminating other spending could improve accessibility to this service. Best estimates suggest that it would cost about $8 billion extra a year (Oxfam, 1999). This is a considerable amount of money, although these funds exist already. Considering that national and community self-reliance and social awareness are among the key factors in human development, and acknowledging that people have the right and duty to participate in the process for the improvement and maintenance of their health, the government should encourage and ensure full community participation through the effective propagation of relevant information, increased literacy, and the development of the necessary institutional arrangements through which individuals, families, and communities can assume responsibility for their own health and well-being. Stressing that PHC should focus on the main health problems in the community, but recognizing that these problems and the ways of solving them will vary from one country and community to another, PHC should at least provide the major services to promote health. Health education is on the top of the list because it is very important in providing adequate service to the people. If individuals are not aware of the services available to them, it is very difficult to take advantage of them.

Societal Concerns

There are things that are controlled by society that can impact the quality of and accessibility to health care. These factors include proper professional training, monitored government expenditures and debt, and the issue of rural versus urban communities. It has been stressed that all levels of the national health system have to support PHC through appropriate training, supervision, referral, and logistic support. High priority should be given to the development of adequate human resources in health and related sectors, suitably trained for and attuned to PHC, including traditional workers and traditional birth attendants, where appropriate. These workers should be organized to work as a team suited to the lifestyle and economic conditions of the country concerned. Attempts to extend health service coverage have led to the increased use of minimally trained health personnel working in often remote rural locations. However, for such workers to function effectively, they must not be isolated from the rest of the health care system (Lee & Mills, 1993). Having them informed on new advances in medicine can keep them up to date with technology even if their training is minimal. Appropriate training of personnel is required to provide adequate service. More sufficient numbers of trained personnel for the support and delivery of PHC are necessary, and governments need to undertake or support reorientation and training for all levels of existing personnel and revise programs for the training of new community health personnel. It is also recommended that special training or an improvement in skills be implemented in order to promote health service.

It is important to train individuals about the specific culture they are located in if it is an unfamiliar area. This will increase the level of care that people receive and possibly decrease any health barriers. Health care providers can learn and benefit from each other's experience and urge all other health providers to cooperate among themselves in the promotion of PHC through the sharing of information, experience, and expertise. Recognizing that all countries can learn from each other in matters of health and development, they can accumulate a technical cooperation among countries, especially developing countries. However, certain health promotion actions such as these can require both time and economic expenditure.

The government is one among many providers of health services in developing countries. Billions of dollars are spent on revision of health care each year, and aggregate expenditure estimates indicate that private spending as a proportion of total health expenditure is highest among the poorest countries. Household expenditure surveys in a number of developing countries suggest that the poorest households may spend a higher percentage of their income on health care than do high-income households, even when free government care is available.

Ways of solving health problems vary from one country and community to another, according to different stages of development, but should provide promotive, preventive, curative, rehabilitative, and emergency care appropriate to meet the main health problems in the community, with special attention to vulnerable groups, and should be responsive to the needs and capacities of the people. The importance of establishing and further developing a comprehensive national health system of which PHC is an integral part, and of encouraging the full participation of the population in all health-related activities, should be affirmed.

Benefits of Primary Health Care

The PHC approach rose out of the perceived inadequacies of conventional health care to meet the needs of people in developing countries. It is an attempt to chart the way toward a more appropriate health care system. However, no one should claim that the PHC approach presents a magic formula by which to solve the numerous problems with the health services and those of ill health in these countries; what it does do is to point the way out of existing difficulties without pretending to have all the answers (Macdonald, 1993). It is especially in so-called developing countries that the failures of the Western model of health care have become increasingly apparent in the last thirty to forty years (Macdonald, 1993). Primary health care offers more cost-effective health care than hospital care, reduces human suffering, and is more accessible.

PHC focus is on prevention rather than on cure; it minimizes preventable human suffering due to diseases. The evidence shows that PHC is effective; however as health budgets are squeezed by economic crises, PHC services are often the first to be cut, since it is politically more difficult to cut spending on hospitals in the cities. Though the staff may be kept on, other items of recurrent expenditure and capital spending will be hit particularly severely. This leads to an acute shortage of drugs and other equipment, a shortage of vehicles (even bicycles), the cancellation of training programs, poor supervision, and low staff morale (Clark, 1991). With primary health care, there is an opportunity to confront the imbalance of the past and to lay the foundations of a better health care system for the future (Macdonald, 1993). PHC programs can meet the original intention of the drafters of the Declaration of Alma-Ata. Benefits can accrue not only to the health status of individuals and communities but also to individual self-confidence, self-reliance, and awareness of the participants (Basch, 1999).

Problems in Primary Health Care

PHC, as envisioned by the Alma-Ata Declaration, has been open to criticism. The Declaration is a normative statement about what should be, and does not actually define how its principles are to be accomplished (Macdonald, 1993). Supporters of the Declaration respond that, since 1978, WHO and other agencies have delineated the specifics for achieving PHC goals. PHC itself defines essential societal changes for more equitable distribution of economic resources.

Evaluation of PHC

The purposes of evaluation are to determine whether a particular PHC program is effective and to identify areas of improvement in planning future PHC programs. All health care programs suffer from the same basic difficulty: It is somewhat simple to measure project inputs (resources) and service outputs (number of health services provided), but it is difficult to measure the underlying goal of improved health. We may compare the number of deaths and cases of specific illness before, during, and after the implementation of a PHC. Nevertheless, to quantify the total health (defined as the mental, physical, and social well-being) of a community in order to demonstrate that positive changes were brought about by specific PHC activities is a challenging task (Basch, 1999). Two basic resources—financial and professional expertise—are needed for such a task. However, in the settings where PHC programs are implemented, it is nearly impossible simply because of the limitation or lack of these two resources.

Cost of PHC

PHC covers a variety of intertwined strategies for financing, delivering, organizing, and administering a set of interventions designed to improve health. PHC is promoted for universal adoption, including the wealthiest and most industrialized countries, but the obvious target for PHC is the poor and underserved developing countries. Therefore, the question of who assumes the cost becomes of great importance for the developing countries. Often, three parties are involved: a foreign donor (which usually is more willing to finance initial investments than to become committed to meeting recurrent costs), the government (at various levels), and the community.

Detailed economic studies of a PHC program in Guinea Bissau have confirmed that such a program is not cheap (Chabot & Waddington, 1987). The recurrent cost alone used up most of the per capita health care service allocation for the project area, but initial investment expenditures more than doubled the PHC project costs, leaving nothing for all the expenses of running the regular health care centers and hospitals.

Community Utilization of Programs

Low utilization rates of services have been found in various programs. Part of the problem may be due to inappropriate allocation of resources by health officials. Some PHC programs spend 59% of the health care budget for hospitals, and only 7% for rural and preventive medicine. Further, usually the local villagers want curative medicine rather than preventive activities, which show no immediate results (Basch, 1999).

The Sociopolitical Roles of PHC Workers

PHC programs operate within the context of a country's sociopolitical dynamics. A government's use of health care inputs as a means of social control may result in the people's suspicion of the PHC workers, particularly in sensitive areas such as family planning. PHC programs and their health care workers may be utilized to further a government's political strategies. The establishment of PHC facilities may be used as a pretext to disseminate a government's viewpoints. Implementation of PHC programs requires PHC workers to critically analyze the local root causes of ill health. These activities may be viewed as hostile acts, and may be subject to reprisals.

Only from the perspective of the twenty-first century we will be able to adequately evaluate what impacts PHC has made in advancing our global health. In spite of all the drawbacks that PHC faces, according to the World Health Report 1999, we made progress. Nevertheless, we still have a long way to go to accomplish the goals that are set forth in previous conferences.

Historical Attributes: The Alma-Ata Conference

In 1977, at the 30th annual World Health Assembly, it was unanimously decided that the main social target issue of governments and of the WHO in the succeeding decades should be "the attainment by all citizens of the world by the year 2000 of a level of health that will permit them to lead a socially and economically productive life" (WHO, 1978). This goal, now known as "Health for All Africans by the Year 2000," has become a major campaign of the WHO (Koivusalo et al., 1998). At the 35th World Health Assembly, conducted in 1982, the plan of action for implementing HFA 2000 was promulgated and adopted.

Much has been written about the need for health services to be oriented toward primary health care if the goal "HFA 2000" is going to be achieved. Health services no doubt constitutes a basic need of people residing in any part of a country. Health service is comprised of complex interrelated elements that also consist of physical and psychological environment. On September 12, 1978, the International Conference on PHC was held in Alma-Ata, USSR. At the meeting (cosponsored by the WHO and UNICEF), 143 representatives from different countries and 67 organizations, including United Nations agencies and nongovernmental organizations, expressed the need for urgent action by all governments, all health and developmental workers, and the world community to protect and promote the health of all the people of the world (WHO, 1997). The Declaration of Alma-Ata was adopted at this conference with the goal of attaining HFA 2000. This declaration states ten essential actions for protecting and promoting health for all the world.

Alma-Ata Declaration

In the Alma-Ata Declaration, PHC was defined as essential health care based on practical, scientifically sound, and socially acceptable methods and technology made universally accessible to individuals and families in the community by means acceptable to them through their full participation; and at a cost that the community and the country can afford to maintain at every stage of their development in a spirit of self-reliance and self-determination. It forms an integral part of both the country's health system, of which it is the central function, and the main focus of the overall social and economic development of the community. It is the first level of contact with individuals, the family, and the community, bringing health care as close as possible to where people live and work; and it constitutes the first element of a continuing health care process (WHO, 1978). The objectives of the conference were stated to provide direction for the policies that were to be developed.

Objectives of Alma-Ata Conference

The key objectives laid out at Alma Ata were as follows (WHO, 1978):

1. To promote the concept of primary health care in all countries;

2. To exchange experiences and information on the development of primary health care within the framework of comprehensive national health systems and services;

3. To evaluate the present health and health care situation throughout the world as it relates to, and can be improved by, primary health care; and

4. To define the principles of primary health care as well as the operational means of overcoming practical problems in the development of primary health care.

The underlying concept of the core components of PHC was to integrate PHC with socioeconomic development so that each would support the other in a context of equity and social justice. Further, decentralization was emphasized in community planning and community implementation by employing local workers and training them to perform these tasks. PHC programs were envisioned to be an integral, permanent, and pervasive part of the formal health care system in any country (Basch, 1999).

Case Studies

Haiti

Haiti, the world's first black republic, fifty miles from the eastern tip of Cuba, shares the Caribbean's largest island, Hispaniola, with the Dominican Republic, occupying 10,714 square miles. The estimated population living in urban areas is 311,124 and the estimated population living in rural areas is 826,466. This country is a prime example of the gap that exists between the health "haves" and the health "have nots." The 1989 health indicators show a total of 944 physicians, or 1 physician per 6,000 people in Haiti. There are 8 hospitals beds per 10,000 people, and the latest public health expenditures show, in United States dollars, $3.60 per capita. It is the lowest per capita expenditure in Latin America (Kurian, 1990). The Haitian life expectancy at birth is 51 for males and 56 for females, the infant mortality rate is 71 per 1,000 live births, and only 39% of the population have access to safe water (WB, 2000).

In 1981, a PHC program was established in rural Haiti serving about 115,000 persons. Surveillance information pinpointed problems such as malnutrition, diarrhea, tuberculosis, tetanus, pertussis, diphtheria, measles, and poliomyelitis. Eight categories of preventive services were offered in the communities. These preventive services include education on nutrition and sanitation, supplemental feeding for children under six, demonstration programs for mothers, oral rehydration therapy education, tuberculosis screening and treatment, deworming, immunization, and support for traditional birth attendants (Basch, 1999). The hospital-based program included 10 physicians, and 30 graduate and 60 auxiliary nurses and technicians. The community-based program included 3 physicians, 2 graduate nurses, 30 full-time auxiliaries, 60 collaborators, and a sanitary officer (Basch, 1999).

More than 50% of expected deaths were avoided. Disease-specific morbidity rates declined drastically, and calculated life expectancy increased from 47.5 to 66.4 years (Basch, 1999). These positive results from the PHC program provide future hope and direction in planning the expansion of PHC program in Haiti. This program was heavily subsidized by funding sources external to the community.

The average annual cost of adding surveillance and health services to hospital services was only United States $1.60 per person (Basch, 1999).

Mali

Mali is located in Western Africa, southwest of Algeria. It had an estimated population of 10,108,569 as of July 1998. Mali is among the poorest countries in the world, with 65% of its land area desert or semi-desert. Economic activity is largely confined to the river area irrigated by the Niger. About 10% of the population is nomadic, and some 80% of the labor force is engaged in farming and fishing (Kurian, 1990). Industrial activity is concentrated on processing farm commodities. Mali is heavily dependent on foreign aid because the population is drastically affected by fluctuations in the economy.

The infant mortality rate (IMR) was 179.5 deaths per 1,000 live births in 1985, and as of 1998 121.72 deaths per 1,000 live births. The three top causes of infant deaths were unexplained cause, diarrheal diseases, and malaria. The three top causes of child deaths between ages 1 to 5 years were malaria, measles, and diarrheal diseases (UN, 1990). The life expectancy at birth was 43 for males and 44 for females, and 56% of the urban dwellers and only 20% of the rural dwellers had access to safe drinking water (WB, 2000). The factors that contribute to the high infant and child mortality and low life expectancy include inadequate maternal nutrition, maternal ailments, unsanitary environment, and local customs and beliefs that are conducive to the onset of ailments and may aggravate the disease (i.e., nonevidence-based traditional healing practices).

The Project Sante Rurale (PSR) in Mali started from a request in 1973 by Mali's Ministry of Public Health to the U.S. Agency for International Development (USAID). PSR created a team to identify health problems that the public health service, operating through volunteer village health workers, could solve. In 1974, the PSR focused on three subsectors of health care: first, maternal and child health; second, training of subprofessional health care providers; and third, drug procurement. The PSR team included officials of the central and regional offices of the National Director of Public Health, the health education unit of the Ministry of Public Health, and health and rural development personnel.

A typical health center that is run by a district physician is staffed by one district physician, one head nurse, two certified nurses, one nurse for leprosy and tuberculosis, 4–5 nurse's aides, one nurse midwife, and 2–3 rural midwives. Mali has 7 regions, 46 districts, and 228 dispensaries (Bang, 1990). In rural populations the nearest public health services are provided by a local dispensary. Oftentimes these dispensaries run short on basic drugs, such as aspirin and antimalaria medications. Ironically, the population that is at highest risk, children and pregnant women, do not receive priority in treatment care.

Traditional healers and herbal medicine are an important primary resource of treatment of illness in this population. More than 80% of this population receives herbal and traditional medicine (Bang, 1990). The PSR's maternal health component was to focus on upgrading traditional birth attendants, providing them a modest kit of tools, and supervising the birth attendants' work after training. Over 90% of births are attended only by these traditional birth attendants (Bang, 1990). When the PSR interviewed village leaders (all adult males) about their perception of priorities for improvement of health services, interestingly, they expressed concern only for improved curative treatment of such illnesses as malaria, infections, and backaches, but no concern was expressed toward their high infant and child mortality and morbidity. Their cultural attitude affects the way they view this; it is their belief that infant and child mortality and morbidity are due to the work of unhappy ancestors or neighbors working through sorcerers to punish the parents for their social misbehavior (Bang, 1990).

The PSR's responsibility for health education was delegated to various directors of the Ministry of Public Health. Health education in rural villages was designed for illiterate villagers, and it includes demonstrations with live subjects or a doll, stories, role playing, and the use of pictures. It covers a wide range of topics such as maternal and child health, including family planning, oral rehydration therapy, nutrition, and sanitation.

Health for All Africans by the Year 2000 aims to improve health for all people in Africa. It defines policies, strategies, and plans by which to establish and strengthen the current health care delivery system via primary health care approaches. The health care coverage will range from immunization, safe water, family planning, and diarrheal disease control. Mali adopted the World Health Organization's goal of Health for All Africans by the Year 2000. With the current PSR in progress, Mali already made a good head start in achieving HFA 2000. However, limited resources and poor coordination in functional organization may be its drawbacks. Primary health care continues to progress and help countries to better their health. As these services continue to grow, the health of the world can possibly make a great turnaround, and the world can be one step closer to reaching its health status goals.

The time has come for primary health care to be firmly implanted in the world political scene. This requires international agreement on the adoption of a worldwide primary health care policy and strategy with the goal of making essential health care available to all the people of the world. It also requires global action to ensure the unstinting support of the international community, and to encourage countries to set primary health care in motion, to maintain its momentum, and to cooperate in overcoming obstacles. Such international determination will provide an outstanding illustration of the practical application of technical cooperation among countries, whatever their level of development. It is important to remember that it is often to the so-called developing world that the industrialized world must turn for examples of the new model of practice. It is in the non-Western countries that the medical model has been most exposed for its inadequacies and where PHC approaches have begun to emerge. As the flaws in the conventional medical model become clearer in Western societies as well, those countries can learn from Africa, Asia, and Latin America, where it is possible to find some examples of the emergence of a more dynamic, rational, and holistic health care model (Macdonald, 1993).

The Overall Analysis of Health Care

Society's economic goal for health is to make service as efficient as possible. The implications of this goal envelop all aspects of health care. The overriding constraint is to offer all the services that society demands of a health care system while providing them at the lowest cost possible, given an acceptable level of quality. This goal can be obtained by either offering existing services at a lower cost, utilizing new technological advances, or improving the current health services while maintaining the existing price level.

Individuals and societies must make these decisions while working in the arena of either preventive or curative medicine. Again, we must ask ourselves which philosophy is more appropriate. There will always be the immediate demands for curative health care required in instances of traumatic emergencies. However, maintaining the continuous and overall health of an individual through preventive techniques might reduce the number and severity of such afflictions.

A new model for looking at personal health issues is to treat health as an investment. The idea that people invest in health just as they invest in schooling or other forms of human capital is an essential part of models of the demand for health (Kenkel, 1994). Given this new role for health care, preventive medicine is quickly being adopted; however, many of the Western health systems are still pushing for high-technology curative medicines at the expense of preventive alternatives (Kenkel, 1994).

Economic Analyses

As health care decision makers, we must decide between preventive and strictly curative treatment for illness. How do we know when it is cheaper and/or more effective to invest in long-term prevention, as opposed to large health care expenditures after an ailment has set in? Standard financing models might be employed to analyze the effectiveness and appropriateness of specific health care procedures. Models such as net present value (NPV), cost-benefit analysis (CBA), and cost-effective analysis (CEA) are used to assist the decision maker in evaluating alternatives.

Net present value (NPV) examines the present value of benefits above the initial resource expenditure for a given investment. When analyzing the preventive health investment, it is not difficult to compare its NPV to another preventive treatment or even to a curative measure expected to be necessary in the future. The health investment strategy chosen must have the highest NPV possible among all viable alternatives. For example, the NPV of regular exercise and a healthy low fat, low cholesterol diet is likely to be much higher than a marginally unhealthy lifestyle that may lead to serious health problems such as heart disease.

Cost-benefit analysis (CBA) is another method of estimating the appropriateness of health care investments. It relies on calculating, or at least estimating, the cost of a procedure and weighing it against the benefits received. Cost-benefit analysis is most effective when used to decide between alternative treatments for the same ailments. Problems with the estimation of cost and benefits might lead to discrepancies in choice. Another problem with CBA is failure to recognize the successes. It is paradoxical that preventive programs are the most valuable, but least visible, precisely when nothing happens. People cannot see the cases of illness that did not occur or miss the money that was not spent.

Cost-effective analysis (CEA) is similar to CBA except that its goal is to compare the cost efficiency and effectiveness of unrelated treatments. For instance, which is a better value: a drug that costs $100 per marginal mm reduction in blood pressure, or another drug that costs $100 per marginal ear infection cure. Cost-effective analysis attempts to standardize these costs in order to make them comparable. The study of the cost effectiveness of pharmaceuticals and health care treatments is known as pharmacoeconomics. When dealing with issues in health care, pharmacoeconomists use the notion of quality adjusted life years (QALY). One QALY is a year spent in perfect health, or 100% health-related quality of life. The cost per QALY is computed among different treatments to determine which investments should be undertaken. That is to say, which treatment decisions would have the greatest benefit to the customers (patients) of the health care entity (hospital)?

These three models, which assist in assessing investment decisions in health treatments, are the most common but not the only alternatives as decision-making tools. Many models are being developed and tested in the field of pharmacoeconomics. In many instances, these decisions are made not with quantitative models but with qualitative knowledge provided by field experts and specialists.

Although these models may seem to provide clear-cut answers to financial issues in health care, they are obviously missing more qualitative and ethical considerations for treatment.

Facilitating Health Care

Facilitating health care is a difficult question that must be considered throughout the world. Along with the economic issues addressed previously in determining the best course of action to battle illness (NPV, CBA, CEA), there are other problems that must also be addressed in terms of management of health care and payment for that health care. These are issues that every country must face, from the least developed countries to industrialized nations. Two basic philosophies have emerged and have been in practice, although they have been altered and are in a constant state of transformation. The two philosophies are fee-for-service health care and managed health care. These ideas have provided the basis for many variations of facilitation in health care throughout the years. However, managed care has become the philosophy of choice—due to society's acceptance that widespread equity in quality health care is mandatory today. However, both philosophies have been important in establishing care, and the transition from fee-for-service to managed care is quite slow. Therefore, this section will explain the two different ideas, the different applications of the ideas, and the transition toward managed care. Also, because managed care is not an exact science, this section will address the problems faced by different nations in using and establishing it.

Fee-for-Service Health Care.   Fee-for service health care's main proponent and facilitator is the United States, which will be used as the example for this facilitation of health care. The fee-for-service system was founded on a payment by the patient, based on the average cost in treating his or her ailment. The charge included the average cost of diagnostic and/or therapeutic procedures done, room, board, nursing services, and generally a price markup (by for-profit organizations). This payment also includes the cost of technology needed for the patient's treatment. The system was based on internal determinations of costs made by physicians and hospital administration derived from the history of prior patients' treatment.

Fee-based health care created an atmosphere in which cost effectiveness for the patient was not really considered. This was the case because charges for health care services were considered to have zero elasticity. Therefore, any diagnostic or therapeutic procedure deemed beneficial was carried out no matter what the cost. The fee-based system also created strange relationships between physicians and hospitals. Presently there are many types of "partnerships" that have been developed in an attempt to consolidate these two entities in the fee-for-service philosophy. These include (1) the traditional doctor's workshop, in which physicians are proprietors of their own practices and are not employed or contracted by hospitals; (2) the integrated delivery system, in which physicians and hospitals are combined into one organization, yet still maintain a fee basis; and (3) the contractual network, in which physicians and hospitals are related through a contractual agreement. The different relationships between physicians and hospitals greatly confused the manner of payment, and in some systems (especially doctor's workshop) created a "medical arms race" in price and patient occupancy in hospitals. Despite existing problems and the creation of new ones, the fee-based philosophy of health care is a legitimate approach to the facilitation of care-giving services. However, with the understanding that quality health care services should be cost effective and offered to all people equally, it became evident that fee-for-service care was geared toward the wealthy. The egalitarian idea of reasonable quality care has caused most countries to use managed health care to facilitate effective services (even in the United States, although the transition is slow).

Managed Health Care.   The basic concept behind managed health care is that the physician is an employee. Instead of billing for services, physicians are paid an annual salary by the facilitating organization. The organization can be private, in which the doctor is an employee of the corporation; or the facilitating organization could be the government, in which case the physician is an employee of the state. This system allows for ease in payment for the patient. It also allows for universal care if the government is the facilitating organization. Managed health care is becoming the choice for the world in facilitating health service.

There are many variations in managed health care organizations. In the United States alone, there are well over 500 different programs (although some are transition programs from fee-based care) represented by managed care organizations that develop the HMO plans. The following is a description of selected programs offered in the United States.

The first plan is the point-of-service (POS) plan. This plan is offered by private HMO organizations and represents a definite transitional product that is assigned to ease into HMOs. POS offers members visits with selected physicians at a nominal out-of-pocket charge, while also offering members the choice of other physicians (non-network providers) for a larger fee. This set-up is similar to the traditional insurance program, which is why it is considered transitional.

Another HMO plan offered in the United States is the preferred provider organization (PPO). This product offers a list of selected physicians who may be used by the patient as his or her primary physician. However, to be examined or treated by another physician without paying directly out-of-pocket, the patient is required to obtain a referral from the primary physician.

Medicare risk and cost contracts are programs offered by almost a quarter of the HMOs in the United States These products are the epitome of managed care. Medicare pays HMOs a total sum on a monthly basis based upon 95% of the estimated cost for beneficiaries who would have remained on Medicare fee-for-service programs.

Managed care is, however, better exemplified in the European nations. Many countries in Europe, including France, Sweden, Germany, and Italy, have socialized medicine. Under this system, any person needing medical attention may be admitted and cared for. These countries are able to do this because each government has apportioned a large budget for this system, appropriated from taxes that are collected from the general population. This is a very positive system with respect to the egalitarian ideal of quality care, no matter the patient's economic circumstance. This contributes to the very low infant mortality rates demonstrated in these countries. Because of this, these countries have become the models for developing countries in creating universal health care services.

Universal health care does not come without significant costs, the burden being carried by individuals and corporations through payroll deductions. Universal coverage by managed care can result in monetary competition between medical research and service. This can cause stagnation in service, and reduce technological advances that might improve the quality of care given. Although managed care is the clear choice of direction in philosophies, there are still problems associated with it in practice. These problems should be recognized and considered in the enhanced facilitation of health care.

Medicare.   Medicare, the health insurance program in the United States for the elderly and the disabled, was funded at $218 billion for 2001, and is expected to grow by an estimated rate of 7.1% from 2001 to 2005, to $309 billion (OMB, 2000). Medicaid, the joint federal and state health insurance program for the poor, was funded at $108 billion at the federal level and $81 billion for states; the federal portion for 2001 is $124.8 billion (OMB, 2000).

Medicare has been very successful in expanding quality medical care for the elderly and the disabled. Part A of Medicare covers almost all Americans over the age of 65, and most persons disabled for two years or more are entitled to Social Security benefits. Part A reimburses health care providers for hospital care, nursing home care, and hospice services. Part B is an optional form of coverage for those over 65 years of age and people who are disabled, and 94% of individuals under Part A also elect for Part B coverage, since it pays for outpatient services, clinical lab work, medical supplies, physical therapy, durable medical equipment, and kidney dialysis. Citizens under Medicare can go either to the traditional fee-for-service option or to a managed care plan. An estimated 83% of Medicare beneficiaries opt for the fee-for-service coverage.

Medicare has significantly increased access to health care for the elderly, from 50% in 1966 to almost 100% in 2000 (OMB, 2000). Medicare coverage has now expanded to include preventive services such as mammography, prostate and colorectal cancer screening, and bone mass measurements for osteoporosis screening. Medicare enrollment is expected to skyrocket in 2010, when the demographic phenomenon known as the "Baby Boom" generation begins to reach age 65 in record numbers, at which time there will be some 46 million enrollees, increasing to 61 million persons by 2030. Since Medicare is funded by the 2.9 percent payroll tax, Part A funding faces severe challenges in the decades ahead. By 2010 the Hospital Insurance Trust Fund, where Medicare monies are stored, is expected become insolvent—with only 2.3 workers paying the payroll tax for every one Medicare beneficiary.

Summary

Primary health care has been defined by the WHO as essential health care made universally accessible to individuals and families in the community by means acceptable to them, through their full participation and at a cost that the community can afford. It is a basic level of health care that includes programs directed at the promotion of health, early diagnosis of disease or disability, and prevention of disease.

Primary health care services vary depending on the location of the health care facility. These services are based around eight core components. The core components are the basis behind the network of PHC, and provide a backbone for the variety of services that are provided. Support for these services greatly impacts how effectively the program is going to work. Public and professional support is necessary to make any system work. The public must unanimously accept PHC as providing the measures that the majority of citizens believe will help increase their health. The support of leaders and decision makers at each level is required to keep the services properly maintained. The personnel who are to be working and providing services should also support these policies in order to ensure that proper procedures are carried out.

Primary health care has been faced with many problems varying from individual concerns—such as limited or no access to health care because of poverty, lack of transportation, and lack of knowledge—to societal concerns—such as the availability of proper professional training, as well as monitored government expenditure and debt. These problems have a solution, although it is up to the individual area and its accessibility to funding. The main benefit of PHC is that it is more cost effective and accessible to the population than regular hospital care. It is also based on prevention rather than on cure. It strives to minimize preventable human suffering due to diseases.

PHC became an international goal at the Alma-Ata Conference in September of 1978. The Conference resulted in the Alma-Ata Declaration to attain "Health for All Africans by the Year 2000." This declaration states actions for protecting and promoting health for the entire world.

Society's economic goal for health is to make service as efficient as possible. The implications of this goal envelop all aspects of health care. Goals can be attained by either offering existing services at a lower cost, utilizing new technology advances, or improving the current health services while maintaining the existing price level. Models such as net present value (NPV), cost-benefit analysis (CBA), and cost-effective analysis (CEA) are used to assist the decision maker in evaluating alternatives to health care. More qualitative and ethical programs for facilitating health care include fee-for-service health care and managed care. These types of programs brought about the ideas of HMOs, Medicare, and Medicaid. Managed care is the clear choice of direction in philosophies, but there are still problems associated with it in practice.

Discussion Questions _____

1. Discuss the origins of PHC.

2. Discuss the key components of PHC.

3. What are the societal benefits of PHC?

4. What is the HFA 2000 goal?

5. What were the four main objectives of the Alma-Ata Conference?

6. Distinguish between CBA and CEA.

7. Why is there a projected shortfall in the Hospital Insurance Trust Fund monies for Medicare?

8. What is the difference between the PPO and POS?

References _____

Anderson, L. (1998). *Mosby's Medical, Nursing, and Allied Health Dictionary* (5th ed.). St. Louis: C. V. Mosby Company.

Atkinson, A. (1970). On the Measurement of Inequality. *Journal of Economic Theory, 2*, 244–263.

Bang, M. (1990). *Primary Health Care in Africa.* Boulder, CO: Westview Press.

Bardhan, P. (1970). On the Minimum Level of Living and the Rural Poor. *Indian Economic Review, 5*, 129–136.

Basch, P. (1999). *Textbook of International Health* (2nd ed.). New York: Oxford University Press.

Bergerhoff, P., Lehmann, D., & Novak, P. (1990). *Primary Health Care*. New York: Springer-Verlag Press.

Buttery, C. (1991). *Handbook for Health Directors*. New York: Oxford University Press.

Chabot, J., & Waddington, C. (1987). Primary Health Care Is Not Cheap. *International Journal of Health Services*, 17: 387–409.

Clark, J. (1991). *Democratizing Development*. Hartford, CT: Kumarian Press.

DC. (1999). Poverty in the United States 1998: Current Population Reports. Washington, DC: United States Department of Commerce, Census Bureau.

Donaldson, M. S., Yordy, K. D., Lohr, K. N., & Vanselow, N. A. (1996). *Primary Care: America's Health in a New Era*. Washington, DC: National Academy Press.

Elling, K. (1984). *Health System Support for Primary Health Care*. Geneva, Switzerland: World Health Organization.

Haines, A. (2000). Joining Together to Combat Poverty. *British Medical Journal, 320*, 1–2.

Kenkel, D. (1994). *The Demand for Preventative Medical Care: Applied Economics*. New York: XYZ Publishers.

Koivusalo, M., Ollila, E., & Ollila E. (1998). *Making a Healthy World: Agencies, Actors, and Policies in International Health*. New York: St. Martins Press.

Kurian, G. (1990). *Encyclopedia of the Third World* (4th ed.). New York: Facts on File.

Kurian, G. (1992). *Encyclopedia of the Third World* (4th ed.). New York: Facts on File.

Lee, K., and Mills, A. (1993). *Health Economics Research in Developing Countries*. New York: Oxford Medical Publications.

Macdonald, J. J. (1993). *Primary Health Care Medicine in Its Place*. Hartford, CT: Kumarian Press.

Miller, R. (1983). *Primary Health Care: More Than Medicine*. New York: Prentice-Hall, Inc.

OMB. (2000). *Budget of the United States Government: Fiscal Year 2001*. Washington, DC: Office of Management and Budget [Online] Available: Http://w3.access.gpo.gov/usbudget

Oxfam International. (1999). *Education Facts Today* [Online] Available Http://www.oxfam.org

Paulanka, B., & Purnell, L. (1998). *Transcultural Health Care*. Philadelphia: F. A. Davis Company.

Seligson, M., and Smith, J. (1998). *Development and Underdevelopment*. London: Lynne Rienner Publishers, Inc.

WB. (2000). Poverty Net: Data On Poverty. New York: The World Bank Group [Online] Available: Http://www.worldbank.org

WHO. (1978). *Alma-Ata Primary Health Care Geneva*. Geneva, Switzerland: World Health Organization.

WHO. (1981). *Global Strategy for Health for All by the Year 2000*. Geneva, Switzerland: World Health Organization.

UN. (1998). *Human Development Report 1998*. New York: Oxford University Press.

UN. (1990). *World Population Policies*. New York: United Nations.

6

Maternal and Child Health: A Global Health Perspective

Matt Flint, Candice Borden, and Lyndsay Graff

The Health of Mothers and Children

Issues involving maternal and child health have long been accepted as global indicators of a country's level of overall health and wellness. Maternal and child health data are collected and reported about populations involved in the early stages of life including infants, children, and women in their childbearing years. Factors that affect maternal and child health include the political environment, socioeconomic levels, and cultural influences. To understand the issues surrounding global maternal and child health, one must better understand the environment, conditions, and cultures throughout the world that influence decision making and behaviors of individuals and communities.

Various governmental and nongovernmental agencies are involved in gathering data, analyzing maternal and child health issues, and providing programs focused on improving health and decreasing risk factors. The World Health Organization (WHO), UNICEF, the World Bank, and the United Nations are leaders in attempting to set standards for providing data that can be useful in making comparisons and evaluating health status. Additionally, many governments, women and children advocacy groups, and community organizations are working to explain the multiple factors involved in maternal and child health.

This chapter has several main purposes. From the perspective of maternal health, first it will discuss issues such as mortality and morbidity. Second, it will identify risks and influences related to these issues in the context of other influencing factors. Third, it will explore interventions that have proved cost effective in reducing health problems. Then, from the perspective of infant and child health, the same three areas will be pursued. Finally, the chapter will address other health issues such as abortion and contraception.

Maternal Health

Maternal health involves the health of women, throughout their entire lives, who anticipate being part of the childbearing process. It is not exclusive to the time when a woman conceives, maintains the pregnancy, goes into labor, and delivers. It also involves lifestyles, behaviors, and issues before and after conception that may influence the health and development of the fetus as well as the mother.

Why is a discussion of maternal health warranted? It is expected that, over the next two decades, the number of women and men of reproductive age will nearly double (WHO, 1997a). This rapid increase in the numbers of women and men with the potential to procreate will increase the need for developing more programs that provide family planning education and prenatal care services. Successful programs will also provide access to skilled health care providers and effective obstetric facilities.

The 1999 World Health Report stated that, in developing countries, *maternal conditions*, HIV/AIDS, and tuberculosis are the three major leading causes of disease burden in adults. The combination of these three conditions accounted for 7% of all disability-adjusted life years in 1998. Not only are maternal conditions being discussed in relationships to disease burden, but they are also part of the larger female experience.

Globally, the experiences of females are beginning to receive much-needed attention. Subjects such as female genital mutilation, "honor-based" abuse, unsafe abortions, nutritional deficiencies, and barriers to health care services are being discussed, often in the context of maternal health. As researchers begin to unravel some of the issues that have been part of female experiences throughout the world, the need for standards of data, effective program planning, and discussion of future direction will become more apparent.

The following sections will attempt to identify the causes of maternal mortality and morbidity, to discuss the risk factors and influencing conditions that contribute to a woman's health status, and to evaluate interventions. Maternal health will be discussed along with other constructs such as poverty, politics, cultural traditions, and social paradigms.

Mortality and Morbidity

To understand maternal mortality and how it is recorded, we must first define what it is and then examine its impact on our global community. Maternal deaths are defined in the *International Classification of Diseases-10* as the disease of a woman while pregnant or within 42 days of termination of pregnancy, irrespective of the duration and the site of the pregnancy, from any cause related to or aggravated by the pregnancy or its management but not from accidental or incidental causes.

Often, maternal deaths are divided into direct obstetric deaths and indirect obstetric deaths. Direct obstetric deaths are those resulting from obstetric complications of the pregnant state (pregnancy, labor, and puerperium), from interventions, omissions, incorrect treatment, or from a chain of events resulting from any of the above. Indirect obstetric deaths include those resulting from a previous existing disease that developed during pregnancy and which was not due to direct obstetric causes, but which was aggravated by physiologic effects of pregnancy.

Of all maternal deaths, obstetric emergencies account for 75% (Kotch, 1997). Among the direct obstetrical causes of death during pregnancy are hemorrhage, infection, eclampsia, and obstructed labor. In 1998, obstructed labor, sepsis (infection of the blood), and unsafe abortions were listed among the top ten leading causes of death and disability in women 15 to 44 years of age in developing countries (WHO, 1999). All of these conditions are found with distressing frequency in developing countries, and most can be prevented at very low cost (see Table 6.1).

Many of these causes, especially infections resulting from contamination during childbirth, can be prevented by observing simple rules of hygiene. It was demonstrated over 150 years ago that having physicians wash their hands could prevent many of these types of fatal infections. However, for various reasons, simple hygiene has not yet been adopted in some parts of the world.

It has been reported that illegal and unsafe abortions for unwanted pregnancies cause some 115,000 to 200,000 of these obstetric deaths (Basch, 1999). The reason for this is simply that women do not have access to the needed family planning services. They also do not have access to safe procedures or treatments for complications from abortions.

The foregoing discussion helps to identify some of the causes of maternal mortality and morbidity, and it also limits what can be reported as a maternal death and what cannot. Though death is defined in very specific terms, one should realize the limitations to maternal death data. These data are often underreported, and there are multiple reasons why this occurs. First, there is incomplete investigation

TABLE 6.1 *Female Mortality and Morbidity Causes, Estimates for 1998*

Maternal Conditions	Mortality	Morbidity
Hemorrhage	123,000 (25%)	3,833,000 (12%)
Sepsis	74,000 (15%)	5,965,000 (18%)
Hypertensive disorders of pregnancy	62,000 (13%)	1,882,000 (6%)
Obstructed labor	38,000 (8%)	7,040,000 (22%)
Abortion	66,000 (13%)	5,498,000 (17%)
Other maternal conditions	131,000 (26%)	8,032,000 (25%)

Source: World Health Organization, World Health Report (1999).

of the death, which affects the information put on a death certificate. Second, there may be a lack of knowledge of the pregnancy status. Third, legal and economic constraints are placed on reporting a death (limited number of days to report, possible fees). Finally, individuals and families may have to travel long distances to a registering office. They may have neither the means of transportation nor the time to actually report the death.

It is also important to examine how extensive the problem really is and what populations are at higher risks. Imagine that, every four hours, day in, day out, a jumbo jet crashes and all on-board are killed. The 250 passengers are women, most in the prime of life, some still in their teens. They are all either pregnant or have just delivered a baby. Most of them have growing children at home, and families that depend on them (Basch, 1999). It is estimated that there are approximately 500,000 to 585,000 maternal deaths every year (The World Bank, 1999; Basch, 1999). However, the true world maternal death rate may be greater than indicated by these statistics due to the fact that most of those who die are poor, live in remote areas, and their deaths are not recorded or accurately accounted for. In those parts of the world where maternal mortality is highest, deaths are rarely recorded, and the cause of death is usually not given (see Table 6.2).

Risk and Influencing Factors

A few statistics quickly reveal who is at higher risk. The World Health Report 1999 identified poverty as the main reason for maternal mortality during childbirth. Complications of pregnancy and childbirth are the leading cause of death and disability in developing countries among women of reproductive age. In fact, nearly 99% of the estimated 500,000 maternal deaths each year occur in developing countries (The World Bank, 1999).

A woman in a developing country has a 1 in 48 chance of dying from pregnancy-related causes compared to a 1 in 1,800 chance for women in developed countries (The World Bank, 1999). More than half of all maternal deaths occur in Asia, where poverty-ridden countries such as Bangladesh, Pakistan, and India have extremely high rates. India has more maternal deaths in one week than all of Europe has in one year (Basch, 1999). The disparities in maternal mortality between developing and industrialized countries are both remarkable and unacceptable.

Poverty plays a major role in maternal mortality, and its influence is seen in a number of different ways. Low-income countries often do not have the medical facilities to perform successful labor and delivery. In addition, so-called "established" facilities may not be capable of supporting pregnancy-related complications. Poverty also affects how many skilled health care providers are available during the labor and delivery processes.

In countries that report fewer than 50% of births being attended by skilled health staff, there is a strong association with a high maternal mortality ratio. The range for maternal mortality per 100,000 live births in those countries is from 170 in Egypt up to 1,500 in Angola and Nepal (WHO, 1999). To put these numbers into

TABLE 6.2   *Mortality Rates for Select Member States of WHO*

Member States	Infant Mortality Rate (per 1,000)		Maternal Mortality Ratio (per 100,000)
	1978	1998	1990
Africa			
Algeria	121	91	160
Benin	122	88	990
Chad	154	112	1,500
Eritrea	123	91	1,400
Kenya	88	66	650
Madagascar	130	83	490
Nigeria	109	81	1,000
Rwanda	133	124	1,300
South Africa	72	59	230
Togo	117	84	640
The Americas			
Brazil	79	42	220
Canada	12	6	6
Cuba	23	9	95
Ecuador	82	46	150
Guatemala	91	46	200
Haiti	139	68	1,000
Mexico	57	31	110
United States of America	14	7	12
Eastern Mediterranean			
Egypt	131	51	170
Iran	100	35	120
Iraq	84	95	310
Kuwait	34	12	29
Europe			
Croatia	21	10	. . .
Czech Republic	18	6	15
Germany	15	5	22
France	11	6	15
Hungary	27	10	30
Israel	18	8	7
Kazakhstan	45	35	80
Kyrgyzstan	55	40	110
Poland	23	15	19
Romania	31	23	130
Russian Federation	30	18	75
Slovakia	22	11	. . .
Slovenia	17	7	13
Switzerland	10	6	6
Ukraine	23	19	50

(continued)

TABLE 6.2   *Continued*

Member States	Infant Mortality Rate (per 1,000)		Maternal Mortality Ratio (per 100,000)
	1978	1998	1990
Southeast Asia			
India	129	72	570
Thailand	56	29	200
Western Pacific			
Australia	13	6	9
China	52	41	95
Japan	9	4	18
Vietnam	82	38	160

Source: World Health Organization, World Health Report (1999).

context, the maternal mortality ratio for some developed countries are Canada, 6; France, 15; Japan, 18; and the United States, 12.

Complications during pregnancy are another major concern in maternal health. Of the approximately 150 million women who become pregnant each year, one out of three is at risk of having complications. Also, one in five deaths for women of reproductive age is due to complications during pregnancy and delivery (WHO, 1995).

These complications may affect the pregnant woman, the fetus, or both. According to the 1999 World Health Report, as stated previously, the three major complications seen globally are obstructed labor, sepsis (infection of the blood), and unsafe abortions. Some of these complications may come about as a direct result of diseases such as tuberculosis, malaria, diabetes, or hepatitis. When a mother has obstructed labor, the infant is at high risk. There can be damage to the brain, causing such disorders as seizures or cerebral palsy, learning disabilities, or even death (WHO, 1993).

Other risk factors are poor nutrition, disease, high parity, and mother age (mortality risk increases for women below 20 or above 35). In Bangladesh, where 50% of women are married by age 15, maternal mortality among women ages 10 to 14 was five times higher compared to women ages 20 to 24. In the United States, the risk of maternal death is tenfold higher at age 44 than at age 24 (Basch, 1999). These maternal mortality risk factors can be reduced through adequate prenatal care, medical and nutritional screening, diagnosis, and treatment, including education.

Many of the risk factors for maternal deaths, disease, and disability are interrelated in vicious cycles. For example, women living in low-income countries have to work in order to help provide food for their families. Because of their concerns for maintaining employment, they report little time to go and receive prenatal care. Also, the nutrients that are provided in the household may not be enough to sustain a healthy pregnancy, increasing the risk for spontaneous abortion or a low birth weight child. When complications occur, or the child is not as healthy as expected, more pressure may be put on the family to meet increased financial costs, forcing the woman to work even more. Interventions must be developed that assist women in becoming aware and educated and that deal with financial, cultural, and social issues.

Interventions

In April 1998, the tenth anniversary of the Safe Motherhood Initiative was celebrated. One of the most crucial interventions for decreasing maternal mortality is safe delivery. In the 1999 report *Safe Motherhood and the World Bank*, it was concluded that interventions focused on children under the age of 5 and interventions for women of reproductive age bring the greatest benefit at the lowest cost (see Table 6.3).

Critical to the reduction of maternal mortality and morbidity is access to skilled individuals before, during, and after delivery. Also, women need to have obstetrical facilities available that can deal with possible complications of labor and delivery. At the minimum the facilities should be able to provide necessary blood transfusions and anesthesia.

TABLE 6.3   *Essential Safe Motherhood Interventions*

Prevention and Management of Unwanted Pregnancies
- Family planning
- Management of complications from unsafe abortion
- Termination of pregnancy where not against the law

Pregnancy-Related Services
Prenatal Care
- Birth planning
- Prompt detection, management, and referral of pregnancy complications
- Tetanus toxoid immunization
- Nutrition promotion, including iron and folate supplements
- Iodine supplements, where warranted
- Management and treatment of sexually transmitted infections, malaria, and tuberculosis

Safe Delivery
- Hygienic, normal delivery
- Detection, management, and referral of obstetric complications
- Facility-based essential obstetric care

Postpartum Care
- Monitoring for infection and hemorrhage
- Child spacing

Source: The World Bank, *Safe Motherhood and the World Bank: Lessons from 10 Years of Experience* (1999).

For women who anticipate becoming pregnant, it is important to develop behaviors that will increase the chances of having a successful pregnancy. Avoiding unhealthy substances (e.g., tobacco, alcohol, and other drugs), improving nutritional habits, and being involved in some form of physical activity are behaviors that will improve pregnancy outcomes. Combining these behaviors with participation in prenatal care and regular medical checkups will reduce risk and prevent mortality and morbidity.

In developing countries, however, access to these women's health and family planning clinics is limited. Nevertheless, trained native or local professional outreach programs can be adapted to effectively accomplish the objectives for a healthy pregnancy. The objectives are to educate and make women aware regarding their behaviors, including reproductive health and disease prevention, and to provide simple and inexpensive health screenings, diagnosis, and treatment. By meeting these objectives, medical, environmental, and behavioral risks that contribute to poor pregnancy outcomes will be reduced.

Empowering women through education and simple preventive measures can significantly improve poor outcomes such as low birth weight infants and birth defects. Health screenings are effective at obtaining information such as weight, height, blood glucose level, hemoglobin level, and phenylketonuria. In addition, a behavioral risk assessment questionnaire screens for eating disorders; alcohol, tobacco, and other substance abuse; and knowledge of contraceptive methods and safe-sex practices.

Effective program planning is a key to reducing the number of deaths attributable to complications during pregnancy. Additionally, some lifelong disabilities that are caused by these complications might be avoided. A good starting point for reducing death and injury from complications is to provide easy access to education and health facilities and to increase the number of adequately trained health personnel. This change could drastically reduce such disorders as pelvic inflammatory disease, infertility, or anemia (WHO, 1993).

To plan programs and implement interventions with the objective of decreasing maternal mortality and morbidity, researchers will have to identify behavioral, social, environmental, and cultural factors that increase risk. Also, significant support (resources) from government and nongovernment organizations will be needed in order to educate and train individuals about better health practices.

Infant and Child Health

Infant and child health is a strong indicator of health and wellness within and between countries and is affected by a number of variables. It is impossible to discuss infants and children without discussing maternal health. In many cases, it is the behaviors before, during, and after pregnancy of the mother that affect the health of the very young more than anything else. Some major maternal behaviors and conditions that become important to proper physical, cognitive, psychological, and social development of a newborn are poverty, nutrition, utilization of health care services, education levels, cultural beliefs and traditions, and social support systems.

Currently, the world population is approximately 6 billion people. As was true in our discussion of maternal mortality, poverty levels are greatly implicated in infant and child mortality and morbidity. Those living in absolute poverty, compared with those who are not poor, are estimated to have a five times higher probability of death between birth and 5 years of age (WHO, 1999).

The *World Health Report 1995* identified poverty as the main reason why babies are not vaccinated, why clean water and sanitation are not provided, and why curative drugs and other treatments are unavailable. More than 12 million children under 5 years of age die in the developing world every year. Most of these deaths are from causes that could be prevented inexpensively. Small financial investments, when used to better manage pregnancies and provide adequate infant care, would have great impact in decreasing the number of deaths in the largest group of infants, ages 1 week to 1 month. The disparity between the developing and the industrialized countries in terms of infant and child survival is striking (WHO, 1995).

The WHO has identified the five major childhood conditions responsible for 21% of all deaths in low- and middle-income countries. These conditions are diarrhea, acute respiratory infections, malaria, measles, and perinatal conditions. Often, because of the mother's behaviors during pregnancy, the newborn child begins life with various health challenges. Poor nutrition, use of tobacco, and consumption of alcohol during a fetus's gestational development can lead to low birth weight, malformation of body systems or organs, birth defects, and other serious health problems.

Mortality and Morbidity

The infant mortality rate (IMR) is often used as one of the key indicators of socioeconomic development, hygienic conditions, and overall health of a population. Infant mortality rate is a useful index for several reasons. First, it is relatively easy to measure. Even in most developing countries, indirect methods can be adapted to estimate the IMR. With reliable estimates, one can effectively compare and assess patterns of infant death around the world. Secondly, the IMR is strongly correlated with adult mortality. In a population where the IMR is high, it is very likely that the population experiences a wide range of health problems due to underlying inadequacies in socioeconomic and hygienic conditions. An example of this is the high proportion of child deaths due to infectious and parasitic diseases that could be reduced by simple preventive and curative public health interventions that cost little. Therefore, the IMR is useful in evaluating the impact of preventive or curative public health interventions and is a sensitive indicator of inequality within a population (Grey & Payne, 1993).

The IMR can be divided into neonatal (within the first 28 days of life) and post-neonatal (after the first 28 days but within the first year of life) mortality rates. The neonatal mortality rate is further subdivided into first-day deaths, early neonatal deaths (from birth to 7 days of age), and late neonatal deaths (from 8 through the 28 days) (Grey & Payne, 1993).

Usually neonatal deaths are due to immaturity, inherent congenital conditions, or circumstances of birth that are independent of postnatal care. On the other hand, postneonatal deaths are often caused by environmental factors such as nutritional deficiencies and infectious diseases. The ratio of neonatal to postneonatal deaths can provide a sensitive measure of adverse environmental conditions (Taylor, 1994). If neonatal deaths are high, women's preconception and prenatal nutrition and their access and use of medical services may be targeted to reduce death rates. If postneonatal deaths are high, environmental causes might be examined to improve the nutrition of the newborn. This could include breast feeding promotion, reduction of infectious disease via hygienic preparation of infant formula, food handling, and other general hygienic practices.

In addition to infant mortality, perinatal deaths have received a great deal of attention in recent years. The perinatal period extends from the gestational age at which the fetus or infant attains 1,000 grams in weight or 35 centimeters crown-heel length, or 28 weeks of gestation until the end of the seventh completed day of postnatal life. The perinatal period is unique because most deaths within it occur due to some influence of the mother on the fetus.

However, collection of data on fetal or prenatal death rates is very difficult, for the following reasons. First, methodological problems make it very difficult to obtain data in the absence of required reporting of miscarriages or spontaneous abortion. Second, criteria for reporting are poorly understood by the medical profession. Third, obstetricians in developing and industrialized countries differ in their reporting. Fourth, the difficulty in deriving fetal death rates is in deciding what to use for the denominator.

With all of these conditions, the international comparability of mortality rates may be in doubt. Maintaining a pregnancy register may be an effective means by which to capture pregnancy-related data; however, currently in many countries this is an unreasonable goal. Even in the industrialized countries where registration systems are maintained, not all pregnant women receive prenatal care. Nevertheless, the collections of data on pregnancies and their outcomes require searching the files of obstetricians and primary-care physicians. Finally, undetected, early, spontaneous abortions and intentional abortions, particularly those with contraceptive intent, are not widely reported, making it difficult to collect meaningful data (Basch, 1999).

There has been improvement in the global figure for mortality among children under 5 years. In 1993, there were 87 deaths per 1,000 live births, an improvement from rates of 215 during the period 1950 to 1955 and 115 in 1980. However, in parts of the developed world only 6 out of 1,000 children born alive die before reaching age 5 compared to over 200 per 1,000 in 16 of the least developed countries (WHO, 1995).

Having explained the different categories of infant and childhood death, it is important to identify some of the major risk factors. Keep in mind that it is in the developing countries that we see more risk factors and where there is an urgent need for programs to be planned, implemented, and evaluated.

Risks and Influencing Factors

Like maternal health, poverty is arguably the most influential condition or factor associated with infant and child death. Families or individuals with low incomes often cannot afford proper nutrition, medical services, transport to medical facilities, and/or access to educational opportunities, especially programs involving family planning.

Nutrition is also a major contributing factor to infant and childhood health. As discussed earlier, the mother's as well as the child's nutritional status impact physiological development and risk for infection of the fetus. Important nutrients that are often not consumed by mothers are iron, folate, iodine, vitamins A, B, and C, and thiamin. High levels of proper nutrition in women of childbearing years can reduce the number of developmental disabilities, infant deaths, and low birth weight infants. In fact, a woman's nutritional status prior to pregnancy is as important for a successful pregnancy as is her diet during the nine months of pregnancy. This, in large part, is because folic acid is important to avoid certain birth defects, and it may take a significant amount of time for a woman to consume enough folic acid for it to be effective.

Nourishment for children begins at birth and is directly proportional to the nourishment or lack of nourishment of the mother (Robinson, 1995). Malnutrition is usually defined as a combination of inadequate nutritional intake and infection. Malnutrition significantly increases risks of childhood disease and death but often goes unrecognized. Malnutrition does not directly cause death, but malnourished children are much more susceptible to illness, and once ill, are more likely to die (WHO, 1999). Almost 2.4 million children under 5 years are still dying every year from diseases such as measles, neonatal tetanus, tuberculosis, pertussis, poliomyelitis, and diphtheria (WHO, 1995).

Malnutrition is implicated in more than half of all child deaths worldwide (UNICEF, 1998). Contrary to what many believe, three quarters of the children who die from malnutrition exhibit no outward signs of problems to a casual observer. They are considered mildly to moderately malnourished. The outcomes of an inadequate diet include lower than normal measurements on height (stunting) and weight (wasting). Stunting and wasting have been shown to have profound effects on cognitive developmental growth, risk for disease, and risk of premature death.

A society's traditions and beliefs can dramatically impact individual behaviors and decision making. For example, in many parts of India there are taboos applied to the women. This is especially true when the woman is pregnant and/or lactating. It is expected that she will not participate in certain activities for fear she will become possessed or that spirits will harm her unborn child. Some of the activities include not going out at night and/or limiting certain dietary items. Eggs, onions, garlic, seafood (shells, clamps, crabs, prawns), certain fish, any kind of sour food, and green leafy vegetables are strictly prohibited during and soon after pregnancy (Bandyopadhyay, 1998).

Interventions

Immunization programs have caused the most significant changes in infant and child health in the last few decades. In fact, the use of vaccines and immunizations at relatively low costs is often referred to as the most significant public health discovery ever. The WHO has identified that 2 million children die each year from diseases for which vaccines are available at low cost. However, even with these wonderful advances in disease prevention, many countries and governments do not take full advantage of having their citizenry immunized. Social and cultural stigmas still exist toward vaccines and toward the health care providers that administer lifesaving medications.

Oral rehydration is also an important intervention, especially in countries where there are high rates of diarrheal diseases. Replacing the fluids and salts lost through diarrhea helps to reduce the risk of malnutrition as well as of serious diseases.

To combat the problem of malnutrition, there are three major organizations that work globally. The World Food Programme is a United Nations organization. It responds to food needs associated with emergencies and development and often works with the Food and Agriculture Organization (also UN) and the International Fund for Agriculture Development. In 1996, the World Food Summit was held in Rome, with 186 countries participating (UNICEF, 1998). The plan of action developed at this conference focused on ways of achieving sustainable food security for all. It also emphasized the need for breast feeding and the importance of ensuring proper family nutrition to children, especially to girls.

For low-income mothers, there are many benefits derived from breast feeding. Children that are typically at a higher risk for problems reduce those risks once they begin breast feeding. With all of the many advantages, one would think there would be few women in the world who did not nurse their children. However, this is not always the case, and many choose to formula-feed their children.

There are several reasons why formula feeding is preferred over breast feeding. Some of those reasons are lack of knowledge, convenience, feelings of inability (to perform the process correctly), and little social support. Recently, there have been a number of marketing plans that have focused on providing formula to developing countries. Of major concern is the promotion of formula feeding in areas where water supplies are highly contaminated. It is critical that the marketing of formulas be accomplished within a comprehensive program that contains an educational component to provide directions on how to prepare the formula and how to decontaminate water sources.

Programs must also be geared toward targeting an individual's support systems, which might include family, friends, health care providers, and community or religious leaders, among others. If positive results from previous pregnancies can be achieved, rates of breast feeding will increase (Sciacca, Dube, Phipps, &

Ratliff, 1995). By getting the whole community involved, new mothers will find support in healthy behaviors and obtain the information necessary to make informed decisions.

Contraceptives and Abortion

Throughout the world, approximately 50 million abortions occur each year. Of these, 90% are unsafe abortions, and many are illegal. These issues contribute to the increase in risks that can lead to infertility, permanent impairment, and even death. In developing countries 1 in 250 procedures result in death, while only 1 in 3,700 occur in developed countries (WHO, 1999). Some of the factors that contribute to the large differences in death rates include access to health care, access to different forms of contraception, and/or proper sanitation (see Table 6.4).

The issues of abortion and contraceptive use raise much controversy. Comparing attitudes and beliefs between individuals in different countries, it becomes obvious that government, religion, social paradigms, and economics play important roles in which types of contraception are used and considered "acceptable." Also, these factors often determine if abortions are legal or illegal. The following describes the experience of Romania with contraception and abortion.

Romania Case Study

Until the revolution in 1989, the strict Romanian government outlawed the use of contraceptives, abortion, and sex education. After the revolution, a number of changes occurred. The total fertility rate dropped from 2.3 to 1.6 lifetime births per woman. The greatest decline was among those aged 35 to 39, with a 48% decrease, and those individuals with higher levels of education. This was due to the repeal of the prohibitions placed on abortion and contraception use.

The rate of total induced abortion increased from 1.7 lifetime abortions in 1987–1990 to 3.4 per woman in 1990–1993. The most common group of women that received abortions was married women. Nonmarried women who had abortions measured at about 1.0 abortions per woman. Among 15 to 19 year olds, the rate rose from 10 abortions per 1,000 in 1987–1990 to 32 per 1,000 in 1990–1993. For women in the age group of 20–34, who are the primary childbearers, rates doubled from 82 abortions per 1,000 to 209 per 1,000 (Remez, 1995).

The change in legalization regarding abortion had a direct role in the decrease of maternal mortality rate, which fell by almost two-thirds. The longer the term of the pregnancy, the more potential for complications. Through early termination, the mother is placed at a lower level of risk than if the child were carried to term.

With the legalization of abortion, changes were evident among the morbidity and mortality rates. Twenty-one percent of illegally induced abortion procedures resulted in complications. After 1989, only 9% of women developed complications. The key factor to the decline in maternal mortality rates was the 60% decrease in abortion-related mortality.

TABLE 6.4 *Abortion and Contraception in Various Countries*

Country	Abortion	Forms of Contraception
Cuba	Legal	Contraceptive failure accounts for the high number of abortions; as many as 3 out of 4 women had an abortion in 12 months while using another form of contraception; small families desired
Dominican Republic	Illegal	Abortion is supported for back-up to contraceptive failure; abortion helps maintain family size goals; 25% of women using a contraceptive method became pregnant unintentionally
China	Legal	Nonuse of contraceptive is main reason for abortion; IUD failure rates contribute to high abortion rate
Turkey	Legal	Most rely on the withdrawal method; women with paid occupations used more effective methods and had fewer pregnancies; abortion performed when contraceptives fail
Mauritius	Legal	Family planning services are available; contraceptives are used by 75% of all married women of reproductive age; abortion is an important part of the available family planning options
Nepal	Illegal	Abortion is a criminal act; sterilization is the leading method; lactation or withdrawal is used to space pregnancies; fear of hormonal methods; even though abortion is illegal, the traditional methods used result in multiple abortions

Source: World Health Organization Data Press Release, May 17, 1999, and World Bank Special Programme of Research (1995).

The other area that added to the impact of the revolution was the legalization of contraceptives. Seventy percent of the Romanian population still relies on traditional methods, with withdrawal being the most common. However, there was a 20% increase in the use of modern techniques between 1987 and 1993. This increase was most noticeable within the higher socioeconomic population. Of the polled individuals, 49% said they would use the traditional method of withdrawal, and 46% said they would use modern methods of contraception.

Knowledge and trust of modern contraceptives were not visible in the Romanian culture. Twenty percent of women did not know what the pill or an IUD was. Ironically, these are the two most common modern methods of contraceptives, with a 3% to 4% usage. Furthermore, the fear of side effects, the questions of partner approval, or lack of places to obtain modern contraceptives seem to impact the way that contraceptives were accepted in the new Romanian world. Although pharmacies and the government provided access to contraceptives, people seem to feel more comfortable using the black market to get these items (Remez, 1995).

Summary

The status of maternal and child health is closely affected by the political, socioeconomic, and cultural factors found in each country. The state of maternal and child health is a good indicator of overall health status and allows for comparisons to be made.

A country's underlying inadequacies in socioeconomic and hygienic conditions reflect in a wide range of nutrition and health problems. In the developing countries, malnutrition and infection are two major causes of the high infant, child, and maternal mortality rates. Both of these conditions can be diagnosed early and cost-effectively treated if attention is given them.

Those programs that will be effective at helping reduce the number of infant and child deaths must include components of awareness, education, and skill development, while at the same time breaking through social and cultural barriers to reach many of the high-risk populations. Such programs will need to involve many organizations that have the overriding goal of improving the health and wellness of individuals and communities. Partnerships working together and combining resources will be able to resolve problems and improve the quality of life for their target populations.

Discussion Questions _____

1. How is maternal mortality defined? Is this important?

2. What are some of the complications that can occur when a woman is pregnant?

3. What age groups are typically involved in infant and child health?

4. What prevention or intervention methods have shown effective in decreasing infant deaths, low birth weight infants, and infants with developmental disorders?

5. At what point during pregnancy is a woman's nutritional status important?

6. What role does malnutrition play in developing countries?

7. Compare the rates of maternal mortality between developing countries and the industrialized world.

8. What is the main reason found in the *World Health Report 1999* that babies are not vaccinated?

9. Define infant mortality rate (IMR).

10. Define perinatal death rate.

11. What roles do ethnicity and culture play in infant and child health?

12. Malnourished children are much more susceptible to what types of diseases?

13. What is the most straightforward approach to prevention of infection?

14. List some of the reasons formula feeding is preferred over breast feeding.

References

Bandyopadhyay, M. (1998). *Women and Health: Tradition and Culture in Rural India*. England: Ashgate Publishing.

Basch, P. F. (1999). *Textbook of International Health* (2nd ed.). New York: Oxford University Press.

Grey, A., & Payne, P. (1993). *World Health Disease* (Rev. ed., pp. 10–11). In A. Grey (Ed.). United Kingdom: Open University Press.

Kotch, J. B. (1997). *Maternal and Child Health: Programs, Problems, and Policy in Public Health*. Rockville, MD: Aspen Publishers.

Remez, L. (1995). Romanian Maternal Death Rate Fell by Two-Thirds after the 1989 Revolution. *Family Planning Perspectives, 2.7* (6), 263.

Robinson, K. (1995). Southeast Asia—Maternal and Child Nutrition in Madura, Indonesia. *Journal of Asian Studies, 54* (3), 902.

Sciacca, J. P., Dube, D. A., Phipps, B. L., Ratliff, M. I. (1995). A Breast Feeding Education and Promotion Program: Effects on Knowledge, Attitudes and Support for Breast Feeding. *Journal of Community Health, 6,* 473.

Taylor, C. (1994). *Child and Maternal Health Services in Rural India, The Narangwal Experiment* (p. 72). Baltimore: Johns Hopkins University Press.

UNICEF. (1998). *The State of the World's Children 1998*. Washington DC: Oxford Press

The World Bank. (1999). *Safe Motherhood and the World Bank: Lessons from 10 Years of Experience*. Washington, DC: The World Bank.

WHO. (1993). *WHO on . . . Making Motherhood Safer. World Health, 46* (5), 30. Geneva, Switzerland: World Health Organization.

WHO. (1995). *World Health Report 1995—Executive Summary*. Geneva, Switzerland: World Health Organization.

WHO. (1997). *Fact Sheet 129*. Available online: http://www.who:int/

WHO. (1999). *World Health Report 1999—The Double Burden: Emerging Epidemics and Persistent Problems*. Geneva, Switzerland: World Health Organization.

7

Comparative National Health Care Systems

Robert W. Buckingham, Zhaohui Zhong, and Edward A. Meister

Health Care Systems and Societal Functioning

Every society manifests forms of health care services because health is a social good needed in adequate amounts to maintain a functioning, productive society. Thus, in some countries the health care system (HCS) is entirely government administered and funded, much like many other public goods and services (e.g., highways, police and fire departments). Most countries have a mixture of public and private health care services, with wide ranges in sophistication of technology and knowledge investment possessed by medical professionals. There are also wide differences in the individual's ability to access medical care, which is a function of both its availability and the extent to which ability-to-pay is required.

Human health frailties are legion, but can be categorized into those that are (1) self-generated, for example, behavior-choice diseases such as tobacco-related heart disease (albeit, the users become nicotine-dependent); (2) quasi-accidents, where people engage in risky behaviors that have very high probabilities of injury (e.g., parasailing, drunk driving, unsafe sexual behaviors); (3) true accidents, where injuries result from simply functioning in societies that are never 100% safe (e.g., E. coli food poisoning); and (4) predestined diseases, such as those that are either part of the natural aging process or that are inherited. The incidence of the first three of these forms of human health frailties can be impacted greatly by population-level public health prevention initiatives, whereas the gene-based diseases are being addressed by molecular biological research. However, the changing of human behaviors to reduce health care needs in any given society is not an easy task, nor is it given much funding priority by central governments.

As with a boat that keeps popping new leaks, everyone is too busy bailing out the incoming water instead of taking preventive actions by actually plugging the holes. Human health care needs, in the absence of strong efforts at primary prevention and health promotion, are virtually infinite. Since no society has unlimited capital resources to address these enormous health care needs, the results are that people either get no medical care and live short or shortened lives, while some get poor quality care or episodic emergency room treatment, or others pay by means of insurance premiums or taxation for the best care available in that particular country.

A harsh reality is that most people around the planet are simply struck with ailments ranging from infectious diseases, mental illness problems, and painful chronic conditions. The quantity and degree of human suffering on Earth are beyond comprehension. Yet there has been tremendous progress over the past 100 years (CDC, 1999). Most of this progress is the result of public health efforts at basic sanitation, potable (safe) water, and population-level immunization (CDC, 1999). Smallpox, polio, anthrax, and many others have been eliminated or nearly eliminated by the development and acceptance of vaccines. Not everyone has access to these vaccines, and the World Health Organization (WHO) estimates that at least 2 million children still die each year from diseases that low-cost vaccines could have prevented (WHO, 1999b).

HCSs are not static, and are constantly evolving and adapting to changing health care needs. Populations get young, they get old, new medical discoveries occur, new technologies emerge, and there are huge profits to be made. Health is one commodity that economists refer to as having an inelastic demand curve. Someone who is ill is willing to forgo many other potential uses of money to enable getting better or cured. The estimates of health expenditures are beyond comprehension. In the United States the annual dollars absorbed into the health care industry are projected to increase from 1 trillion to 2.2 trillion dollars by 2008 (HCFA, 2000).

According to the WHO, the goals for health system development in the twenty-first century need to include reducing health care inequalities; increasing efficiency; protecting individuals, families, and communities from financial loss; and enhancing fairness in the financing and delivery of health care services (WHO, 1999b). The WHO delineates two important health care themes common to most countries. The first is to redefine the roles of the government, health care providers, consumer, and health care financing agencies. The second is to find new financing methods that will generate additional resources and bring greater efficiency in health care. Addressing preventable childhood diseases and those of women is a priority goal that can bring about many positive changes in the functioning of the society and reduce population growth. The equitable allocation of health care resources, coupled with the emphasis on the individual and community empowerment, are the keys to bettering the level of population health.

This chapter will review how countries decide the essential questions about health care services. Who pays the health care costs of a nation—the government, the private sector, or individuals? What proportion of monies come from each sector? How the HCS is funded has a lot to do with answering the question: How is it organized? These are the key questions that will be addressed in the review of HCSs around the world. It is not simply a matter of getting more health by spending more money. Money can be wasted in inefficiencies, or health care services can be overpriced as reflected in high medical salaries, procedure costs, or pharmaceutical expenses. Health care systems to a great extent also reflect the political ideology of the country. Countries with universal health coverage are typically organized within social democracies, while countries such as the United States, which has an emphasis on individual responsibility ethos, are more inclined to private for-profit systems.

Often the adjective "crisis" is used in regard to the operations of HCSs. In the United States, for example, it means ever-spiraling costs; in Russia it means organizational disarray and lack of essential services; while in such African countries as Ghana, it can mean the systematic collapse of medical services (the majority of physicians trained there have immigrated to other countries for a better life). HCS has a pivotal role in each society, and this review will present standardized measures of health for making a comparative analysis on how well each system works. The two key health indices that can assist in this comparison process are the infant mortality rate (i.e., the number of infant deaths per life births) and the life expectancies in that country.

The countries reviewed in this chapter represent a cross-section of the health care systems from around the world. The countries include Australia, Canada, Peoples Republic of China, Germany, Japan, Mexico, Russia, the United States, and South Africa. The country health care systems range from those with a long history of universal health coverage, to some with a mix of private and public payers and to others that exhibit a collapsing infrastructure and grossly underfunded health care systems.

The Health Care System of Australia

Australia is a large country that occupies an entire continent. In 1996, it had a population of over 18 million, of which 85% lived in urban areas (Peabody et al., 1996). About 8.4% of its gross domestic product (GDP) was spent on health services (AIHW, 1996). Despite universal health insurance, Australia's per capita spending is lower than that of most developed countries. In 1996, Australia spent $32.2 billion (all monies are in USD) on health services, equivalent to a rate of $1,775 per person (OECD, 1997). The health indicators of Australian people are among the best in the world (see Table 7.1).

Health Care System Structure

Australia has a complex HCS that involves many providers of medical service. The system is financed by both public and private sources. The public resources are mainly from the tax revenue of federal, state, and local governments. Australian government has an important role in health care system: In 1996–1997, it provided

TABLE 7.1   *Australian Health Indicators in 1999*

Life expectancy at birth (years)	80.14
Male	77.22
Female	83.23
Infant mortality rate	5.11/1,000 live births
Annual population growth rate	.90%
Total fertility rate	1.81 births/woman
Birth rate	13.21/1,000
Death rate	6.90/1,000

Source: World Factbook (1999).

almost 69% of funding for health expenditure (AIHW, 1998). The federal Commonwealth Department of Health has a leading role in forming policies, especially in the public health area, research, and national information management. State and local governments are responsible for delivering and managing health services. The private sector also plays an important role in providing health services, insurance, and public health. Some health services—such as nursing home long-term aged care beds—are mostly privately owned.

The Commonwealth Department of Health was established in 1921, yet it did not have much power until 1946. An amendment of the Constitution in 1946 gave the Commonwealth authority to make laws about pharmaceutical, sickness and hospital benefits, and medical and dental services. State and territory governments have the major responsibility for delivering public hospital services and a wide range of community and public health services, including public and psychiatric hospital systems.

Private insurance provides additional benefits in addition to Medicare. Because of the success and popularity of universal coverage under Medicare, private insurance has constantly decreased each year. Approximately 50% of Australian population had private insurance at the end of 1984; the rate had reduced to 31.6% in 1997 (AIHW, 1998). In 1999, hospital insurance coverage further declined to 31.2% (PHIAC, 2000). Insurance purchases are not tax deductible, even when provided by employers, so insurance is usually not included in wage-compensation packages. Therefore, most private insurance purchasers are individuals rather than employers. Most of the private health insurance funds are used to finance private hospital sectors. Private hospitals are increasing in importance in providing health services, from providing only less complex health care in the past to today's complex, high-technology services.

Financing Health Care

In 1996–1997, Australian governments provided 68.7% of the funding for health expenditure: 45.5% from the Commonwealth and 23.2% from local governments;

the remaining 31.3% provided by private sector (AIHW, 1998). Over time, the proportion of total expenditure provided by governments has been decreased, from 71.9% in 1984–1985 to 68.9% in 1996–1997. In the same period, the private sector's proportion in total health expenditure has risen from 28.1% to 31.3% (AIHW, 1998) (see Table 7.2).

The Commonwealth is the major funding provider for nursing homes, medical services, and pharmaceuticals. Private insurance funded about 11.4% of total health expenditure in 1995–1996 (AIHW, 1998). Its funds were largely concentrated in the private hospital sector. The coverage by private insurance includes using standard facilities for private inpatients in public hospitals receiving private hospital care, and supplementing benefits to Medicare. Some insurance may also have ancillary benefits that include dental care and optical, therapeutic and other nonmedical services.

Medicare

Australian Medicare is a universal health insurance system that was established in 1984. It generally covers all permanent residents. By arrangement with Medicare, patients receive free medical services, including inpatient and outpatient care. However, the choice of doctors is limited, and it does not cover private room stays.

The Medicare system is partially financed by a federal income tax (called the Medicare levy) which initially contributed about 15% of the total costs of physician and hospital services (Collopy, 1991). The Medicare levy has been increased several times since the introduction of Medicare, and it is currently set at 1.5% of taxable income (AIHW, 1998). In recent years, the Medicare levy has funded about 20% of Medicare total costs. The rest of the medical service costs of Medicare (about 80% of total costs) is financed by state and federal grants from other revenue sources plus fees paid by patients (Peabody et al., 1996).

Specific Medicare items covered are grouped under three basic categories as follows: hospital, medical, and pharmaceutical. Medicare patients can be treated,

TABLE 7.2   *Comparison of Australian Health Indicators in 1986 and 1996*

Indicators	1986	1996
Total expenditure on health as % of GDP	8	8.6
Public expenditure on health as % of GDP	5.6	5.9
Total expenditure on health per capita in $	1,072	1,775
Practicing physicians per 1,000 population	2	2.5
In-patient care beds per 1,000 population	NA	8.7
In-patient care average length of stay (days)	NA	15.5

Source: OECD (1997).

at no charge, in a public hospital by a doctor appointed by the hospital, not chosen by the patient. Medicare covers up to 75% of the medical costs associated with being a private patient in a hospital. For outpatient care Medicare will reimburse 85% of the costs of treatment. For physicians billing directly to Medicare there will be no charges for the patient. Under the pharmaceutical benefits provisions the patient pays only a part of the cost of most prescription medicines purchased at pharmacies.

Private patients, whether insured or not, can choose their own doctor and decide whether to go to a public or a private hospital at which the physician attends. Treatment in a private hospital can be very expensive, and private health insurance will cover some or all of these costs.

Hospital Care.   Hospital health care consists of three sectors: public acute care hospitals, private acute care hospitals, and psychiatric hospitals. There were 1,027 acute care hospitals in Australia in 1995–1996, and over two thirds of them were public hospitals, the rest being private hospitals (AIHW, 1998). The acute care hospitals provide medical, surgical, and obstetric services. The length of a patient's hospital stay has decreased due to advances in patient care, drug usage, and medical technology. The sizes of hospitals are quiet different: from as few as about 10 beds in a community hospital to as large as over 1,000 beds in hospitals in large cities. The National Health Ministers Benchmarking Working Group developed an indicator called "casemix" for measuring hospital cost performance. This indicator measures the average cost of patient care, adjusting to the patients' condition and hospital services provided. The cost per casemix-adjusted separation for acute hospital care varies from $2,261 to $3,466. About 46% of those costs are nursing and medical staff costs (AIHW, 1998).

Mental Health Services.   In recent years, reform in mental health services has led to a trend wherein only those people with severe mental problems are hospitalized. The majority of the less severe patients who need only custodial institutional care were moved into community care settings. The number of psychiatric hospital decreased from 59 to 36 between 1989–90 and 1992–93 (AIHW, 1998). However, the demand for health care services is increasing over time, mainly due to the growth and the aging of population. According to *Australia's Health 1998* statistics, between 1986 and 1991, the population aged 70 and over—the highest consumers of health services—increased by 18.1% (AIHW, 1998).

Physicians

Physicians in public hospital are paid either by salaries or on a per-session basis. Physicians in private practices are usually paid by fee-for-services, but they have to accept a fee schedule for Medicare set by government. The number of female doctors underwent a major increase during the 1980s and 1990s. The proportion of female doctors rose from 19.0% in 1981 to 30.3% in 1996 (AIHW, 1998).

New Changes.   In October of 1999 the government passed the National Health Amendment Act, which created the Lifetime Health Cover program. Lifetime Health Cover recognizes the length of time that a person has had private hospital coverage and rewards that loyalty by offering lower premiums. Younger people who join will be charged lower premiums throughout their life compared to people who join later. For example, after 1 July 2000, someone joining at 30 years of age will pay lower premiums throughout his or her years of membership than someone who first joins at 50 years of age.

The Health Care System of Canada

Canada had a population of 31,006,347 people in 1999 (CIA, 1999). The health care expenditure of Canada was 77.1 billion for 1997 and is continuously increasing (CIHI, 1998). Despite multiple concerns with their health care system, Canadian citizens experience a high level of care. The mean life expectancies for Canadians are 82.79 years for females and 76.12 years for males (CIA, 1999) (see Table 7.3). One hundred percent of expectant mothers receive prenatal care. The leading causes of death for all Canadians are heart disease (53.0 deaths per 1,000 people) and accidents (35.3 deaths per 1,000 people) (Frenk et al., 1994).

Health Care System Structure and Financial Schemes

The Canadian health care system is one of social insurance with public funds and private delivery. It is a universal and comprehensive insurance system with no financial access barriers. Each Canadian citizen can receive medical care in any of Canada's 10 provinces and have free choice of health care providers (Iglehart, 1986). Universal hospital insurance began in all Canada's provinces and territories in 1961, and universal medical care insurance came into effect in 1971 (Vayda, 1986). In Canada, health care is the provinces' responsibility, so its national program is actually composed of 10 provincial and two territorial plans.

TABLE 7.3   *Health Indicators for Canada in 1999*

Life expectancy at birth (years)	79.37
Male	76.42
Female	82.79
Infant mortality rate	5.47/1,000 live births
Annual population growth rate	1.05%
Total fertility rate	1.65 births/woman
Birth rate	11.86/1,000
Death rate	7.26/1,000

Source: World Factbook (1999).

The idea of the universal insurance was first discussed in 1919, but the serious legislative steps toward that goal were started in 1945 (Vayda, 1986). The first national HCS model that was proposed by the federal government was rejected by the provinces. The Canadian federal government funding commitment was finally written into federal legislation in 1958. By 1961, all the provinces had joined the plan to take advantage of federal cost sharing. Although the basis of the cost sharing was 50–50, the federal government provides more than 50% of the cost in the poorer provinces and less than 50% for the wealthier provinces.

The Canada Health Act of 1984 established five principles for the foundation of the health care system: (1) Comprehensiveness requires coverage of all medically necessary health services provided by hospitals and medical practitioners. (2) Universality requires that 100% of the population be insured for health services under uniform terms and conditions. In effect, this principle ensures that services are provided without regard to race, income, age, sex, and origin. (3) Portability requires that persons who move from one province to another be covered. (4) Public administration requires that administration will be by a public nonprofit authority, subject to audit, and responsible to the provincial government. (5) Accessibility requires that there must be reasonable access by insured persons to insured health services unimpeded either directly or indirectly by charges or other means. The nature of financing health insurance was specified by the Canada Health Act of 1984. The Canadian government therefore retains a high level of control in this system. It controls the budgeting of things such as additional hospital beds, new programs, resource distribution, costs, and advanced technology (Rakich, 1991). Yet, Canada's health care system is the nation's most popular publicly financed service.

Canada's 10 provinces and two territories each have their own rules within a broad national framework. Most Canadians have private insurance through their employers, which covers only what the government does not, such as private hospital rooms and dental and vision care (Topolnicki, 1993). All of the plans are essentially universal; all residents are covered for all medically necessary inpatient and outpatient hospital and physician services. There's no direct cost to patients for physician visits or hospital stays. There is 100% coverage for prescription medication dispensed by pharmacists (Akaho et al., 1998). Public agencies in each of the provinces pay for all costs of necessary hospital and medical care of their residents. These payments are made from general government revenues, from both provincial and federal branches, which are raised through taxation. The public sector pays the majority of total health care costs. In 1993, 72% of total health care expenditure was paid by the public sector (Akaho et al., 1998) (see Table 7.4). Canada's payer model is based on provincial governments being single-source payers of health care, with a centralized source of control. These provincial governments reimburse both hospital and physician services on a prospective budgeting basis. The total health expenditure includes spending from both public and private sources. The public sector includes funds from governments and government agencies. The private health sector includes primarily third-party insurers and out-of-pocket expenses by Canadians.

TABLE 7.4 *Comparison of Canadian Health Indicators in 1986 and 1996*

Indicators	1986	1996
Total expenditure on health as % of GDP	8.7	9.2
Public expenditure on health as % of GDP	6.5	6.4
Total expenditure on health per capita in $	1,289	2,065
Practicing physicians per 1,000 population	2	2.1
Inpatient care beds per 1,000 population	6.7	5.1
Inpatient care average length of stay (days)	13.9	12

Source: OECD (1997).

In 1996, spending on health care by the public sector was $52.9 billion, accounting for 70.3% of total health care expenditure in Canada. Private sector spending was $22.4 billion for the same year, representing 29.7% of total health care expenditure in Canada (CIHI, 1998). Private health care spending in Canada basically is the spending not specifically covered by the Canada Health Act—such as dental services and vision care. Hospitals use the largest portion of total health expenditure, while physician services and drugs rank second and third. In 1996, Canada spent 34.3% of total health expenditure on hospital care, while the cost for physician services was 14.3% and the spending for drugs was 13.6% of the health expenditure (CIHI, 1998).

Provincial funding for health care mainly comes from the tax system. Although there's no direct payment by patients for their health care insurance, 75% of health care system cost is paid for through taxes (Akaho et al., 1998). Unemployed and low-income Canadians are not required to pay premiums for their health insurance but are covered for all health services.

Current Problems

The Canadian HCS today is facing problems because it sets a high priority on basic patient care yet limits the use of advanced medical technology. Access to advanced technology is based on medical priority, with all individuals categorized according to their "need" basis. Consequently, patients often must wait longer for advanced technological services than in a system that requires only the financial ability to pay. More and more Canadians are coming to the United States for immediate medical care and access to highly advanced technology. High demand also creates long waits by patients for even basic services. Canadian physicians often immigrate to the United States for higher salaries. Recently, large debt has forced the government to close hospital wards with a loss of 11,000 hospital beds. The government also reduced nursing staff as well as the number of positions available in medical schools. Severe medical staff shortages are only going to worsen as the population grows older.

The Health Care System of PRC
(Peoples Republic of China)

PRC is the world's most populated nation, with an estimated 1,246,871,951 people as of 1999 (CIA, 1999). It is also a large country with a landmass of 9,600,000 square km that is divided into 31 provinces. There were 314,097 medical/health institutions and 4,569,000 medical professionals reported in 1998 (CNBS, 1999). The life expectancy in PRC was 69.92 years in 1999, 68.57 for males and 71.48 for females (World Factbook, 1999) (see Table 7.5). PRC still has considerable morbidity and mortality associated with infectious diseases, nutrient deficiencies, and increasing trends of heart disease, strokes, malignant tumors, and respiratory diseases related to tobacco use and poor ambient air quality.

Overpopulation

With one-quarter of the world's population, the Chinese government has adopted strict policies and controls in order to regulate population growth. Such emphasis has been placed on this that severe measures are currently in effect. The implementation of the one-child policy encourages couples to limit family size in the best interest of the future of PRC. The one-child policy is based on the constitutional provision that permits the national government to regulate matters of family planning. The policy of one child per couple is strictly enforced in the urban centers, but is relaxed somewhat in the rural areas. The government has established a set of incentives and consequences in order to steer couples to observe the policy. Parents with one child have priority housing, receive monthly subsidies, have higher pensions upon retirement, and are allowed free education for their child. Families with more than one child face consequences such as exclusion from benefits and financial penalties.

The Chinese government has attempted to limit fertility rates for 20 years and is achieving increased success. In 1998, the population growth rate was .89%. The government provides population education that covers delaying marriages,

TABLE 7.5 *Health Indicators for PRC in 1999*

Life expectancy at birth (years)	69.92
Male	68.57
Female	71.48
Infant mortality rate	43.31/1,000 live births
Annual population growth rate	.77%
Total fertility rate	1.8 birth/woman
Birth rate	15.1/1,000
Death rate	6.98/1,000

Source: World Factbook (1999).

as well as birth control education including abortion education; it also provides free services related to birth control.

Health Care System Structure and Financing Methods

The Director of Medical and Health Services, the Director of Urban Services and the Urban council, the Commissioner of Labor, and the Secretary for the New Territories are responsible for the administration of health care services in PRC. All Chinese clinics offer primary care, outpatient care, preventive services, family health services, and a maternity ward. Some clinics have a full-time chest clinic. Special clinics are designed for the diagnosis and treatment of venereal diseases. All medical staff in government hospitals and clinics are employed by the government on a full-time basis and are not permitted to offer their services elsewhere. However, some physicians engage in private practice and directly charge the patient the fees they choose and are not controlled by the government.

The Chinese government emphasizes prevention. Government measures include developing additional medical and health services, increasing the number of maternal and child health facilities, and training qualified medical personnel. In 1989, the government allocated one-half of central and local government funding for preventive and public health programs, medical education, and research. The budget for disease prevention and public health was about 5% of the total health expenditures, but comprised 23% of government health expenditures (Hsiao, 1995). This preventive approach has yielded major improvements in health status for the people at very low cost.

There are two sets of health care methods in most hospitals: the Chinese traditional medicine and Western-style medicine which has the same diagnosis and treatments as in the Western world. The traditional Chinese doctors get education from Chinese medical schools, and the Western doctors are the graduates of Western-style medical schools. Students go directly from high school to medical school, and obtain a five-year degree that qualifies them to be physicians. In order to specialize in a field of medicine, the doctor must obtain either a masters or Ph.D. degree in that specialty. There are significant differences in the provisioning of primary care facilities when comparing urban with rural locations (see Table 7.6)

Universal Health Care System: From the 1950s to the 1980s

From 1952 to 1982, PRC achieved major improvement in people's health status. Although PRC had a limited number of well-trained professionals and hospital beds, and an expenditure $5 per capita for health care, within 30 years the country increased the average life expectancy from 35 to 68 years and reduced infant mortality from 250 to 40 deaths per 1,000 live births (Hsiao, 1995). The health services and disease prevention programs were both effective and low cost to people and also to the economy. The success was partially attributed to political attention and

TABLE 7.6   *Supply of Beds and Health Care Providers in PRC*

	Total Number	*Urban*	*Rural*
Beds			
Hospital beds	1,901,209	6.56/1,000	NA
Township health center beds	722,877	NA	0.79/1,000
Health Care Providers			
Physicians	1,302,977	3.80/1,000	0.54/1,000
Assistant physicians	422,352	0.78/1,000	0.28/1,000
Nurses	974,541	3.00/1,000	0.37/1,000
Village doctors	1,231,510	NA	1.34/1,000
Midwives	58,397	0.12/1,000	0.04/1,000

Sources: Hsiao (1995).

priority given to funding of disease prevention and health promotion, as well as very low payment to the health care providers.

The traditional universal HCS was an enterprise-based system of social welfare, operated through central planning, community organization, and cooperative financing of health care. Although there are many problems in the health care system, especially in rural areas, the health status of Chinese people has not declined.

Over several decades, there was no health insurance system in PRC. People enjoyed nearly free health services financed by the central government. The only citizens of the country who were exempt from free health care were the 10% of the Chinese population who could afford private care. The length of hospital stay in PRC is about three times that of the United States, according to Diagnostic Related Grouping (Hsiao, 1995). Very often patients are admitted into the hospital several days before having surgery and there's no rush to leave after the operation.

The government has always provided an important share of health care financing, and now it has shifted its financing to mostly capital investments, which include buildings and equipment. This has led to extensive underfunding of the operational costs of hospitals and reduced patient care and has contributed to a two-tier hospital system. Those who can afford the care, with ready cash, get faster and better-quality health care services, while the poorer segment of the population has enormous difficulties.

The traditional Chinese medicine (TCM) of herbs and acupuncture has rebounded from its days of being suppressed during the period of the Cultural Revolution. Chinese leaders thought that TCM was retarding social development because it was based not on any science but on folklore and tradition. With such a huge population demanding some form of medical care, and a paucity of doctors trained in Western medicine, the leadership reversed course and began promoting TCM. Today the Ministry of Public Health regulates it through the State Administration of TCM office.

Health Care Reform

In the past two decades, PRC has changed its economic system from central planning to a market-driven economy. The central government has given more freedom and power to the provincial governments. With changes in economy policy, health care policy also has changed. The PRC government has cut back public funds for health care. It established a laissez-faire policy by which the private market would cover the costs that were not covered by the government. Especially in rural areas, when collective farming was replaced by individual household responsibility, collectively financed and organized village health stations collapsed due to lack of funding. Rural health services are now largely provided by fee-for-service private practitioners, and patients' ability to pay determines supply and demand (Hsiao, 1995). Government financing basically covers only health care workers' wages and new capital investments. Hospitals have to get the rest from patients. The government has permitted the private ownership of health facilities and private clinical practices. Even foreign joint ventures are allowed in some pharmaceutical companies and hospitals.

The largest portion of health care spending is for drugs. In 1989, this amounted to about 45% of health care dollars (Hsiao, 1995). The government financed most investments in new capital equipment and facilities, and the remainder was financed by industrial enterprises. In 1989, 78% of capital investment funds was provided by local governments and 5% by central government (Hsiao, 1995).

In 1989, the central government funded only about 1% of total health expenditures. The provincial and local government paid about 19%. The main finance sources for health expenditure were direct patient payments through fee-for-service (36%) and labor insurance and industry's direct provision (32%) (see Table 7.7).

TABLE 7.7 *Chinese Health Care Financing Sources: 1989*

Source	Percentage of Contribution
Government employee insurance	7%
Labor insurance and industry's direct provision	32%
Central government direct support	1%
Provincial and local government direct support	19%
Cooperative medical insurance	5%
Self-pay	36%

Sources: 1. Hsiao (1995); Wei (1991).

As a way to compensate for reduced government financing, hospitals have had an incentive to buy the most advanced equipment and to sell more medicine. Each year, PRC spent more than $1 billion on medical equipment, more than half of it imported (Lipson & Pemble, 1996). Since economic reform, some Western pharmaceutical companies have established factories and market in PRC. The Western medicines are usually much more expensive than those made by Chinese pharmaceutical companies, which has resulted in an increase in health care costs.

Hospitals in PRC are primary suppliers of both medical care and medicines. With a doctor's prescription, patients can get all kinds of medicines (even drugs for the common cold) from hospitals. People can also get any medicines from drug stores without a doctors' prescription, including antibiotics. In the past, the government reimbursed 100 percent of all drug expenses. But in 1992, the Ministry of Health began developing a National Essential Drug List (NEDL) by which to set reimbursement for medicines prescribed to patients under state insurance plans. The local and central governments reimburse for drugs based on the NEDL.

The Chinese HCS is undergoing major changes in response to the shift of the economic system from a state-planned to a more free-market orientation. The result is that many people who do not have sufficient financial resources must rely on the less expensive TCM, and lower-quality health care, compared to those who have private insurance or the money to pay for Western-type medical services. One should never judge PRC policy without understanding the simple magnitude of the population (five times larger than the United States) which makes any provisioning of public goods and services very difficult. Hence, the PRC Health Ministry has consistently placed an emphasis on the prevention of illness and basic public health improvements that are of lower cost. The difficulty is that the PRC is also undergoing industrial modernization, and many of the environmental and occupational safety provisions are often given secondary or no consideration. In view of widespread increases in the use of tobacco, PRC is on track to experience millions of lung cancer cases resulting in widespread suffering and death.

The Health Care System of Germany

The Federal Republic of Germany is a densely populated country estimated at 82,081,361 people (World Factbook, 1999). The average life expectancy for males is 74.01 years and 80.50 years for females (see Table 7.8). With a low birth rate and a growing life expectancy, the German population is shifting toward an older age structure. One out of five people is older than 60, and the figure is projected to be one out of four in 2030 (Selbmann, 1996). Infectious and parasitic diseases are low in Germany, and the main causes of death are diseases of the circulatory system, cancer, stroke, and accidents (Sonderdruck, 1994).

TABLE 7.8 *Health Indicators for Germany in 1999*

Life expectancy at birth (years)	77/17
Male	74.01
Female	80.50
Infant mortality rate	5.14/1,000 live births
Annual population growth rate	.01%
Total fertility rate	1.26 birth/woman
Birth rate	8.68/1,000
Death rate	10.76/1,000

Source: World Factbook (1999).

Welfare-Oriented Health Care System

The history of the German health care system dates back to the Industrial Revolution in Europe. Otto von Bismarck's conservative government was being threatened by German socialists (Stassen, 1993), and in an effort to satisfy this group of primarily blue-collar workers, Bismarck developed the first modern, universal, comprehensive, and publicly funded health insurance program in 1881. This program would eventually cover most Germans (Stassen, 1993). The Health Insurance Act of 1883 paved the way for more improvements such as accident insurance (1884), retirement funds (1889), public assistance programs (1924), and unemployment insurance (1927) (Schulenburg, 1992). Revised in 1911, the Health Insurance Act is still in effect today (Schulenburg, 1992). This first period of government-influenced health care ended with Bismarck in 1914 (Iglehart, 1991). Between World War I and the establishment of the Weimar Republic (1914–1932), there were no significant changes in health care policy. From the end of World War II to the present, most of the pre–Third Reich acts and insurance programs were restored (Iglehart, 1991).

In 1961, the West German legislature established the Federal Department of Health and Human Services. This department has the power to set statutes determining the fees for dentistry and physician services, employers' liability for employee illness, the medical profession requisites, laws concerning the financing of hospitals, and cost containment statutes (Schulenburg, 1992). The old German system of the former East Germany has put additional strain on modern (West) Germany. In the past, all physicians in former East Germany were paid by the state, and health services were solely the responsibility of the government (Schulenburg, 1992). The German Hospital Association estimates that it will cost tens of billion of dollars to raise the standards of the hospitals in former East Germany to those of the modern state (Iglehart, 1991).

Today, unified Germany has a welfare-oriented system of health care (Roemer, 1991). The government supports medical care for most, but not all, of the population (Roemer, 1991). Usually, this support is limited to payment of health-related bills; a higher value is placed on the health of the general public rather than on the results of operating on the capitalist system of supply and demand (Roemer, 1991). The German system receives over half of its total health expenditures from government sources. Some aspects remain traditional. For example, most of the physicians remain in private practice (Roemer, 1991). Having a system of collective and organized coverage, Germany is proud of its base of solidarity and mutuality (Stassen, 1993). The head of a household contributes to a sickness fund, and then the spouse and any handicapped children are covered for life. All other children are covered until the age of 25. Coverage includes all office visits, house calls, treatments as a result of diagnostic procedures, and rehabilitation services. Coverage also includes any physician in any situation (such as emergency, outpatient or inpatient centers), all long-term illnesses, pregnancy expenses, all prescriptions, transportation to and from health care facilities, and all funeral expenses. Included in coverage were spa-rejuvenation centers (Stassen, 1993). Recently, however, the funding for treatment in spa-rejuvenation centers has been cut. In addition, the criteria to qualify for a paid treatment have been strictly increased. With the former Christian Democratic Union government one was obliged to contribute some days of vacation in order to receive treatment. This enforcement has been made obsolete by the new SDP (Social Democratic Party) government. Several health reforms have occurred in the decade of the 1990s as western Germany grappled with the vastly underestimated costs of German unification. However, the costs for the medication (prescriptions) are covered by the Krankenkasse, except for a small fee the patient has to pay (the amount of the fee depends on the size of the prescription but does not exceed DM 15 per medication). There have been long and continuous public discussions about the correct level of these contributions following the takeover by the SDP in 1999.

The Federal Parliament and the Federal Government only provide the necessary framework of laws and regulations for the health care system (Selbmann, 1996). The health care system largely relies on the "self-administration" of its components: the health insurance funds, the hospital association, the medical professions, the governments of the Federal States, and other suppliers of related services. Insurance is mandatory. Anyone whose income is below a certain level has to belong to a health insurance system. About 88.5% of the population have mandatory insurance provided by the statutory health insurance funds; 11.4% have private insurance or are civil servants who get their health care costs back from their employers (Selbmann, 1996).

Health expenditure has increased in recent years (Federal Statistical Office Germany, 1998). The majority of health expenditure was for medical treatment, and only a very small portion was used for preventive care. In 1996, 59% of the health expenditure was spent on medical treatment; about 8.4% was for preventive care (Federal Statistical Office Germany, 1998) (see Table 7.9).

From the 1970s to the 1990s, the number of physicians increased by more than 100%. There was one physician per 615 inhabitants in 1970, and the ratio was one to 290 in 1997 (Federal Statistical Office Germany, 1998). About 41% of physicians work in private practice (see Table 7.10).

TABLE 7.9   *Comparison of German Health Indicators in 1986 and 1996*

Indicators	1986	1996
Total expenditure on health as % of GDP	9.2	10.5
Public expenditure on health as % of GDP	7.1	8.2
Total expenditure on health per capita in $	1,014	2,278
Fertility rate (children per woman)	1.35	1.26
Infant mortality per 1,000 live births	8.6	5
Practicing physicians per 1,000 population	2.1	3.4
Inpatient care beds per 1,000 population	8.7	9.6
Inpatient care average length of stay (days)	16.9	14.3

Source: OECD (1997).

TABLE 7.10   *The German Health Care System, 1997*

Physicians	282,737
Working in private practice	114,995
Hospital physicians	115,734
Dentists	62,024
Hospitals	2,258
Beds	580,425
Average length of stay (days)	11.0
Prevention/rehabilitation facilities	1387
Beds	188,869
Average length of stay (days)	27.3

Sources: World Factbook (1999); Federal Statistical Office Germany (1998).

It is important to note that insurance will not cover an abortion, unless it is proved to be necessary on medical grounds (Tuffs, 1993). Although the German Supreme Court decided in 1993 to make abortion an illegal act, neither the doctor nor the woman involved will be prosecuted if an abortion is performed within three months of conception (Tuffs, 1993).

Financing Health Care

How is the German health care system financed? Originally, contributions were made by citizens and based on income, and benefits were not dependent upon the amount contributed. Sex, age, health situation, and race had no part in determining the amount of money paid (Kaps, 1993). The moneys were tax-based.

Krankenkasse, or sickness funds, are legal private, not-for-profit institutions that collect money from employees and employers (Kaps, 1993). The description of the system is well broken down by Stassen (1993), who examines five key features. All public and private employers were required to identify with one of six varieties of sickness funds. These varieties are local health insurance funds (40% of the population), company health insurance, guild health insurance (for artists and other skilled workers), agricultural health insurance (for self-employed farmers), national health insurance (for merchant navy members), and government-accredited private health insurance (for those wealthy enough to not qualify for another plan). The second feature explains that all Germans (except those in the private sector) are covered by the system. Next, Stassen explains that benefits also apply to citizens of other European Community countries who have moved to Germany. Fourth, the German citizen has a choice of hospitals and physicians. Finally, all citizens have access to free information and advice relating to health care (Stassen, 1993).

Today much of the manner in which German health care is financed has changed. The Krankenkasse have been privatized, so although the old ones still exist (and new ones evolved), one can choose in which sickness fund to be a member since they are all public. An individual can change from the guild health insurance to the local health insurance, no matter what his or her profession is. The interesting part is that each individual now has competition within the Krankenkasse Sector (meaning that there are slightly different contribution margins of gross income). All public Krankenkasse are required by law to guarantee the same service. If a person decides, however, to change from a public Krankenkasse to a private insurance (in case of high income), he or she can decide upon the amount of service that is wanted. However, the individual who decides to change to private insurance (and the spouse and children) is not able to return to a public Krankenkasse ever! This is because, in the case of children, a public Krankenkasse is very attractive (since only one family insurance rate is paid), and thus many people (88.5%) are not willing to change. Once the children are older than 25 years old, it is very expensive for the parents to change into private insurance, so people stay within the public Krankenkasse.

In the German health care system, ambulatory and hospital care are strictly separated, brought about by different responsibilities and ways of financing. The government funds major hospital investments, and statutory health insurance funds pay hospital operating costs (Selbmann, 1996). Diagnosis-related groups and fees for specific treatments have been introduced in hospitals since 1995. In only two years, the new financing methods applied to about 30% of the hospital budget (Selbmann, 1996).

How is financing distributed? A general description of financing is a blend of obligatory financing by employers and employees, controlled expenditures by hospitals and not-for-profit insurance organizations, and private action by physicians (Iglehart, 1991). The government puts limits on physicians' charges and hospital fees, along with prescription drug costs. These limits are determined by the government, the medical association, private sector hospitals, and the pharmaceutical industry (Stassen, 1993). This system has helped to control many costs (Kaps, 1993).

The Health Care System of Japan (Nippon)

Japan believes in the philosophy of universal health care coverage for all its citizens, and it has been successful in achieving this goal at a relative low cost. Only 7.3% of its GDP is spent on health care, which is the lowest, after the United Kingdom, among seven major developed countries (Arai & Ikegami, 1998). The infant mortality rate and the life expectancy at birth are among the best in the world (Ikegami & Campbell, 1995). Japan has a population of 126,182,077 (CIA, 1999). The life expectancy at birth for male was 77.02 and 83.35 for female (World Factbook, 1999) (see Table 7.11).

The main cause of death in Japan is cancer, the cause of some 280,000 deaths per year, followed by heart disease at 143,000 deaths per year (MHW, 2000). These are related to high smoking rates, stressful occupational and societal conditions, and limited exercise practices.

Health Care System Structure

Every Japanese citizen must belong to an insurance plan. There are two types of insurance, an employee-based system and the national health insurance plan. Four different groups are covered under the employee-based system: (1) employees of large firms covered by a corporate-managed insurance program, (2) employees of small firms covered by a government-managed health insurance plan, (3) local and national civil servants and staff of teaching institutes who belong to a mutual aid association, and (4) day labor and seamen under a government-managed health insurance plan (Akaho et al., 1998).

The national health insurance system covers those people who are not covered by the employee-based system. There are two groups under the national

TABLE 7.11 *Health Indicators for Japan in 1998*

Life expectancy at birth (years)	80.11
Male	77.02
Female	83.35
Infant mortality rate	4.07/1,000 live births
Annual population growth rate	.20%
Total fertility rate	1.48 birth/woman
Birth rate	10.48/1,000
Death rate	8.12/1,000

Source: World Factbook (1999).

insurance system: agricultural workers and the self-employed, and retirees who were originally covered by employee health insurance (Akaho et al., 1998). All dependents are covered under their sponsors' health program.

Regardless of the various health plans, there is a nationalized fee schedule. No matter what patients' health plans are and where they receive care, the fees for the procedures are the same. The fee schedule lists all procedures and products that can be paid for by health insurance and sets their prices (Ikegami & Campbell, 1995). The national fee schedule defines the structure of the health care system. Since the fees are the same, patients are not distinguished according to their health program.

The administration of health care in Japan is divided into general public health, school health, and industrial health. Health administration services, based in Tokyo, are conducted by the Bureau of Public Health, with eight divisions: General Affairs, Public Health, Environmental Health, Medical Affairs, Health and Welfare, Pharmaceutical Affairs, Hospital Administration, and Hospital Buildings. The Ministry of Health and Welfare sets national standards for reimbursement fees for medications, procedures, hospital stays, and clinic visits (Tierney & Tierney, 1994).

Health Care Financing

The costs of health care in Japan are low. The average cost of health care per capita was $1,677 in 1996, while the cost was $3,898 in the United States (OECD, 1997). The Japanese public expenditure on health care covers the cost for the care and treatment of diseases and injuries. Other services such as pregnancy, childbirth, health examinations, vaccinations, vision care, artificial limbs, private hospital rooms, and some dental charges are paid privately or by other insurance.

People with employee health insurance pay 10% of the fee when they visit hospitals or clinics, and the rest is covered by insurance programs. The coverage includes fees related to hospital stay, procedures, and prescription drugs. The coverage for dependents, which is lower, is 80% of inpatient services and 70% of outpatient services (Arai & Ikegami, 1998).

There are two main financial resources: insurance premiums and national support. With the employee health system, about 8% of salaries of insured people are paid for insurance premiums (Akaho et al., 1998). The national government gives a subsidy to each insurance program; for example, the government-managed health insurance program and the day laborer's health insurance program each receive a 13% subsidy. In 1992, private insurance received Yen 4.85 billion of benefit costs from the government, and seamen's insurance received Yen 3 billion (Akaho et al., 1998).

The national health insurance is administered by local governments. The local government is responsible for collection of payments by the insured individuals in their jurisdiction. The insured individuals can go by either an income-based payment system or a fixed-amount payment system. The national financial system subsidizes the agricultural group 50% of the cost of benefits and for the self-employed group, 32 to 52% (Akaho et al., 1998) (see Table 7.12).

TABLE 7.12   *Comparison of Japanese Health Indicators in 1986 and 1996*

Indicators	1986	1996
Total expenditure on health as % of GDP	6.6	7.2
Public expenditure on health as % of GDP	4.8	5.7
Total expenditure on health per capita in $	853	1677
Fertility rate (children per woman)	1.72	1.41
Infant mortality per 1,000 live births	5.2	3.8
Practicing physicians per 1,000 population	1.5	1.8
Inpatient care beds per 1,000 population	14.9	16.2
Inpatient care average length of stay (days)	54	43.7

Source: OECD (1997).

Health Care for the Aged

With the longest life expectancy of the countries compared here, Japan is becoming an aged society. There were 6% of people aged 65 and over in 1970; the proportion increased to 12% in 1990 and is projected to reach 25% in the year 2020 (Arai & Ikegami, 1998). Japan created a pooling fund through the Geriatric Health Act to pay for all health care costs of citizens aged 70 and older regardless of the insurance plans they have. It also covers bedridden patients aged between 65 to 69. The pooling fund is contributed to by each insurance plan so as to share the burden of the health care costs of the elderly.

Hospitals

National or local governments, voluntary organizations, and universities own most large hospitals. The majority of hospitals in Japan are small, family enterprises that developed from physicians' offices, and no for-profit, investor-owned hospitals are permitted (Ikegami & Campbell, 1995).

Physicians

More than 90% of doctors are private practitioners, and about 80% of the hospital are private (Ikegami & Campbell, 1995). Office-based doctors and hospital doctors are the two basic types of care providers. There are no functional differences between them. Doctors are not acting as gatekeepers to secondary care; anybody can go to a hospital without obtaining a referral in advance.

Problems.   Japan's Ministry of Health and Welfare oversees the system of socialized medicine, and there are many problems associated with minimal patient care and profit making over prescription drugs. Tight price controls have kept health care costs at 7% of gross domestic product, roughly 50% less than in the United States, but at a heavy cost in unmet patient needs. Since consultation fees are kept as low as $8 per office visit, doctors look for other means of compensation (Weinberg, 1997). Operating their own small hospitals and expanding the time of patient hospitalization from several days to several weeks can do this. Thus, outpatient service for minor surgery is virtually nonexistent in Japan (Beason, 1999).

About 80% of physicians in private practice and 89% of hospitals dispense their own medicines (Ikegami & Campbell, 1995), which generates substantial income. Since those providers purchase medicine at wholesale, the prices are much lower than the reimbursement specified by the fee schedule. Therefore, the doctors end up overprescribing prescription drugs, increase the price, and pocket the difference. As a result, the country spends 28% of its health care budget on prescription drugs. As a country, Japan has always been restrictive on permitting importation of technology from other countries, with the result that surgeons complain that the health ministry will not let them import many of the latest medical devices from abroad. This holds down costs, yet not without reduction and sacrifice of health care innovation and advancements.

The Health Care System of Mexico

Mexico has a population estimated at 100,294,036 (World Factbook, 1999). The average life expectancy in Mexico is 68.98 for males and 75.17 for females (World Factbook, 1999) (see Table 7.13). In 1990, the main causes of death in Mexico were diseases of the circulatory system, diseases of the endocrine system, and poor nutrition. Next listed are diseases of the respiratory system, tumors, infectious and parasitic diseases, diseases of the digestive system, and diseases of the reproductive systems (Garcia de Miranda and Falcon de Gyves, 1993). Mexican children under the age of one are at severe risk of death from infectious and parasitic disease. Only 50% of mothers in Mexico receive adequate prenatal care (Pan American Health Organization [PAHO], 1994). Although 90% of Mexico's urban population has a "safe" water supply, only 66% of the rural population has what is considered a "safe" water supply. Often, waste disposal methods are questionable and considered dangerous, especially in rural areas.

The History of the Mexican Health Care System

The history of the Mexican health care system dates back to the Constitution of 1917, when the right to health care was established (Marquez & Sherraden, 1994). Like Germany, Mexico has a welfare system of health care (Roemer, 1991). However, the system is officially termed socialistic. The rule of Cardenas between 1934

TABLE 7.13   *Health Indicators for Mexico in 1998*

Life expectancy at birth (years)	72.00
Male	68.98
Female	75.17
Infant mortality rate	24.62/1,000 live births
Annual population growth rate	1.73%
Total fertility rate	2.85 births/woman
Birth rate	24.99/1,000
Death rate	4.83/1,000

Source: World Factbook (1999).

and 1940 marked an era when the government began to take control of many industries. As a result, special medical services were given to the workers (Roemer, 1991). Social security was adopted in 1943, and the Mexican Institute of Social Security was established the following year as the main social security agency (Marquez & Sherraden, 1994). The legislature began to include more of the Mexican population over the following decades. The Ministry of Health, COPLAMAR, private services, or nothing covers those not covered at all by the Mexican Institute of Social Security. The Ministry of Health was founded in 1917 and is the oldest institution that operates a web of clinics and hospitals throughout the country. Minimal fees are charged to those (including foreigners) who use their services. COPLAMAR was established in 1979 as a federal rural program, with the purpose of bringing health care to the large, isolated, impoverished rural areas. This program also subsidizes food, roads, clean water, schools, electricity, and farming assistance. The rest of the population (10%) either uses private services or has no access to health care (Frenk et al., 1994).

The Mexican Health Care System Today

Poverty is a major issue in Mexico today. Many problems arise in health care in a country that is monetarily poor. Mexico has a large native population, and many indigenous populations are not recognized by the government. It faces many problems such as malnutrition, poor sanitary conditions, limited resources, poorly trained workers, and infectious diseases (UN, 1991)—problems that are often characteristic of developing countries.

During the past two decades, government expenditures have decreased (Marquez & Sherraden, 1994). With an increasing population, the government still seeks to provide adequate, low-cost health care, yet in reality there is a large population without any coverage. Mexico spends about 4% of its gross national product on health care (Frenk et al., 1994) (see Table 7.14). Fortunately, due to Mexico's long Catholic history, numerous charitable health services have been provided for

TABLE 7.14   *Comparison of Mexican Health Indicators in 1986 and 1996*

	1986	1996
Total expenditure on health as % of GDP	NA	4.6
Public expenditure on health as % of GDP	NA	2.7
Total expenditure on health per capita in $	NA	358
Fertility rate (children per woman)	3.82	2.73
Infant mortality per 1,000 live births	24	17
Practicing physicians per 1,000 population	0.9	1.5
Inpatient care beds per 1,000 population	0.8	1.1
Inpatient care average length of stay (days)	4.2	4.1

Source: OECD (1997).

many years, and sometimes these church-affiliated health service organizations are subsidized by the government of Mexico (Roemer, 1991). As shown in Table 7.14 the fertility rate decreased over the 10 years between 1986 and 1996, and the infant mortality rate also decreased significantly. Practicing physicians per 1,000 population increased from 0.9 to 1.5 per 1,000 population.

Roemer (1991) describes a general overview of Mexican health objectives—including decentralization of responsibilities, modernizing administration, integrating the health sector, intersectional coordination, and community responsibility. Decentralization means thrusting responsibility from the federal level in Mexico City to the state and local levels. Coordination intersectorally refers to greater communication and cooperation between health administrations and pharmaceutical industries.

The Health Care System of Russia

Russia is the largest country in the world in terms of landmass, with an area of 17,075,200 square km (6,592,800 square miles). The population of Russia is about 146,393,569 and has been experiencing a decline as a result of the breakup of the Soviet Union (CIA, 1999). The Soviet Union breakup in 1991 resulted in tremendous changes in all aspects of the society, including the health care system. Due to changes in economic and other factors, health status indicators have been getting worse in recent years. The life expectancy in Russia is declining, particularly for males. The annual population growth rate is –0.31% (CIA, 1999). Infant mortality rate increased to 23.26 per 1,000 live births (World Factbook, 1999), which is more than twice that in the high-income countries. The life expectancy at birth has been declining over the past decade, particularly for males (see Table 7.15).

TABLE 7.15   *Health Indicators for Russia in 1998*

Life expectancy at birth (years)	64.97
Male	58.61
Female	71.64
Infant mortality rate	23.26/1,000 live births
Annual population growth rate	−.31%
Total fertility rate	1.34 births/woman
Birth rate	9.57/1,000
Death rate	14.89/1,000

Source: World Factbook (1999).

History of the Soviet Health Care System

The Russian health care system was rooted in the Soviet health care system, which lasted over 70 years. It was organized with three levels of general state administration: the federal level, the state level, and the local level. Hospitals, clinics, and other facilities were structured into an integrated network run by different levels of health institutions and authorities.

For decades, the Soviet health care system provided universal health care access to its entire population, financed by government and maintained by government ownership and management. The Soviet Union health care system achieved continuous improvement in a wide array of health indicators such as life expectancy and the infant mortality rate (Twigg, 1998). There were some problems with the structure, such as patients' choice of physicians and hospitals and the quality of care; however, it was effective until the late 1950s. By the end of the 1980s, it could not keep up with the demand, which lead to a massive nationalized reform (Chernichovsky & Potapchik, 1999). However, various initiatives of health care system reform must take into account the existing system, so it is important to understand its origin.

Structure and Financing of the Soviet Health Care System

The management of the Soviet health care system was completely centralized, with a vertical structure. At the top of the hierarchy were several federal organizations, including the Federal Ministry of Health (FMOH), the State Committee for Sanitary and Epidemiological Surveillance (SCSES), the Russian Academy of Medical Sciences, and some other federal-level ministries. Each federal-level authority was empowered to oversee the state-level and local-level authorities. The selection of heads of state-level authorities and institutions had to go through the approval of the FMOH. It was the FMOH's responsibility and authority to determine the investments and development needs of hospitals and clinics, based on the number of hospital beds and patient visits that were at capacity (Twigg, 1998). Although health care facilities were mainly financed by state budgets, FMOH had the power to allocate the financial resources (Chernichovsky & Potapchik, 1999).

Each federal-level institution was in charge of state-level health ministries and authorities. Under the local-level authorities, there were rural central hospitals and city health authorities. From the federal level to the lowest health care facilities, there were several vertical "panels" in the management of the Soviet health care system. Though each panel, the federal ministries had the power to regulate even the lowest-level health facilities or education/NS (nursing school). There were also patient care facilities, research centers, and education/NSs at each level (Chernichovsky & Potapchik, 1999). The health care facilities at federal level mainly provided highly specialized care, and the state and local levels mainly provided general medical care.

FMOH, as a federal institution, also directly controlled some care facilities. It regulated the state-level hospitals, research centers, and education/NSs via state-level health ministries and authorities. Each state-level health ministry and its authorities were in charge of certain parts of local-level called rural central rayon hospitals and city health authorities. SCSES was another federal institution that leads a panel all the way to local-level facilities (Chernichovsky & Potapchik, 1999).

Some federal-level institutes and academies that were directly funded by the FMOH provided only medical education. Continuing education for physicians was mainly provided by the FMOH, but the training of paramedical personnel was provided by all management levels—federal, state, and local (Chernichovsky & Potapchik, 1999).

Physicians were all government employees; they were paid with state-specified salaries, which varied only according to their years in service and level of specialty and training. Russia always has had a high per capita number of physicians. Physicians were paid with low salaries, only about 75% to 80% of the average Soviet skilled worker's wages. Patients had to go to specific care facilities, without a choice of physicians (Twigg, 1998).

The Soviet health care system was constantly underfunded, as only about 3% of GNP compared with 8% to 12% of GNP in the Western industrial countries (Twigg, 1998). The funding for all levels of health care facilities was mainly allocated by the FMOH. As the result of the funding deficiency, hospitals were severely underequipped, extending even to such basics as disposable syringes. In order to get funding from the government, hospitals had the incentive to keep patients for the maximum possible length of stay, and patients who were sick usually got fully paid salaries for sick leave. These circumstances tended to increase the consumption of the already inadequate health care resources, and Soviet health care eventually reached its limits. In the later 1980s, it was almost impossible for it to provide adequate access and quality services to the entire nation. Improvements in health care vanished, and the quality of Soviet health care started to deteriorate—even with its huge network of medical facilities and high number of physicians (Twigg, 1998). Russians started seeking new models of health care that were more efficient and cost effective.

Health Care Reform

The first experiment was started by the new economic mechanism (NEM) in the City of St. Petersburg, the Kemerovo state, and Kuibyshev (now Samara) state. The goal was to encourage more efficient and higher-quality medical care by changing health care financing methods. Instead of funds being allocated by the FMOH, now most money was attributed directly from state budget to health care facilities in those three areas, on a weighted capitation basis of payments per registered client, regardless of the frequency or intensity of the client's use of the facility (Twigg, 1998). The idea was that since clients could choose their clinics and general practice physicians, the clinics would have the incentives to provide more efficient and user-friendly service (Twigg, 1998).

Problems

In the post-Soviet era the Russian HCS has been drastically set back to almost the standards of a developing country. For example modern heart monitors (from Germany) are installed in only five out of the over 100 hospitals in Moscow. Basic health care needs are simply not being met. The Russian Health Ministry recently reported that 50% of all hospitals had no hot water and 25% lacked sewage systems.

Left with insufficient funding by the central government, and with the shift of funding to local resources, many medical organizations have tried to operate in the market economy, which means that people now have to pay for services that they had previously received for free. This has led to some expansion in health care options, with people paying directly for services, yet for most people the increase in prices makes services essentially unattainable. The quality of care simply declines, as hospitals and clinics can no longer afford to obtain new medical technology. The emphasis on charging for services rendered (fee for services) together with the simultaneous cutting of government budget support to medical organizations has forced these organizations to restrict technological development and to cut the more expensive services, which tend to be the highest-quality services.

The dismal conditions of Russian health care and the decline in the public health infrastructure clearly have contributed to the overall reduction in life expectancies that has occurred since the breakup of the Soviet Union. Premature mortality is related to many social ills that beset Russian society, including high levels of both alcohol and tobacco use. However, it is artificial to separate out these factors from the society as a whole. High unemployment, social stresses, low wages, labor force turnover, as well as increasing income disparity and crime, all contribute to deteriorating social conditions and poorer health (Walberg et al., 1998).

The Health Care System of the United States

The United States had a population of about 274, 301,705 in mid-2000 (U.S. Bureau of Census, 2000). The indicators of people's health status are comparable with other high-income countries (see Table 7.16). U.S. healthcare expenditures and the amount per capita are the highest in the world. In 1997, the health expenditure in the United States was $1,095.1 billion, while the second-place country, Japan, spent $219.6 billion. For the same year, health care expenses per capita were $4,090, but the second-place country, Switzerland, spent only $2,547 per capita. See Table 7.17.

The Health Care System

The United States health care system of today is neither universal, comprehensive, nor publicly funded, except for the 41.3 million participants in the Medicaid pro-

TABLE 7.16   *Health Indicators for the United States in 1998*

Life expectancy at birth (years)	76.23
Male	72.95
Female	79.67
Infant mortality rate	6.33/1,000 live births
Annual population growth rate	.85%
Total fertility rate	2.07 births/woman
Birth rate	14.3/1,000
Death rate	8.8/1,000

Source: World Factbook (1999).

TABLE 7.17   *Comparison of United States Health Indicators in 1986 and 1996*

Indicator	1986	1996
Total expenditure on health as % of GDP	10.8	13.6
Public expenditure on health as % of GDP	4.4	6.3
Total expenditure on health per capita in $	1,917	3,898
Fertility rate (children per woman)	1.84	2.06
Infant mortality per 1,000 population	10.4	7.8
Practicing physicians per 1,000 population	2.3	2.6
Inpatient care beds per 1,000 population	5.4	4
Inpatient care average length of stay (days)	9.3	7.8

Source: OECD (1997).

gram and the 39 million participants in the Medicare program (Iglehart, 1999a & b). About 180 million United States residents have privately financed health insurance, with 82% receiving it from employers. This multiple-payer model creates a fragmented locus of control and allows cost shifting (Rakich, 1991). Health care is a patchwork ranging from minimal to full coverage, with premiums, copayments, and/or deductibles. Citizens of the United States pay for health care through Medicare/Medicaid government entitlement programs, Blue Cross and Blue Shield, other commercial carriers, through employers who are self-insured, or by self-payment.

Medicare and Medicaid

During the 1950s and 1960s, major health care reform moved from the margins of American policy discussions to the top of the government agenda. Policy makers became more sensitive to public attitudes, largely due to the 1960 presidential campaign. By November 1960, many were willing to pursue health care reform. John F. Kennedy had formally established his position favoring health insurance for the elderly by sponsoring legislation in the Senate during the spring and fall of 1960. Eisenhower, as the Republican president, was then pressured to take a stance on health care. Both parties emerged with the accepted idea that the federal government had a responsibility to assist the aged who were sick and too poor to pay for medical care. The political struggles with health care reform continued to become stronger in the support of Medicare. Finally, between November 1964 and July 1965, the Medicare Bill was signed into law.

Medicaid is the largest health insurer in the United States, covering medical service and long-term care for about 41.3 million people (Iglehart, 1999a). About 12.4% of total national health care expenditures was on Medicaid in 1997 (Iglehart, 1999a). Medicaid covers low-income people who are usually not covered by an employment-based insurance system. The number of people who become eligible for Medicaid has increased rapidly in recent years, from 28.3 million in 1993 to today's 41.3 million people (Iglehart, 1999a). Medicare beneficiaries include 34 million people over the age of 65, 5 million of all ages who are permanently disabled, and 284,000 with end-stage renal disease (Nissenson & Rettig, 1999).

Both Medicare and Medicaid are administrated by a federal agency—the Health Care Financing Administration (HCFA). The federal government funds Medicare, while both the federal and state governments fund Medicaid. Medicaid expenditures represent about 40% of all federal funds received by the states (Iglehart, 1999a).

The HMO Revolution

In the 1980s a new form of health care services began, called the health maintenance organization (HMO). The concept was simple enough: Patients would pay, either directly or indirectly through their employer on a regular basis, into an HMO whether they were sick or not. The HMO would organize networks of physicians and relatively lower-cost primary care providers who would serve as "gatekeepers" to the expensive specialists. The HMO physicians would all get paid, whether or not patients were sick, and hence there would be an emphasis toward prevention (Donatelle & Davis, 1999). This whole HCS is now referred to as "managed care." The HMO revolution has enveloped the country, with some 60 million Americans covered by the system. The problems with the HMO approach are mainly associated with three issues: (1) patients must use the doctors who are within their particular HMO network, which limits choice, (2) a patient cannot get to a specialist unless he or she is first referred by a primary care physician (known as the gatekeeper), and (3) the HMO sets strict rules that the doctors must follow regarding procedures and tests for a particular disease, thus it is not uncommon for procedures to be denied by the HMO.

These interrelated issues have lead to horror stories of patients being denied service by their HMOs and having major health consequences—even death—occur. HMOs are striving to provide service while keeping costs down—meeting the bottom line. Some of the cost-cutting strategies involve increasing doctor-patient loads, which results in fewer minutes spent with each patient. Thus, the initial claim that the HMO service would be more predisposed to prevention has not been been realized. Less time per patient means less time for a wellness emphasis. HMOs even pay doctors bonuses when they cut costs by, for example, ordering fewer diagnostic tests, a practice found legal by the U.S. Supreme Court. Patients are restricted as to what specialists they can see, since every time they must first have an appointment with the gatekeeper to obtain a referral. Since many specialists are very booked (e.g., dermatologists), an appointment can takes months to schedule, and by then the gatekeeper referral has expired. The patient must make a return appointment to get a renewed referral, with more delays in obtaining a gatekeeper appointment.

Physicians want the best treatment for their patients, and they are even willing to use deception of the insurance companies in order to get their patients to the appropriate specialists and secure reimbursement. The willingness to deceive varies, based on the seriousness of the patients' conditions as follows: for coronary bypass surgery 57.7%, for arterial revascularization 56.2%, for intravenous pain medication and nutrition 47.5%, for mammography screening 34.8%, and for psychiatric referral 32.1% of the primary care physicians were willing to lie in order to secure third-party approval in a study of hypothetical vignettes (Freeman et al., 1999). The ethical dilemma between professional medical responsibilities and contractual obligations to the HMO to cut costs forces physicians to choose every day. Deception has become so common a practice that in the trade it is called "gaming the system" (Freeman et al., 1999).

The core problem is the fact that people within an HMO are typically there because their employer contracted with the provider for this service. Thus, the employer is the actual customer (i.e., the agent buying the service) rather than the future patients, and the employees are not and never were part of the purchasing negotiations. Granted, most places have a sort of "cafeteria" style plan that permits employees to pick and choose the services they want, but they are still constrained within that defined benefit plan. There is no doubt that managed care is going to undergo major restructuring: Patients are unhappy and anxious over the issue of accessibility, doctors feel overworked and constricted in treatment options, and many of the major HMOs in the United States are reporting severe monetary losses (Bodenheimer, 1996; Hellinger, 1998). A recent proposal suggests that primary care physicians need to dump their role as gatekeepers, allow freer patient access to specialists, and take on the role of coordinating patient care (Bodenheimer et al., 1999). This may necessitate a restructuring of the payment process such that financial incentives occur for a balanced approach between over- and underreferral to specialists.

The Future of U.S. Health Care

The HCS in the United States is an enormous and very costly enterprise that is financed by a mixture of public and private monies. Overall real income disparities steadily increase, as wealth concentrates in ever fewer hands. The crucial issue is access—who gets the care. Today 1 in 6 Americans, or 43,000,000, are without health insurance coverage (U.S. Census Bureau, 2000). This results in the uninsured delaying treatment, getting fewer potentially life-saving screening tests done, fewer vaccinations, and greater levels of morbidity and mortality. The prevalence of the uninsured is projected to reach 1 in 5 or 55,000,000 by the year 2008 (SoRelle, 2000a; So- Relle, 2000b).

Given the ideological climate in the United States that historically has emphasized individualism, efforts at universal coverage that have been developed in social democracies appear unlikely in the near term. The so-called "baby boom" generation will soon reach the age of sixty and will be a major political force that will be demanding access to and better facilities for long-term care. The major change that is desperately needed is to place much greater emphasis within medical care on primary prevention. A tiny 3% of all health care expenditures goes to prevention and health promotion (Woolf, 1999). The culture of medical education creates physicians who are trained to be rescuers and fixers of pathology, and they perceive little drama in preventing a disease or injury. No one lives indefinitely, just yet, but a strong and pervasive commitment to primary prevention can reduce human suffering and shortened life spans.

Health Care in South Africa

South Africa has a total land of 1,219 thousand square kilometers, and a population estimated at 43,426,386 (World Factbook, 1999). South Africa is relatively prosperous relative to other countries in the African continent. The life expectancy at birth is 52.68 for males and 56.90 for females (see Table 7.18).

TABLE 7.18   *Health Indicators for South Africa in 1998*

Life expectancy at birth (years)	54.76
Male	52.68
Female	56.90
Infant mortality rate	56.90/1,000 live births
Annual population growth rate	1.32%
Total fertility rate	3.09 births/woman
Birth rate	25.94/1,000 population
Death rate	12.81/1,000 population

Source: World Factbook (1999).

Health Care in South Africa

The health care system in South Africa is supported by both the public and the private sectors, and it features modern Western standards of hospital care and technology. In the public sector, there are various health authorities: the Department of National Health and Population Development, the provincial directors of health, local authorities, and others. The Department of National Health is the agency in charge of health policy making and public health services planning. South Africa spends approximately 9% of total GDP on heath care (Ministry of Health, 2000b).

Inequity is one of the major characteristics of South African health care. People with economic power have sophisticated health care, while many poor people do not even have adequate access to the basics. The AIDS epidemic placed a major burden on the South African health care system. In many hospitals, about half of acute care pediatric and adult medical beds are occupied by patients with HIV-related illnesses (Health Systems Trust, 1999). The inequity exists in all aspects of the health care system: allocation of health care funding, access to health care providers, service delivery, and quality of care. The greatest inequity is between the users of private care and those who must rely on the public sector. About 18% of South Africans (about one in every five) get health care in the private sector, and those 18% of people access 85% of all pharmacists and 60% of medical specialists (Simon, 1999). Health care personnel are concentrated in better-funded urban provinces. In Gauteng there are 2,000 people per one pharmacist, but in Northern Province there 160,000 per pharmacist (Simon, 1999).

Private Health Sector Care

The 18% of people in the private health sector consume more than half of all health resources (Health Systems Trust, 1999). People with private health insurance or medical scheme coverage are the major consumers in the private health sector. To be eligible to become members of medical scheme, people need to have a certain income level. About 60% of those who have top income (>R11000 per year) in South Africa have medical scheme coverage. But those who have low income (<R5000 per year) are largely unable to get medical scheme. Private health care in South Africa is composed of two sectors. The larger sector comprises corporate, private, for-profit hospitals and the smaller one is composed of various health services in the private not-for-profit sector. The smaller sector includes workplace health services and nongovernmental organizations.

For-profit hospitals, the largest section of non–state hospital provision, can be independent organizations or can belong to large hospital groups. The for-profit hospitals usually do not employ their health care professionals. Doctors just use those hospitals and charge insurance companies separately. From 1990 to 1998, the number of private hospitals increased by 33%. The number of hospital beds increased 50% over the same period of time. The majority of health care professionals are employed by the private sector (see Table 7.19).

With the end of apartheid in South Africa there have been many efforts to redress the history of inequalities and mistreatment of black citizens. To this end and to ensure the right of access to health care services as guaranteed in the Constitution of the Republic of South Africa (Act No. 108 of 1996), the Department of Health has adopted a patient rights charter that contains the following key precepts (Ministry of Health, 2000a):

1. Everyone has the right of access to health care services that include receiving timely emergency care at any health care facility that is open regardless of one's ability to pay.

2. Treatment and rehabilitation must be made known to the patient to enable the patient to understand such treatment or rehabilitation and the consequences thereof.

TABLE 7.19 *Health Personnel Practicing in the Private Sector*

	Total Number of Registered Personnel		Proportion of Each Category in the Private Sector	
	1989/90	*1998*	*1989/90*	*1998*
General practitioners	12,889	15,376	61.7%	52.7%
Specialists	3,595	6,136	66.2	76.6
Nurses	109,236	125,349	21%	NA
Pharmacists	8,262	9,599	89	85
Dentists	3,111	3,482	93	NA

Source: South Africa Health Review (1998).

3. Provision will be made for special needs in the case of newborn infants, children, pregnant women, the aged, disabled persons, patients in pain, persons living with HIV, or AIDS patients.

4. There will be palliative care that is affordable and effective in cases of incurable or terminal illness.

5. Everyone has a right to choose a particular health care for services or a particular health facility for treatment, provided that such choice shall not be contrary to the ethical standards applicable to such health care providers or facilities and the choice of facility is in line with prescribed service delivery guidelines.

Nurse-Oriented Primary Health Care

Nurses play an important role in providing primary health care services in the public sector. Community nurses, who mainly work in clinics, have responsibilities of diagnosing and treating common diseases and ordering medicines. Today, clinic nurses are expected to provide ongoing care for chronic diseases such as hypertension and diabetes, as well as management of tuberculosis and STDs, and HIV/AIDS counseling and care (Strasser, 1999).

There are three types of nurse training programs: basic training, post-basic formal training, and post-basic informal training programs. The basic training is practical training that usually occurs in tertiary hospitals. Nurses get hands-on training in curative services under doctors' supervision. The basic training in South Africa does not provide nurses adequate knowledge to provide primary health care. The hospital-based training provides them skills for working in a hospital environment, but it does not give them the necessary analytical and problem-solving skills to deliver primary health care in clinics. Some nurses seek post-basic training in order to make the move from hospital to clinic nursing. The post-basic formal training programs include such courses as nursing administration, nursing education, psychiatry, midwifery, community health, and primary health care. The post-basic informal training programs are in-service training programs.

Problems

Clearly there still remain wide discrepancies in access to high-quality health care within the South African population. There are regional differences in accessibility and level of care. South Africa also shares with the whole of Africa the AIDS epidemic, which necessitates strong efforts for behavioral/educational interventions and costly palliative care. By the end of 1996 it was estimated that 2.4 million adults were infected, and that 156,000 babies born since 1990 had been infected with HIV. There is also the burden of TB cases. The transition to representative democratic governance in South Africa has been far from miraculous in its speed and relative peacefulness. Efforts are under way to improve the quality of life and health care for all citizens, which will no doubt take time and require financial commitment by the government. The government is currently undertaking massive reorganization and restructuring based on the principle that private health practitioners should be integrated with the public sector in the provisioning and management of health services. The central emphasis remains to enhance the capacity of the National Health Service to deliver affordable quality health care to all citizens of South Africa (Nkosazana & Zuma, 1999).

Summary

Health care systems in different countries all have their unique yet similar organizational structures. Each health care system has to provide answers to some basic questions: How accessible are the health services to all citizens? How is the health care system financed? Who pays for the health care? What structure and management style does the health care system have? And so forth.

In this chapter, we examined health care systems in nine different countries. In some countries, the health care systems are very similar, such as in Japan and Canada: Both have universal health care coverage. In other countries, the differences are quite large. The extent of private versus public financing is the major factor that defines the differences in health care systems. All countries are working on cost control—that is, attempting to be more cost effective while trying to provide adequate health care to their citizens. Countries around the world are making efforts to improve their health care systems; they are paying more attention to different systems and trying to learn from each other. Each health care system has its own strengths and weaknesses; there is no perfect one to serve all. Countries with universal coverage struggle with increasing costs driven by (1) changing patient needs, as demographic patterns manifest older populations, and (2) technological advances that improve treatment choices. Health care needs are seemingly infinite, and efforts at rationing access continue. Russia represents a dramatic example of a society that once provided quality universal coverage but has lost enormous ground because of larger societal changes as it transitions from a planned economy to a market-driven system. Each society must organize a system of health care to provide for the productive functioning of its citizens. Historical precedent, ideological issues (i.e., politics), and societal resources all combine to determine the extent to which each citizen must pay for health care needs. HCSs must also be in constant flux, adapting and changing to different societal demographic trends (i.e., the world's aging population), advances in biotechnology, and new acute and chronic diseases. Diseases that were once unknown—such as Alzheimer's and prostate cancer—now burden millions, simply because humans are living long enough to develop these diseases (we are victims of our own successes). The future holds great promise for extending human life through biomolecular research, and those societies with greater wealth need to commit to biomedical knowledge transfers to low-income countries.

Discussion Questions

1. Considering infant and maternal mortality rates, what factors of the HCS seem to be most relevant in explaining the observed differences?

2. What is "gaming the system," and why does it occur?

3. Name three key problems each country is having regarding its health care system.

4. Which health care systems are getting worse and why?

5. How do advances in technology impact health care costs?

6. What is happening to the Russian health care system?

7. What are the advantages and disadvantages of the universal coverage health care system?

8. Why is primary prevention such a marginalized component of most health care systems, and why is it more prominent in China?

References

Akaho, E., Coffin, G. D., Kusano, T., Locke, L., & Okamoto, T. (1998). A Proposed Optional Health Care System Based on a Comparative Study Conducted between Canada and Japan. *Canadian Journal of Public Health, 89*(5), 301–307.

Arai, Y., & Ikegami, N. (1998). Health Care Systems in Transition. Japan, Part I. An Overview of the Japanese Health Care Systems. *Journal of Public Health Medicine. 20*(1), 28–33.

AIHW. (1996). *Health Expenditure Bulletin*, No. 12. Canberra: Australian Institute of Health and Welfare.

AIHW. (1998). *Australia's Health 1998.* Australian Institute of Health and Welfare [Online] Available: Http://www.aihw.gov.au/publications/health/ah98.html.

Barron, P. (1998). Equity in 1998—an overview. Found in: Ntuli, A. *South Africa Health Review* [Online] Available: Http://hst.org.za/sahr/98.htm

Beason, T. (1999). Japan Looks to USA for Health-Care Reform. Seattle: *Seattle Times*, April 27.

Basch, P. F. (1999). *Textbook of International Health* (2nd Ed.). New York: Oxford University Press.

Bodenheimer, T. (1996). The HMO Backlash: Righteous or Reactionary? *New England Journal of Medicine, 335*, 1601–1604.

Bodenheimer, T., Lo, B., & Casalino, L. (1999). Primary Care Physicians Should Be Coordinators, Not Gatekeepers. *Journal of the American Medical Association, 281* (21), 2045–2049.

Canadian Institute for Health Information (CIHI). 1998. Canada to Spend More on Health Care in 1998 Says Canadian Institute for Health Information. [Online] Available: Http://www.cihi.ca/facts/canhe.htm

CDC. (1999). Achievements in Public Health, 1900–1999: Decline in Deaths from Heart Disease and Stroke—United States, 1900–1999. *Morbity, Mortality, Weekly Report, 48*(30), 649–656.

Chernichovsky, D., & Potapchik, E. (1999). Genuine Federalism in the Russian Health Care System: Changing Roles of Government. *Journal of Health Politics, Policy and Law, 24*(1), 115–134.

CIA. (1999). United States, The World Factbook [Online] Available: Http://www.odci.gov/cia/publications/factbook/country.html

CNBS (China Bureau of Statistics). (1999). China Statistical Yearbook 1999. [Online]. Available: Http://www.stats.gov.cn/yearbook.htm

Collopy, B. T. (1991). Audit Activities in Australia. *British Medical Journal, 303*, 1523–1525

Commonwealth of Australia. (1999). Australia Now—A Statistical Profile [Online]. Available: http://www.abs.gov.au/websitedbe.html.

Donatelle, R., & Davis, L. (1999). *Access to Health,* (6th Ed.) Needham Heights, MA: Allyn and Bacon.

DOH. (2000). Patients Right Charter. Pretoria, South Africa: Department of Health. [Online] Available: Http://www.health.gov.za/

Federal Statistical Office Germany (1998). Health Expenditure [Online] Available: http://www.statistik-bund.de/basic/e/gesu/healtab4.htm.

Francis, D. (1990). A Radical Proposal to Cure Health Care. *Maclean's, 103,* 19.

Freeman, V. G., et al. (1999). Lying for Patients: Physician Deception of Third-Party Payers. *Archieves of Internal Medicine, 159*(19), 2263–2270.

Frenk, J., Gomez-Dantes, O., Criuz, C., Chacon, F., Hernandez, P., & Freeman, P. (1994). Consequences of the North American Free Trade Agreement: A Perspective from Mexico. *American Journal of Public Health, 84*(10): 1591–1597.

Garcia de Miranda, E., & Falcon de Gyves, Z. (1993). Atlas-Nuevo Atlas Pomea de la Republics Mexicana. Mexico City: Editorial Porrua.

Grumback, K., et al. (1999). Resolving the Gatekeeper Conundrum: What Patients Value in Primary Care and Referrals to Specialists. *Journal of the American Medical Association, 282* (3), 261–266.

HCFA. (2000). National Health Expenditures Projections: 1998–2008. Health Care Financing Administration [Online] Available: http://www.hcfa.gov.

Health Services; A Perspective from Mexico. *American Journal of Public Health, 84* (10), 1591–1597.

Health Systems Trust. (1991). South African Health Review 1998. [Online]. Available: Http://www.hst.org.za/sahr/98/

Hellinger, F. J. (1998). Regulating the Financial Incentives Facing Physicians in Managed Care Plans. *The American Journal of Managed Care,* 4(5), 663–674.

Hsiao, W. C. L. (1995). The Chinese Health Care System: Lessons for Other Nations. *Social Science Medicine, 41*(8), 1047–1156.

Iglehart, J. K. (1986). Canada's Health Care System. *The New England Journal of Medicine, 315,* 202–208.

Iglehart, J. K. (1991). Health Policy Report: Germany's Health Care System. New *England Journal of Medicine, 324*(7), 503–508.

Iglehart, J. K. (1999a). Health Policy Report: the American Health Care System—Medicaid. *The New England Journal of Medicine, 340*(5), 403–408.

Iglehart, J. K. (1999b). Health Policy Report: the American Health Care System—Medicare. *The New England Journal of Medicine, 340*(4), 327–332.

Ikegami, N., & Campbell, J. C. (1995). Special Report: Medical Care in Japan. *The New England Journal of Medicine, 333*(19), 1295–1299.

Kaps, C. (1993, April). Health Care in Germany: A Model for the United States? *Europe: Magazine of the European Community,* 10–11.

Kransy, J. (1992, February). The Wrong Health Care Model. *National Review, 2,* 43–44.

Lipson, R., & Pemble, L. (1996). Reshaping the Medical Equipment Landscape. *The Chinese Business Review, 23*(4), 8–17.

Marquez, V. B., & Sherraden, M. S. (1994). Political Change and the Welfare State: The Case of Health and Food Policies in Mexico. *World Development, 22*(9), 1295–1312.

MHW. (2000). *Statistics and Other Data.* Nippon: Ministry of Health and Welfare [Online] Available: http://www.mhw.go.jp/english/

Ministry of Health. (2000a). Patients Rights Charter. Pretoria, South Africa: Dept. of Health [Online] Available: http://www.health.gov.za

Ministry of Health. (2000b). Transformation of the health system. Pretoria, South Africa: Dept. of Health. [Online] Available: http://www.health.gov.za

Nissenson, A. R., & Rettig, R. A. (1999). Medicare's 2nd-stage Renal Disease Program: Current Status and Future Prospects. *Health Aff (Millwood), 18*(1): 161–79.

Nkosazana, C., & Zuma, D. (1999). White Paper for the Transformation of the Health System in South Africa. Pretoria, South Africa: Ministry of Health [Online] Available: Http://www.health.gov.za/hlthwhit.htm

OECD Health Data 97. (1997). Frequently Asked Data—Inputs and Throughputs [Online] Available: http://www.oecd.org/els/health/fad_2.htm

PAHO. (1994). *Health Conditions in the America.* Washington, DC: PAHO Scientific Publication No. 549.

Paine, L. (1978). *Health Care in Big Cities.* New York: St. Martin's Press.

Peabody, J. W., Bickel, S. R., & Lawson, J. S. (1996). The Australian Health Care System. *Journal of the American Medical Association, 276* (24), 1944–1955.

PHIAC (2000). Coverage of Hospital Insurance Tables. Private Health Insurance Administration Council [Online] Available: http://www.phiac.org.au/phiac/tr_index/htm

Rakich, J. S. (1991). The Canadian and United States Health Care Systems: Profiles and Policies. *Hospital & Health Administration, 36*(1), 25–39.

Roemer, M. (1991). *National Health Systems of the World* (Vol. I). Oxford: Oxford University Press.

Schulenburg, J. M. (1992). Germany: Solidarity at a Price. *Journal of Health Politics, Policy & Law, 17*(4), 715–738.

Selbmann, H K. (1996). Germany: Health Care. *The Lancet, 348*(9042), 1631–34.

Simon, J. (1999). The Health Review in Depth. *The South African Health Review* [Online] Available: http://www.hst.org.za/update/40/policy10.htm

Soderlund, N., Schierhout, G., and Heever, A. (1998). Private Health Sector Care. *South Africa Health Review* [Online] Available: http://www.hst.org.az/sahr/98.htm

Sonderdruck fur Presse-und Informationsamt der Bundesregierung. (1994). *Zahlen Kompass.* Wiesbaden: Statistisches Bundesamt.

SeRelle, R. (2000a). Study predicts 55 million people uninsured by the year 2008. *Circulation, 101*(4), E61.

SoRelle, R. (2000b). Numbers of uninsured increases. *Circulation, 101*(22), E9048–9049.

Stassen, M. (1993). The German Statutory Health Insurance System. *Social Education, 57*(5), 247–248.

Strasser, S (1999). Nurse Oriented Primary Health Care: The Needs of Nurses. *South Africa Health Review* [Online] Available: http://www.hst.org.za/sahr/98/chap8.htm

Tatsachen uber Deutchland. (1993). Frankfurt am Main: Societats-Verlag.

The World Bank Group (1997). Poverty in Africa [Online] Available: http://www4.worldbank.org/afr/poverty

Topolnicki, D. M. (1993). How to Get Medical Care for All. *Money, 22,* 87–89.

Tierney, M. J., & Tierney, L. M. (1994). Nursing in Japan. *Nursing Outlook, 24*(4), 210–213.

Tuffs, A. (1993). Germany: Illegality of Abortion. *The Lancet, 341*(8858), 1467.

Twigg, J. L. (1998). Balancing the State and the Market: Russia's Adoption of Obligatory Medical Insurance. *Europe-Asia Studies, 50*(4), 583–602.

United Nations. (1987). *World Population Policies.* New York: United Nations.

United Nations. (1991). *Overcoming Obstacles to Institutional Development in the Least Developed Countries.* New York: United Nations.

U.S. Census Bureau. (2000). United States Census 2000. [Online]. Available: Http://www.census.gov

Vayda, E. (1986, Summer). The Canadian Health Care System: An Overview. *Journal of Public Health Policy,* 205–210.

Walberg, P., McKee, M., & Shkolnikov, V. (1998). Economic Change, Crime, and Mortality Crisis in Russia: Regional Analysis. *British Medical Journal, 317,* 312–318.

Wei, Y. (1991). China's Current Health Care Financing, Utilization, and Future Policy Direction. Beijing: Ministry of Public Health.

Weinberg, N. (1997). Bad Medicine. *Forbes.* 160(14): Page 46.

Woolf, S. H. (1999). The Need for Perspective in Evidence-Based Medicine. *Journal of the American Medical Association, 282* (24), 2358–2365.

World Health Organization. (1995). The World Health Report 1995: *Bridging the Gaps.* Geneva, Switzerland: Office of Publications, World Health Organization.

World Health Organization. (1996). *Most Recent Values of Global Health-for-All Indicators.* South Africa [Online] Available: http://www.who.int/whosis/hfa/countries/sou3.htm.

World Health Organization. (1999a). WHO Estimates of Health Personnel—Physicians, Dentists, and Nurses/midwives [Online] Available: http://www.who.int/whosis/healthpersonnel/index.html

World Health Organization. (1999b). The World Health Report 1999: *Meeting the Challenges: Health Systems Development* [Online] Available: http://www.who.int/whr/1999/en/report.htm

World Health Organization (1999c). The World Health Report 1999: Basic indicators for all member states [Online] Available: http://www.who.int/whr/1999/en/indicators.htm

8

Epidemiology: Methods and Global Practice

Edward A. Meister and Robert W. Buckingham

Epidemiology

Epidemiology is the study of disease (and injury) patterns in human populations to enable preventing them. Today, epidemiology is a well-established academic and highly expert profession throughout the world. It has blossomed into a plethora of specialties covering genetic, nutritional, clinical, molecular, psychiatric, environmental, and occupational forms. The newest specialty is called social-behavioral epidemiology, which seeks to understand the behavioral components to lifestyle-related diseases such as infectious diseases that are sexually transmitted (STDs). This is because human behavior is both a biological and cultural phenomenon, and as a result the societal context that contributes to the spread of STDs must be included in the analysis.

Epidemiology began forming as a discipline in the nineteenth century with the work done by Dr. John Snow, who studied the cholera outbreaks in London and found a link between the disease and the consumption of fecal-contaminated sources of drinking water. In the 1950s Doll and Hill produced the now famous British doctors' smoking study, which found a positive linear association between the annual number of lung cancer deaths and the average number of cigarettes smoked per day (Beaglehole, Bonita, & Kjellstrom, 1993). Today, epidemiologists around the world are still undertaking their basic mission: to identify the occurrences and risk factors for human diseases and injuries, and to formulate preventive strategies. This chapter will provide an introduction to basic concepts, methods, and the global practice of epidemiology.

Defining Epidemiology

Epidemiology, considered a branch of public health, is formally defined as the study of the nature, cause, control, and determinants of the frequency and distribution of disease, disability, and death in human populations (Timmreck, 1994). There is considerable debate as to whether the profession of epidemiology is a science or simply a system of data collection and analysis techniques. However, most would agree that epidemiology does embrace, to a considerable extent, the scientific method of empirical (observation-based) testing of hypotheses to support etiological theory.

Epidemiology also seeks to characterize the distribution of health status in terms of person, place, and time. Characteristics of the person can be categorized as follows: (1) acquired or hereditary characteristics—age, gender, ethnicity, marital status; (2) activities—work, play, recreational activities, religious activities, customs; and (3) living circumstances—economic, social, political, and environmental (Stone et al., 1996). Characteristics of place are geography, climate, population densities (urban, rural), social and cultural-political dimensions, and a variety of environmental factors such as water sources and air quality. Time is the crucial dimension of epidemiological studies, since at its most essential level epidemiology is about measuring change over time in the occurrence of some phenomenon adverse to human health. The enterprise of epidemiology is uncovering the etiology (causality) of human morbidity and mortality to enable future efforts of primary prevention.

Basic Epidemiological Concepts

Epidemiology rests on two basic assumptions: Human diseases do not occur by chance, and underlying factors that cause or contribute to diseases and injuries can be identified by means of systematic investigation (Hennekens, Buring, & Mayrent, 1987). The defining characteristic of epidemiology is that it takes a population or subpopulation focus. Its unit of measurement may ultimately be the individual, in some fashion, but its perspective is to measure and compare population-based aggregate occurrences of the disease of interest.

Epidemiology begins by assessing the frequency of the disease of interest as it occurs in populations, which thus makes relative comparisons possible. For example, the frequency of infant deaths on an annual count basis can be compared from one community to the next, or even among countries, to ascertain which countries are doing relatively well in preventing infant deaths, and which are in need of taking stronger actions to reduce their occurrence.

There are essentially four recognized levels of prevention: primordial, primary, secondary, and tertiary (see Table 8.1). Primordial prevention attempts to avoid the development of social, economic, and cultural patterns of living that have been established as contributing to increase the risk of various diseases. Primary prevention seeks to avoid the occurrence of a disease in a population or individual that is presently free of the disease of interest. A good example would be childhood immunizations for measles, mumps, and rubella. Secondary prevention is for individuals whose disease status is currently unknown. Examples would include screening tests for prostate cancer, or breast cancer mammography testing, whose results can then be used to determine treatment options to enable curing the individual. Finally, tertiary prevention occurs when the individual has the disease, is no longer curable, and is referred to treatment practices geared to reduce the suffering or slow the eventual decline associated with the condition. A good example would be physical therapy for a rheumatoid arthritis patient.

The Search for Causality

The essential enterprise of epidemiology is determining and assessing the causal relationship between some exposure and some disease outcome. There are several key factors that can muddy the analysis of causality (Dardis, 1993). Epidemiological research begins with an observed association—such as ultraviolet sun radiation (UVR) exposure and a skin cancer. It is observed that people that have UVR exposures are also developing skin cancer. This is known as an association between an exposure and a disease outcome. However, this association could be explained by factors other than a causal relationship. For example, skin cancer patients may be overreporting the amount of UVR that they have had, known as recall bias. Perhaps there was a bias in the selection of subjects for the study, or maybe patients were even incorrectly diagnosed with skin cancer, know as misclassification bias. Another major problem that characterizes every epidemiological study is the problem of confounding. The association between UVR and occurrence of skin cancer may be the result of a powerful third factor that impacts both the exposure and the outcome of interest. Such factors are called *confounding variables*, because they can truly distort the causal relationship being studied. For example, a person's hereditary background, smoking status, previous cancer history, or immunocompetency status could all "interfere" with the linear causal relationship observed between UVR and skin cancer. The third possible explanation

TABLE 8.1 *Levels of Prevention*

Level of Prevention	Phase of Disease	Target
1. Primordial	Underlying conditions predisposing to disease	Total populations
2. Primary	Presently not diseased	Total healthy populations and selected groups
3. Secondary	Early stage of disease	Patients
4. Tertiary	Postcurability, late stage	Patients

Source: Beaglehole, Bonita, & Kjellstrom (1994).

for the observed association is that it is due purely to chance alone. People with skin cancer may just by chance happened to engage in more sun-exposure activities than those people without skin cancer. Random chance is always a possible explanation that must be considered in any observed correlation. For example, 99% of all people who have died in fatal car crashes have eaten raw carrots. Hence, the epidemiological mantra "correlation is not causation."

Criteria for Judging Causality

Over the years, epidemiologists have come to rely on the causation criteria developed by Austin Bradford Hill, a famous British medical statistician (see Table 8.2). When Hill's criteria are achieved, researchers can move to a more confident position regarding the cause and effect relationship that they have been observing.

The last criterion reveals a fundamental dilemma of epidemiological causality. Since it is unethical to expose humans to agents, either alive or inert, that could potentially cause harm, only those exposures that have potential benefit (e.g., vaccines, fluoride) can be used experimentally. Thus, when tobacco industry executives assert that it has never been proved that smoking causes lung cancer, technically they are correct because researchers cannot randomly assign people to smoke. However, based on the first eight of Hill's criteria, and a new criterion of preponderance of evidence (i.e., thousands of studies obtaining the same resultant association), it has been conclusively established that smoking does cause lung cancer.

TABLE 8.2 *Bradford Hill's Causality Criteria*

Criteria	Explanation
1. Strength of association	The stronger the association the more likely it is cause and effect.
2. Consistency	Same association is found everywhere.
3. Dose-response relationship	The more the exposure the greater the response.
4. Time sequence	Exposure always precedes the outcome.
5. Biological plausibility	Association fits with previously known biological understandings.
6. Specificity	The exposure alone can induce the outcome.
7. Coherence	The evidence fits with related facts.
8. Analogy	Similar exposures should produce similar outcomes.
9. Experimentation	Experimental control of exposure produces predicted outcome.

Basic Epidemiological Measures

The practice of epidemiology is divided into two main domains—descriptive and analytical. The former is concerned with counts and rates of diseases, while the latter undertakes significance tests of the hypothesized relationships between particular exposures and outcomes.

Counts, Proportions, and Percentages

Counts are the most elementary of epidemiological measures and refer to the number of individuals who have a certain disease or exposure (Friedman, 1994). In 1984 in Bhopal India, when the Union Carbide pesticide factory exploded, the first measures taken were the number of immediate fatalities (3,000 deaths), the number of casualties (13,000 injured), and the number exposed to toxic fumes (a 200,000 community-wide estimate). Proportions are a way of assessing some member's status relative to the entire group. In the Bhopal example, the proportion of immediate deaths is equal to 0.015, calculated as

$$P = 3,000/200,000 = .015$$

The percentages of people experiencing immediate death is 1.5%, calculated as

$$P\% = [3,000/200,000] \times 100 = 1.5\%$$

Percentages are simply proportions multiplied by 100, accomplished by moving the decimal place over two places in the number. Counts and proportions, as the most basic epidemiologic measures, are quantitatively very useful.

Frequency Rates

There are two basic frequency rates that take into consideration the size of the source population and the time period at which specific events have occurred. The first is called prevalence rate, which is the total number of cases, both new and old, divided by the population at risk over a given period of time.

$$\text{Prevalence} = [\text{Existing cases}/\text{Population at risk}] \times 1,000 =$$

Notice that the denominator is defined as the population at risk, which means that it excludes those people not at risk for the disease. For example we would exclude women from the denominator when calculating the prevalence of testicular carcinoma, since they are obviously not at risk. Secondly, we multiple by 1,000 (or some other level of counting) to enable expressing the prevalence at a rate, such as 15 per 1,000, or 15 per 100,000. The rate multiplier is somewhat arbitrary, but is usually contrived to enable expressing a whole number for the answer.

The next important frequency measure is referred to as the incidence rate (IR), and is the number of new cases divided by the population at risk over some specified period of time.

IR = [New cases/Population at risk] × 1,000 =

Suppose we followed 1,000 students over their freshman year and counted five new cases of herpes simplex II. For the freshman year the incidence would be calculated as

IR = (5/1,000) × 1,000 = 5 per 1,000

Thus, incidence rate can be interpreted as a measure of the current probable risk of getting a particular disease (if one is at risk), while prevalence is the societal burden of the disease. Incidence generates new cases that add to the overall prevalence, while prevalence declines by means of case recoveries and/or deaths.

Epidemiologists often can agree on what constitutes a case, that is, the numerator, but there can be considerable disagreement over what is the population at risk. To resolve some of the denominator debate, some epidemiologists have gone to using a more precise measure of population at risk called "person-years." Person-years are calculated as the sum of the total disease-free months for each individual, and divided by 12 to convert the total to years.

Another form of the incidence rate is called cumulative incidence (CI), and quantifies the number of persons who become a case for some disease or disability during a specified period of time. The CI estimates the probability or risk of a person's becoming a case during some specified period of time, and is calculated per the formula (Portney & Watkins, 2000):

CI = [No. New cases during specified time/Population at risk] × 1,000 =

Crude Mortality Rates

The most basic of the mortality rates is called the crude mortality rate, and is calculated as;

CMR = [Number of deaths/Population] × 1,000 =

The United States has a population of 275,000,000, and annual deaths of 2,000,000, thus the

CMR = [2,000,000/275,000,000] × 1000 = 7.2 per 1,000

The CMR means that for every 1,000 persons in the United States there are 7.2 deaths per year. There are several rates that epidemiologists commonly use relating to infant mortality, specified by the time of life the infant had. These rates are as follows: infant mortality rate (children <12 months), neonatal mortality rate (children <28 days old), postneonatal mortality rate (children 28 days to 12 months), perinatal mortality (dead at 28 weeks of gestation to 7 days of life), and fetal death rate (number of fetal deaths for one-year period). These mortality rates can be calculated using the following formulae (Friedman, 1994):

Infant MR = [No. deaths <12 months of age/Total population] × 1,000 =

Neonatal MR = [No. deaths <28 days of age/No. live births-year] × 1,000 =

Postneonatal MR = [No. deaths 28 days to 12 months of age/No. live births-year] × 1,000 =

Perinatal MR = [Dead at 28 weeks of gestation to 7 days of life/Total fetal deaths + live births-year] × 1,000 =

Fetal Death Rate = [Number of fetal deaths for 1-year period/Total fetal deaths + live births-year] × 1,000 =

One of the crude mortality measures that are often used by world health agencies to preliminarily assess the health status of the population is the infant mortality rate, and the maternal mortality rate (MMR). During the Middle Ages a women typically died in childbirth with every fourth birth, given the limited medical assistance that was available.

MMR = [Number of puerperal deaths-year/No. live births] × 1,000 =

Another rate of importance is the age-specific mortality rate, which calculates the number of deaths per year for a particular age group; an example is as follows:

ASMR = [No. Death-specific age group/ Total no. in age group] × 1,000 =

For example, if one-year deaths for the group aged 65 to 74 were 10,000 and a total population in that age group was 5,000,00, then the ASMR would be:

ASMR = [10,000/5,000,000] × 1,000 = 2 per 1,000 population

Similarly the case fatality rate is the rate of deaths per cases, and is calculated as follows:

CFR = [(No. deaths per specific disease)/No. of cases per specific disease] × 100 =

Finally, the proportional mortality rate is the proportion of all deaths attributable to a particular disease, and is calculated by:

PMR = [(No. deaths per specific disease)/Total deaths] × 100 =

Adjusted Rates

These crude rates are called *crude* because they do not take into consideration a great variety of population characteristics such as age, gender, ethnicity, educational level, and/or occupation (Stone et al., 1996). Crude rates include all the potential factors that may influence the disease or death under study. Epidemiologists often want to "control" for these other factors—that is, remove their influence on the rates—to better understand the causal process underlying the disease and make more meaningful comparisons among populations. When rates are adjusted, they are often referred to as standardized rates.

For example, suppose we wanted to compare the death rates for Shanghai and St. Petersburg. If we calculated the crude death rate and the age-specific death rates, could we then compare the two cities? We could, except that the underlying populations are vastly different; Shanghai has a much younger overall population, while St. Petersburg has a much older population structure. There are two basic approaches to standardization. In the direct method a death rate is used from an arbitrarily chosen population to serve as a standard with a known age structure. Thus, one uses a population that presumably exemplifies typical death rate patterns. The indirect method of standardization is more appropriate for comparing two populations of one age-specific rate, by means of calculating the SMR or standardized mortality ratio (Mausner & Kramer, 1985).

SMR = [Observed deaths/Expected deaths] × 100 =

The SMR conveys the ratio of observed deaths in a community (or country) adjusted by the expected deaths in a standard population, and is usually expressed as a percentage (Lilienfeld & Stolley, 1994). The SMR is useful in occupational settings when attempting to determine whether certain industrial exposures have greater mortality compared to people with similar age (and other background factors, minus the industrial exposure) in the general population. When the SMR exceeds 100, then there is greater risk of mortality associated with the exposure under study. The concern with all adjusted rate procedures is that it creates a "fictional rate" because the calculated rates are dependent upon the particular "standard" population that was selected (Mausner & Kramer, 1985).

Specialized Epidemiological Measures

An epidemiological measure that is becoming more popular is called years of potential life lost (YPLL), which measures the number of lost years of life due to some cause based on a projected life expectancy (Gordis, 1996). For example, if a male dies of AIDS in the United States at age 35, and would have been expected to live to age 72, then the YPLL = 72 – 35 = 37 years of lost potential life. YPLL can be done that is age specific. Suppose 3,000 people aged 17 died in Rome, Italy, due to motor scooter accidents each year. Then the YPLL would be calculated as: YPLL = [(3,000 × (72 – 17)] = 165,000 years of potential life.

Epidemiologists calculate what is referred to as the dependency ratio (DR) for a given society as follows: DR = [No. <18 + >64]/[>18 + <65] × 100 = _____%. The DR is the proportion of dependents in a society based on the ratio of children (under 18) and elderly (over 64) to the number of adults (between 19 and 63). DR can provide a useful indicator of changing demographics and social needs for that country. For example, the DR for China was 73 in 1978 and 47 in 1998, while for Oman it went from 89 to 90, hence Oman has a greater proportion of its population that is considered "dependent" upon the adult segment (WHO, 1999).

Assessing Risk

Relative Risk Calculation

One can hardly read the news on any given day without being advised of a new study that found increased risk associated with some activity or condition. For example, researchers in Sweden recently found that infants born to snoring mothers had reduced birth weights (growth retardation), lower Apgar birth outcome scores, and greater risk of induced hypertension (Franklin et al., 2000). What epidemiologists are trying to find are measures of associations between a particular exposure (e.g., tobacco, fatty foods) and a particular health outcome (e.g., lung cancer, coronary heart disease). When they find an association between exposure and outcome, this is reported as an identified risk factor for that outcome (i.e., disease or injury). Recent examples include increased risk of adult-onset asthma (outcome) in women who gained weight from age 18 depicted by increasing BMI (body mass index) (exposure) (Camargo et al., 1999); increased risk of coronary heart disease mortality (outcome) associated with the habit of cigar smoking (exposure) (Jacobs et al., 1999); increasing risk of dental cavities (outcome) associated with increased blood lead levels (outcome) (Moss et al., 1999), and increased risk of Type II noninsulin dependent diabetes (outcome) associated with low cardiorespiratory fitness (exposure) (Wei et al., 1999). These risk associations are based on comparing the ratio of the frequencies among the diseased who have the exposure compared to those diseased without the exposure of interest. Thus, relative risk (RR) can be conceptualized in the formula as follows:

RR = Risk in exposed/Risk in unexposed

The calculation of RR is greatly facilitated by organizing the data into what is called a two-by-two contingency table, with exposure status in the rows and outcome status in the columns. Each cell of the two-by-two table, as demonstrated in Table 8.3, is labeled with a letter.

TABLE 8.3   *Two-by-Two Contingency Table Example*

Exposure Status	Disease Status: YES	Disease Status: NO
YES	a	b
NO	c	d

Relative risk is calculated as follows: RR = [(a/a+b)]/[(c/c+d)]. Relative risk is actually the ratio of the incidence rate in the exposed to the incidence rate in the unexposed, represented as follows: RR = IR_e/IR_o. Thus, the incidence rate represents the absolute risk of a disease in the population for those with the exposure of interest, whereas relative risk is the odds or probability of getting the disease based on having the exposure (Stone et al., 1996).

Let us do an example using the contingency table with data from a recent study on the risk of coronary heart disease (CHD) and degrees of baldness (Lotufo et al., 2000). The study classified subjects from moderate to severely bald, and determined their CHD status (yes or no) (see Table 8.4).

Thus, we calculate RR as follows: RR = [a/a+b]/[c/c+d] = [79/554]/[40/324] = 1.15. Interpreting RR results is actually fairly easy. When RR = 1, then there is no increased risk of the disease when comparing the exposed subjects with the unexposed; when RR is great than 1 then the exposure is associated with increased risk; and finally when RR is less than 1, then the exposure of interest has a protective effect (as is typically the case for a vaccine). Putting the RR results for the baldness study into words would be as follows: Severe baldness among males over age 55 was associated with a 1.15 times greater risk of coronary heart disease.

Relative risk is calculated when epidemiologists employ a study design called cohort design. A typical cohort design begins with subjects who are free of the disease of interest, but do have the exposure of interest, and then follows them forward in time, along with another disease-free group of subjects who do not have the exposure of interest. After a disease-appropriate period of time (cancer takes a long time, whereas rhinovirus colds are quick) has elapsed, a count is made of who has the disease and who does not in each of the two groups (i.e., the exposed and unexposed). During the analysis of RR, epidemiologists may control for what are termed "effect modifiers," which are conditions that can distort the risk association that is being researched. In the pregnant snoring study, the researchers controlled for age, weight, and smoking status of the expectant mothers. Another

TABLE 8.4   *Two-by-Two Table for Severely Bald Males and CHD*

Severely Bald Men over age 55	CHD (Yes)	CHD (No)
Yes	79 (a)	475 (b)
No	40 (c)	284 (d)

potential effect modifier could be parity status of the expectant mothers, which is the number of previous births each has had.

There are several advantages with the cohort design: it uses real incidence cases, is very valuable when the exposure of interest is rare, and has the strength of incorporating a temporal structure—that is, linking exposure and outcome by time. The cohort is also useful for rare exposures, because exposure status is where each subject begins. The disadvantages are that it is very inefficient for rare diseases, and it can be costly both in resources and time to follow subjects throughout their lives.

Exposure Odds Ratio Calculation

An alternative to the cohort design that epidemiologists often use is called the case-control design. The case-control design permits the calculation of an approximated relative risk, referred to as the exposure odds ratio (EOR). Using the familiar two-by-two table, we calculate EOR as follows: EOR = ad/bc.

Subjects are selected into the study who already have the disease of interest, and then are separated by exposure status. Hence, the distinct advantage of the case-control design is that since subjects already are cases (i.e., people with a disease), this design is very useful for rare diseases and common exposures. The disadvantages with case-control design are that the temporality dimension is lost for assessing causality, direct incidence rates are not computable, it is inefficient for rare exposures, and it is vulnerable to subject selection and recall bias (Hennekens et al., 1987). Table 8.5 displays the research orientation for both the prospective cohort design and the retrospective case-control design. There can also be combinations of these designs, such as a cohort with a nested case-control design.

Let us illustrate the EOR calculation with a recent study that looked at the exposure of leisure-time physical activity levels and the risk of primary cardiac arrest (Lemaitre et al., 1999). Table 8.6 presents the two-by-two table construction from the study, and EOR is calculated as: EOR = ad/bc = $(128 \times 18)/(293 \times 45) = .17$.

TABLE 8.5 *Epidemiological Study Designs Relative to Time*

Design Type	Past	Present	Future
Cohort		Exposure status →	Disease frequency
Case-control	Exposure status	←Disease frequency	

TABLE 8.6 *Two-by-Two Table for Level of Exercise and Cardiac Arrest*

Level of Exercise	Cardiac Arrest (Yes)	Cardiac Arrest (No)
Moderate exercise	128 (a)	293 (b)
No exercise	45 (c)	18 (d)

In this study the EOR is less than 1 and can be interpreted the same as for RR; thus moderate leisure-time exercise has a protective effect against cardiac arrest.

Interpreting Confidence Intervals

Associated risk for either RR or EOR is typically presented in the research literature with confidence intervals (CI). When RR or EOR is calculated, it is termed a point estimate of the association between exposure and outcome; that is, it is a single value depicting the level of risk. The CI is a calculation that conveys an estimate of effect size or range of risk that goes from lowest level to highest level. Secondly, CI also conveys whether the risk calculation is statistically significant. Statistical significance is a concept that implies that the results obtained are not likely to be due to chance alone (i.e., the results obtained are meaningful). The rule for CI interpretation is simple: If the CI range includes 1, then the RR or EOR is not considered statistically significant. The opposite is also true; if the CI does not include 1 in either direction, then the RR or EOR is considered statistically significant (Page et al., 1995). Biostatisticans measure statistical significance by calculating a point estimate statistic that enables obtaining a p-value. The rule with p-value is also simple to employ: When it is equal to or less than .05, the p-value is interpreted to be statistically significant (and conversely, if greater than .05, it is not significant).

Table 8.7 displays the results from a case-control study that compared mothers who exhibited depressive symptoms and the risk for three different types of hospital visits for their infants. To recapitulate, the case-control begins with cases, and in this study it was mothers exhibiting depression symptoms. Then the researchers count retrospectively the number and types of hospital visits for both depressive and nondepressive mothers. Overall, infants of depressive mothers were at increased risk for a hospital visit; this is evident since all three of the EORs are greater than 1. The confidence intervals are displayed and indicate the effect size or range effect for the risk of infant hospital visits based on a depressive mother. The final column displays the p-values.

Applying our two rules, if the confidence interval contains 1, then there is no statistical significance, and if p-value is greater than .05, then there is no statistical significance. This is easily confirmed by the results in Table 8.7; both Type 1 and 2

TABLE 8.7   *Maternal Depressive Symptoms and Infant Medical Visits*

Type of Infant Visit	EOR	Confidence Interval	P-value
1. Problem visit	1.9	1.1 to 3.8	.04
2. ER visit	3.3	1.7 to 6.7	<.001
3. Well-child visit	1.3	.7 to 2.4	.46

Source: Mandl et al. (1999).

infant hospital visits were statistically significant because the CIs did not contain 1 (this is also evidenced by the p-values since they were either equal to or less than .05). Notice that EOR for well-child visits was not statistically significant, even though the EOR was greater than 1 (i.e. 1.3). This study demonstrates an important consideration regarding statistical significance. The RR or EOR may exhibit increased risk associated with a particular exposure, yet fail to meet the criterion of statistical significance. When that occurs, does it always mean that the results have no research importance? The answer is, not necessarily. The epidemiologist always needs to consider whether the results have some practical significance that warrants further investigation. Finally, RR and EOR are estimates of risk of some particular exposure from a study population, and the CI, since it is a range of potential risk, may actually reflect the true population risk more adequately.

Sources of Error: Bias

Epidemiologists work very hard to reduce and eliminate error in their research. Sources of error can be addressed in both the design stage and in the analysis stage, yet these attempts are not always completely successful. The most important source of potential error is referred to as "bias." This term is not used in the ordinary meaning of some manner of prejudice. Bias for epidemiological researchers is some condition or set of conditions that exert a distorting influence on the data. The following will discuss each of the key types of bias that can cause this distortion of results:

1. *Selection bias* occurs when cases and controls (those not diseased) are differentially included into the study based on some factor related to the exposure of interest. The result is that the individuals do not have a common underlying mean value for the measurement of interest (Selvin, 1996). An example of selection bias would be as follows. Suppose a physician knew that certain patients had low T-helper cell counts and then proceeded to selected these patients (who are more at risk for AIDS) to receive the active test drug in a clinical trail. The patients with high T-helper cell counts were selected to received the inert placebo drug. This would certainly create the potential for distorting the safety and efficacy findings that are the core objective of any such study. Another form of selection bias is called self-selection bias, where subjects choose exposures or degrees of exposure, which can also distort the research findings because of unequal representation in the study groups.

2. *Misclassification bias* occurs when there are mistakes made regarding what a subject actually is. A subject may be designated a case, when in fact the diagnosis was incorrect, or incorrectly indicated on the individual's chart. If these misclassifications are equally represented in both groups of subjects, this is referred to as nondifferential misclassification (Portney & Watkins, 2000).

3. *Observation bias* happens when there is a systematic difference in the manner in which information about the subjects' disease or exposure is gathered from the study groups. This can take the form of *interview bias,* when subject information gathered is in some way altered either intentionally or accidentally by the interviewer himself or herself (e.g., excessive prompting or coaching the answer out of a subject). *Recall bias* results when the subjects for whatever reason distort the information they provide to the researchers. In nutritional studies it is well documented that subjects often report more healthful diet history recalls if they think the interviewer or survey taker will think better of them. At other times, recall bias is purely unintentional, as, for example, subjects try to recall when a child's illness occurred or was resolved.

Addressing Bias

Epidemiologists address the potential for bias by establishing a careful design at the outset, and carefully following the established protocols of the study. The first step is to develop a percise definition of exactly what characteristics constitute a case—that is, a subject with the disease of interest. For example, a case of skin cancer must be explicitly defined as to which type of skin cancer the patient has, and may even involve malignancy typing or severity of the cancer. For a prospective cohort design, where subjects will be followed over time, it is important that all subjects in all regions enter the cohort simultaneously.

When choosing the study population, it is crucial to get a representative sample, one that is indicative of the population. No two people are exactly the same, yet the researchers strive to include subjects who approximate the level of sameness or differences in the exposure and the control group. Collection of data is least biased when protocols are standardized and adhered to by those administering questionnaires or extracting information from patient charts. These protocols are best when written out, and periodically reviewed with study personnel to ensure they are being followed.

Finally, bias can be minimized when researchers use multiple sources for cross-checking the accuracy of data. For example, getting independent confirmation of a subject's exposure status from sources other that the subject's own self-report serves to increase confidence in the measure. Eliminating bias is a crucial aspect of any epidemiological study, because once it is introduced, it is very difficult to extricate it from the study.

Another form of bias is referred to as "publishing bias," which has to do with the fact that scientific journals are more interested in publishing positive findings, rather than what is called null (or nonsignificant) study results (Friis & Sellers, 1999). Thus, researchers experience subtle pressures to find positive results to better their chances of getting published. This can take the extreme form of actual data doctoring or manipulation, or more subtle strategies such as dropping certain "odd" subjects from the study (referred to as extreme outliers) in order to achieve better results. The "signficant findings" emphasis in the scientific publishing world then leads to a bias in the literature favoring positive findings rather than the true picture.

The Practice of Epidemiology

Infectious Diseases

The practice of epidemiology began historically, as the old saying goes, by "doctors who could count." What they counted was mostly corpses resulting from the litany of infectious diseases that ravaged human beings from the dawn of time. Rubella, smallpox, diphtheria, tuberculosis, leprosy (Hansen's Disease), malaria, cholera, plague, anthrax, mumps, rubeola, syphilis, typhoid fever, and typhus are some of the major communicable diseases that have swept across the human time line filling the cemeteries and funeral pyres with the dead of all ages and social strata. Millions upon millions suffered and died while humans searched in vain for explanations that were sometimes theological (i.e., the wrath of divine beings) and as other times political (blaming of other countries or various ethnic groups).

Black Death and the Search for Etiology

Bubonic plague, known as Black Death, is a horrific example of the search for answers. The Black Death was one of the great epidemic scourges of human kind that went across Europe and Asia in a series of devastating pandemics during the Middle Ages (albeit it attacked Constantinople during the sixth century of Justinian). In fourteenth-century Europe an estimated 24 million people died—equal to 25% of the entire population (Cartwright, 1972). Entire countries were socially paralyzed, wars halted, villages and farms emptied, ships drifted haplessly in the Mediterranean and North Seas for lack of sailors, and trade virtually ceased. Those who lost their loved ones also lived in panic and fear for their own lives, and answers were sought. Jews were often blamed for this disease. In Basel and Freiburg, Germany, in 1348 A.D., the Jews were rounded up and either burned alive, beheaded, or hanged by the thousands. Other strategies included self-flagellation, a form of public whipping as a means of achieving religious penance, that even Pope Clement ordered in an effort to abate the plague. This practice was based on the idea among Christians in the Middle Ages that the Black Death was a punishment from God for their sins. Thus, flagellation was used by these people in a bid to pay retribution for their sins and thereby be saved from the grim reality of the Black Death. Physicians and priests alike were helpless against the disease. The only partial efficacy was pursued by public health officials in Venice, who ordered foreign ships to be in quarantine for 40 days before unloading their cargo. If only there had been an epidemiologist afoot.

Plague is caused by Yersinia pestis, a bacteria, and is typically spread by Xenopsylla cheopis (the Oriental rat flea), a species of flea that lives on the black rat (Rattus rattus). This black rat, as opposed to its cousin the brown rat, prefers residing in close proximity to humans, in their ships and dwellings (Benenson, 1995). When the flea bites a human for a blood meal, some of the Yersinia pestis bacteria in the flea's saliva is then regurgitated into the human blood stream, thus transferring the infection to a new host. Today plague is still around, yet the disease is treatable with antimicrobial drugs, and prevented by controlling the vectors—rats and fleas.

Infectious Disease Concepts

The example of bubonic plague illustrates several key concepts in epidemiological investigations. The first is referred as the agent-host-environment triad. The agent of an infectious disease is the specific pathogenic cause, which can be any of the following: bacteria, rickettsia, virus, mycoses (fungi), protozoa, helminthes (worms), and prions. The host is the victim who develops the disease, and the environment the domain where the agents of disease exit (Friis & Sellers, 1999). All three of these factors dynamically interact with each other. In another example, India has had a long-standing custom of river burial of human corpses in the Ganges. These corpses then pollute the river, which is subsequently used as a source of water for bathing and consumption. The plague bacillus lived inside the guts of fleas that traveled around on the backs of the black rat, finally infecting humans who were treated as a food source by the fleas. Epidemiologists refer to the flea as a vector, because it actually spreads the plague disease, while the black rat is an intermediate vector of the fleas. Another term used in the infectious disease process is "reservoir," which refers to an entity that carries the agent but does not develop the disease (Walker, 2000). For example the agent of typhoid fever is Salmonella typhi, which can reside in shellfish reservoirs and is conveyed to humans upon consumption of the shellfish (but shellfish do not develop typhoid fever). Humans are one of the most efficient reservoirs, spreading a myriad of infections such as hepatitis B and C, chlamydia, or Giardia. The concept of "etiology," previously alluded to, entails the rigors of ascertaining the precise causal agent of a particular disease. Finally, the level of population disease dispersal is typically expressed as one of four types:

1. Endemic: The typical or normal level of disease occurrence in a population.
2. Epidemic: A major increase and spread of the disease throughout a population.
3. Pandemic: The spread of the disease beyond its normal population of occurrence, sometimes approaching a worldwide distribution (e.g., TB, AIDS).
4. Sporadic: The disease occurs only episodically, for example typhoid fever in the United States.

Properties of Infectious Agents

Infectious diseases can occur with different duration patterns or natural history. Some are acute, with rapid onset and severe symptoms, yet last only a short time (such as many of the bacterial food poisonings). Others are chronic and develop slowly, such as hepatitis B and C, HIV/AIDS, tuberculosis, and mononucleosis. Diseases can also occur in a subacute form, for example, sclerosing panencephalitis that is somewhere between the acute and chronic forms. Finally, some diseases can be latent or quiescent, a stage in which the agent remains inactive for long periods of time and then manifests symptoms. Examples of the latter would include varicella-zoster, or even syphilis.

Infectious agents have distinct characteristics as follows:

1. Pathogenicity is the ability of the agent to cause disease once it gains access to the host.

2. Toxigenicity refers to the ability of the agent to produce toxins that cause the host to be sick. Microbial toxins come in two forms: Endotoxins release upon microbial death (mostly Gram-negative bacteria), and exotoxins are released by the microbe into the body (mostly Gram-positive bacteria).

3. Infectivity refers to the ability of the agent to enter and multiply in the host.

4. Virulence is the ability of the agent to do harm to the host. For example, the rabies virus and Ebola virus cause rapidly fatal diseases once the host is infected. Evolutionary biologists observe that pathogens spread from person to person tend to be less virulent (because they need the host to be up and making contact with other hosts in order to get transmitted), while those pathogens transmitted by insects or other vectors tend to be more virulent because the agent does not need an active host in order to replicate (Nesse & Williams, 1996).

When the bacteria gain access to the bloodstream, this is referred to as bacteremia, and when they colonize and multiply, the condition is referred to as septicemia. Toxemia is a condition in which the bacterial toxins have entered the bloodstream. Agents of disease, that is pathogens, gain access to human hosts by various portals of entry—respiratory tract, gastrointestinal tract, skin breaks, and genital and mucous areas (Burton, 1992). Once they have gained entry, they typically go through several specific periods of infection as follows: incubation, which is the time from entry to initial symptoms; the prodromal period, which is a fairly short time characterized by the very first mild symptoms; then the period of the illness; the period of decline; and finally a period of convalescence (Tortora et al., 1998).

The Essence of Epidemiology: Surveillance

Globally infectious diseases still account for 25% of all mortality, estimated at some 13 million deaths per year, and they account of 45% of all annual mortality in low-income countries (WHO, 1999). Diarrhea disease accounts for 1.8 million annual deaths for children under 5 years of age, while malaria kills close to 700,000, and measles deaths are estimated at close to 1 million per year (WHO, 1999). Acute respiratory infections and pneumonia cause close to 2 million deaths for children under age 5, and 3.5 million deaths per year overall.

Noncommunicable diseases—typically thought of as injuries, cancers, and tobacco- and diet-related cardiovascular diseases—account for 55% of all annual mortality in the world. These noncommunicable diseases are becoming a major concern in low-income countries because of the increasing cultural penetration of unhealthy fast foods and tobacco usage, originating from the high-income countries.

Incidence rates and prevalence rates of both the communicable and noncommunicable disease counts originate in the quintessential function of epidemiology, that of surveillance. Surveillance is the systematic recording and documenting of cases, and is of vital importance in the global efforts to reduce the mortality and disability associated with human disease. Surveillance serves several key functions:

1. Documenting total disease burdens by geographical areas
2. Communicating disease intervention needs in both money and personnel
3. Identifying disease changes from endemic to epidemic
4. Identifying newly emerging diseases
5. Contributing to further understanding of disease patterns, risk factors, and the potential for primary and secondary prevention
6. Providing laboratory services for isolating etiological agents from specimen samples

Infectious disease surveillance stories in the news of late include West-Nile-like virus, dengue fever, and influenza A. In September of 1999 an outbreak of West-Nile-like virus occurred on the East Coast of the United States for the first time. This particular virus is a member of the flaviviruses that are endemic in Africa and the Middle East, and are reemerging in Eastern European countries like Romania and Ukraine (Hubalek & Halouzka, 1999). The virus was apparently transported to the United States by migratory birds, and this potentially fatal disease is transmitted to humans via mosquitoes. Public health authorities responded by arial insecticide spraying of New York City. Given the potential for further migratory bird dispersions, the West-Nile-like virus may be introduced to the Caribbean and South America (CAREC, 1999).

The State of New Jersey health department has begun using chickens for tracking the spread of the virus. Chickens do not develop the disease, unlike crows, but do develop antibodies to the virus, which can be detected by means of a blood test. Public health workers periodically visit their strategically located chicken pens and collect blood samples to determine of the virus has been spread via mosquitoes to the chickens.

Texas recently has its first fatality due to dengue fever, and Florida has had several cases. The dengue virus is transmitted via mosquito bite and can cause widespread morbidity and mortality (CDC, 1999). Hong Kong recently had an outbreak of influenza A (H5N1) flu virus that leaped from chickens and other birds to humans. Hong Kong health authorities took the seemingly drastic action of slaughtering over a million chickens and other domestic birds, since this strain of influenza A was particularly virulent and fatal cases had been reported.

Yellow fever cases are reported in Brazil, typhoid fever cases are reported in Jamaica, 31 European countries have joined the Legionnaire's Disease surveillance network, and Lyme disease surveillance is maintained in Switzerland and throughout central Europe. Sporadic suspected cases of Marburg hemorrhagic fever have been reported from Durba, Democratic Republic of Congo, and a new case of Marburg has been confirmed by virological tests performed by the National Institute for Virology (NIV), South Africa. Cases of cholera in Madagascar, particularly in Mahajanga Province, brought the 1999 total to 6,983 cases, with 433 deaths. In Hungary, the Ministry of Health informed WHO of an outbreak of meningococcal disease that began in early December 1999, in the Bàcs-Kiskun area (in Kecskemet City and Szabadszallas Town) with, thus far, a total of 30 cases and 4 deaths. The Hungarian National Epidemiology Center in Budapest has confirmed that the agent is Neisseria meningitis groups B and C.

From samples collected in the western area of the country, Sierra Leone has confirmed an outbreak of dysentery in November 1999 caused by Shigella flexneri. The Ministry of Health reports that from December 6, 1999, to January 16, 2000, a total of 3,094 cases of shigellosis occurred, with 132 deaths. The outbreak appears to be spreading, and a rapid epidemiological assessment of the situation is being planned through a WHO mission to the affected areas (WHO, 2000).

These are just a few example of infectious disease that illustrate the necessity of epidemiological surveillance operations. Outbreaks can be identified, along with strategies to abate the spread of the pathogen. New diseases are constantly emerging, and old diseases erupt in new parts of the world that they had previously never inhabited. This is the globalization of disease phenomenon that characterizes the modern world. International travel increased from 20 million in 1945 to 450 million in 1995 (WHO, 1999), which has contributed to the removal of physical barriers that used to help contain outbreaks, at least by continent. Hence, national and international disease surveillance is a vital function of epidemiological agencies in order to enable rapid and long-term effective responses to disease threats to human life.

The surveillance function also involves specialized registries for such chronic diseases as cancer. In the United States, the National Cancer Institute operates a national cancer registry program called SEER (Surveillance Epidemiology End Result). SEER began tracking cancer events in January 1973, for the states of Connecticut, Iowa, New Mexico, Utah, and Hawaii and the metropolitan areas of Detroit and San Francisco-Oakland. In 1974–1975, the metropolitan area of Atlanta and the 13-county Seattle-Puget Sound area were added. In 1978, 10 predominantly black rural counties in Georgia were added, followed in 1980 by the addition of American Indians residing in Arizona (SEER, 2000). The SEER cancer database is available for researchers, and the public can access extensive data online. Approximately 160,000 new cases of cancer are added to the registry each year, including patient data on demographics, primary tumor site, morphology, stage of diagnosis, initial therapies, and follow-up.

Conducting Investigation of a Disease Outbreak

Field epidemiology is probably the most recognized form of the profession, partially because it is occasionally glamorized in Hollywood movies, for example, the virus-hunting character Sam Daniels portrayed by Dustin Hoffman in the film *Outbreak*. Field epidemiology also gets much media and news attention when there is an outbreak of E.coli infection from contaminated meats or strawberries, or from episodes of mosquito-contracted meningitis. Field epidemiologists work throughout the world responding to and investigating disease outbreaks, which can be detected by identifying unusual disease clustering in the routine analysis of surveillance data or by rapid communications between local health officials and surveillance staff.

In 1999, some 19 different states in the Sudan experienced an outbreak of meningococcal disease that involved over 22,000 cases and 1,600 fatalities. The Federal Ministry of Health of Sudan responded to the outbreak by means of a special task force. The international community responded with money and expertise from WHO and UNICEF. A total of 10.7 million doses of meningococcal vaccine were administered in the affected states, along with case management and public health information education.

The example of meningococcal disease helps to explain the process of outbreak response. The basic goal of the outbreak investigation is to control and prevent the spread of new cases of the disease. The sequence of events for the outbreak investigator is as follows:

1. The existence of an outbreak is confirmed. This entails determining whether the observed cases are more than the expected endemic level of occurrence. For example, every fall/winter is flu season, and there will be many cases of influenza; the question to be addressed is whether there is really an epidemic beyond the normal levels. This confirmation process can involve rechecking surveillance records, examining hospital records, or even telephone surveys of primary care providers. Above-normal cases of the disease may not necessarily mean an outbreak, since there may have been recent local changes in the ability to diagnose the disease or better means of reporting the cases. There may also be seasonal fluctuation in population that may be explanatory for the increased number of cases (Page et al., 1995).

2. A similar companion step is verifying the diagnosis or detection of the disease. This may involve repeating laboratory testing of specimens to confirm the initial clinical diagnoses. These clinical findings need to be summarized in frequency tables, with a timeline of case occurrence.

3. Criteria are established as to what characteristics are sufficient in order to define what constitutes a "case." This process is called establishing the case definition. Fortunately, for most existing diseases the symptomatology is fairly well established, along with reference measures of body temperature, white blood cells count, and elevated antibodies. The important caveat with case definition is that it cannot include any of the possible exposure risks. For example, the case definition cannot include attendance at a summer picnic or hotel convention, which are possible sites of certain agents' transmission.

4. The next step is identifying the counts of the cases, the date being reported, date of onset, number of case-definition symptoms occuring laboratory test results, and relevant demographic measures such as age, weight, and gender. In addition, all relevant risk-factor information for each case needs to be documented.

5. Conducting the descriptive epidemiological phase is next, which involves identifying all the characteristics of time, place, and person. Geographical maps of the investigation area, whether state, city, or building, need to be organized and counts or rates per area need to be identified. At the most basic level is a pin map, on which all cases are placed to aid in identifying possible risk factors.

6. Once these descriptive data have been collected as described above, the outbreak investigators can begin to formulate hypotheses of the causal agent. These hypotheses can be further studied using a cohort or the case-control design (previously articulated). Epidemiologists often use a variant of the incidence rate called the "attack rate" to enable comparing different exposures, such as food menu items at a restaurant outbreak. The attack rate is calculated as follows: AR = [No. Cases/(No. cases + No. noncases)] × 100 =

7. Albeit the mission of the epidemiological investigation is to ascertain causation, very often control and prevention measures take priority before understanding the etiology of the outbreak. Cases and/or areas can be isolated and quarantined as the first defense. Water and other food sources can be altered, and person-to-person contacts can be restricted.

8. Finally, an outbreak investigation needs to transmit its findings to relevant neighboring public health authorities and the world community. For example, the WHO maintains an Internet Website for the purpose of reporting initial outbreak findings. Peer-reviewed journal publication is ultimately the goal for reporting the investigation results.

Field epidemiology is thus a vital frontline practice that functions to investigate outbreaks. These investigations are not only for acute infections but also for injuries and disease-related morbidity, and new emphasis is being placed on social-behavioral factors that interact with the outcomes of interest (particularly with sexually transmitted diseases).

Epidemiology in Action

International Salmonellosis Outbreak. Between December of 1995 and the early months of 1996, an unusually steep increase of foodborne illnesses occurred simultaneously in Oregon and British Columbia that were being caused by Salmonella enterica serotype Newport (Beneden et al., 1999). Epidemiologists in the

United States and Canada identified a total of 133 cases of salmonellosis, and the investigation began to determine the source of the bacteria. A case-control design was used that was comprised of identified cases and healthy controls (from the Portland and Vancouver area).

Descriptive plotting of cases for each week of onset indicated that the outbreak period (i.e., epidemic, rather than endemic, levels of salmonellosis) occurred between late December of 1995 and the ninth week of 1996. Detailed interviews were done of all cases to determine individuals' recent dietary food exposures. Risk association was done by calculating the exposure odds ratios.

The first finding was that cases were more likely to to have eaten meals away from home compared to controls; EOR = 6.7 (CI = 1.5 to 61.0). Alfalfa sprouts were the only consumption item from a list of 70 foods and drinks that was a common link among the cases; EOR = 5.4 (CI = 2.0 to 15.0). The alfalfa sprouts were eventually traced back to a farm in West Virginia, where the seeds had been purchased from a Dutch distributor. The investigators eventually found that the alfalfa seeds had come from a single seed-grower source in Europe and had made their way to North America. What was most unusual about this outbreak is that the incubation period (the time from exposure to symptoms) was greater than normal clinical expectations. Had the researchers restricted the case food histories to three or fewer days, alfalfa sprouts would not have been statistically implicated.

Traveler's Diarrhea in Jamaica.   International tourists to Caribbean countries often experience a short-lived illness known as traveler's diarrhea (TD). Although TD is rarely fatal, considerable acute morbidity, discomfort, and lost vacation activity time can occur. Epidemiologists of the Jamaica Ministry of Health undertook a thorough and yearlong investigation of TD among tourists in their country. A total of 30,369 short-term tourists were surveyed at Sangster International Airport, and at ten hotels in the Montego Bay area. Laboratory evaluation of stool samples was also done to identify potential pathogens and microbial toxins. The survey consisted of 25 questions that assessed the quality of life in relation to contacting TD. The total TD incidence was 18.9%, with an attack rate of 24.1% (Stefffen et al., 1999).

What researchers found interesting was that TD risk differed based on country of origin as follows: United Kingdom, EOR = 3.4; Canada, EOR = 3.2; United States, EOR = 2.6; and various European countries, EOR = 1.3. Other interesting findings included increased risk of TD when couples were on their honeymoon (EOR = 1.7) and for those tourists who took their meals in their rooms (EOR = 1.58). The lab work found that 11.9% of TD was caused by E. coli, 7.8% by Salmonella, 9.2% by rotavirus, and the majority of cases, 68.3%, had no detectable pathogen. Finally, it was not surprising that quality of life was reduced by the severity of TD.

Web of Disease Etiology

Nothing stunned the world more than the developments that emerged from the germ theory developed by Louis Pasteur and Robert Koch in the nineteenth century. Vaccines for anthrax and then rabies were developed for diseases that absolutely terrified people because of helplessness to cure and prevent them. These vaccines changed the world and brought a new sense of confidence to microbial researchers. The success of epidemiology was in part due to the efficacy of the germ theory, which is based on the premise that each disease has one and only one specific etiological agent. This paradigm worked very effectively, until the development of the chronic so-called "lifestyle" diseases that began to predominate in the high-income countries. These diseases, like the cancers and coronary heart disease, do not have a single etiological agent, but rather a whole panoply of interrelated factors that both predispose to and cause the disease. Subsequently, epidemiology moved to a multifactorial approach to disease research, identifying so-called "risk factors" for each disease process. This has lead to the new etiological paradigm called the "Web of Causation" model (Timmreck, 1994).

Take, for example, Alzheimer's disease, for which many interrelated factors are used to attempt to explain its etiology—such as genes, endocrine hormones, herpes simplex virus, aluminum exposure, glucose and energy metabolism, and oxidative stress (Post, 1999). The old linear model of X causes Y, which began with the germ theory (and is still efficacious in many circumstances), is not sufficient to explain chronic and complex disease phenomena such as Alzheimer's disease, cardiovascular disease, environmental lead contamination, maternal mortality, or various forms of cancer. To cope with these more complex diseases and risk processes, epidemiologists often use more sophisticated statistical techniques such as multiple regression analysis, logistic regression analysis, multivariate statistical analysis, and forms of structural equation modeling and path analysis (Daniel, 1998; Fisher & Van Belle, 1993; Zar, 1999).

Summary

The quest to reduce human suffering and death from communicable and noncommunicable diseases and injuries is constant and yet ever changing. Demographic transitions in the low-income countries will necessitate shifting their efforts to the prevention of the great panoply of chronic debilitating afflictions related to importation of tobacco addiction and Western fat-based fast-food diets. Epidemiology is also a maturing scientific discipline and not merely a collection of data-dredging methods. What began primarily with John Snow's work on the London cholera epidemics of the nineteenth century is now a highly structured field of study and application. New areas of epidemiological application are constantly emerging. The standard modus operandi of comparing the frequencies of disease conditions in different communities and calculating exposure risk ratio is now shifting to genetic and molecular levels of identifying risk (Adami & Trichopoulos, 1999; Susser, 1999).

Molecular epidemiology seeks to find risk prior to the onset of any disease symptoms by means of measuring what are referred to as molecular "biomarkers" in association with exposure status (Friis & Sellers, 1999). This new approach does not rely on a subject's recall of exposures, or wait until a full-blown disease

TABLE 8.8 *World Wide Web Box: Epidemiology*

1. University of Pittsburgh: Epidemiology Super Course	http://www.pitt.edu/~super1/main/epi.htm
2. Johns Hopkins School of Public Health: Department of Epidemiology, Center for Epidemiology and Policy	http://www.med.jhu.edu/cep
3. Infectious Control and Hospital Epidemiology	http://www.slackinc.com/general/iche/ichehome.htm
4. China Epidemiology Net	http://www.epinetchina.com
5. Journals of Epidemiology	http://www.jhsph.edu/Departments/Epi/journals.html
6. Epidemiology Data Center: University of Pittsburgh	http://www.edc.gsph.pitt.edu
7. International Clinical Epidemiology Network	http://www.inclen.org
8. Global Environmental Epidemiology Network	http://www.who.int/peh/geenet/index.htm
9. International Epidemiological Association	http://www.dundee.ac.uk/iea/Home.htm
10. Centers For Disease Control, Morbidity, Mortality Weekly Report	http://www2.cdc.gov/mmwr/
11. Surveillance, Epidemiology, and End Results Cancer Registry	http://www-seer.ims.nci.nih.gov
12. Epidemiology Virtual Library: University of California, San Francisco	http://wwwepibiostat.ucsf.edu/epidem/epidem.html
13. Epidemiology Supercourse, University of Pittsburgh	http://www.pitt.edu/~super1

is present, or treat all forms of a particular cancer as the same. A gene typing can be done preclinically—such as with the genes BRAC1 and BRAC2 that predispose for breast cancer (Hopper et al., 1999). Risk of some cancer can be assessed by such useful biomarkers as PCNA (proliferating cell nuclear antigen), which predicts risk of laryngeal cancer (Sarac et al., 1998). Both of these new fields of epidemiological investigation are still undergoing growing pains (Bogardus et at., 1999); however, the complete Human Genome Project (the mapping of all the genes of the 46 human chromosomes) will no doubt intensify gene and biomarker investigations.

Epidemiology has certainly changed since the London haberdasher John Graunt (who devoted his entire life to the keeping of vital statistics) published the now-famous Bills of Mortality in 1662. He attempted to distinguish the acute from the chronic diseases, and urban versus rural differences in mortality. In 1775, Percival Pott was the first to identify an environmental cause of a cancer—that of testicular cancer among London chimney sweeps who were exposed to chimney tar and soot. In 1747, James Lind did the first controlled experimentation among British sailors and discovered the powers of citrus fruits in preventing scurvy. Semmelweis (the Hungarian physician working at the General Hospital in Wein, Austria) in the 1840s conducted a retrospective study on maternal mortality due to childbed fever (puerperal fever), and advanced the notion of physical hand washing by physicians prior to the delivery of babies.

These examples serve to highlight the important historical contributions to the betterment of humankind that epidemiologists have made. They also demonstrate that one of the real powers of epidemiology is that the exact agent does not need to be delineated prior to the taking of public health actions that save lives. James Lind never knew he has stumbled upon vitamin C deficiency as the cause of scurvy, and Semmelweis was not able to culture and examine the microbial pathogens passed from physician to delivering woman.

The practice of epidemiology will continue to excel into the future through meticulous adherence to sound research methodology and population-based science (Pearce, 1999). Epidemiology is foundational to all population-based community interventions that are directed at prevention and health promotion. These efforts at societal change must be rooted in epidemiological understanding, to best ensure that time and effort are not wasted or misdirected, and that substantive contributions are made to the betterment of human life and well-being.

Discussion Questions

1. What are the advantages and disadvantages of the cohort design and of the case-control design?

2. Why is the incidence rate the probability of getting a disease in a population while prevalence is the probability of having the disease?

3. Give intervention/treatment examples of each of the four levels of prevention.

4. What is the ethical dilemma associated with epidemiological causality?

5. Which disease would have the greater YPLL, AIDS or prostate cancer? Why?

6. Which is a better measure of risk, relative risk or the exposure odds ratio?

7. What would be the p-value if the confidence interval for RR did not include the null value of one?

8. Discuss the steps to address the problem of bias in epidemiological studies.

9. Name three disease vectors and their reservoirs.

10. Discuss why epidemiological surveillance is so vitally important.

11. Name two new fields of epidemiological investigation.

References

Adami, H. O., & Trichopoulos, D. (1999). Epidemiology, Medicine and Public Health. *International Journal of Epidemiology, 28,* S1005–S1008.

Beaglehole, R., Bonita, R., & Kjellstrom, T. (1993). *Basic Epidemiology.* Geneva, Switzerland: World Health Organization.

Beneden, C. A. V., et al. (1999). Multinational Outbreak of Salmonella Enterica Serotype Newport Infections Due to Contaminated Alfalfa Sprouts. *Journal of the American Medical Association, 281*(2), 158–162.

Benenson, A. S. (1995). *Control of Communicable Diseases Manual* (16th ed.). Washington, DC: American Public Heath Association.

Bogardus, S. T., Concato, J., & Feinstein, A. R. (1999). Clinical Epidemiological Quality in Molecular Genetic Research. *Journal of the American Medical Association, 281*(20), 1919–1926.

Burton, G. R. W. (1992). *Microbiology for the Health Sciences* (4th ed.). Philadelphia: J. B Lippincott Company.

Camargo, C. A., Weiss, S. T., Zhang S., Willett, W. C., & Speizer, F. E. (1999). Prospective Study of Body Mass Index, Weight Change, and Risk of Adult-Onset Asthma in Women. *Archives of Internal Medicine, 159,* 2582–2588.

CAREC (1999). CAREC Surveillance Report. Republic of Trinidad and Tobago: Caribbean Epidemiological Center Vol 21 (1). [Online] Available: Http://www.CAREC.org

Cartwright, F. F. (1972). *Disease and History.* New York: Barnes & Noble Books.

CDC (1999). Fatal case of dengue fever in Texas. *Morbidity and Mortality Weekly Report, 48,* 1150–1152.

Daniel, W. W. (1998). *Biostatistics.* 7th Edition New York: John Wiley & Sons, Inc.

Dardis, A. (1993). Sunburn: Independence Conditions on Causal Relevance. *Philosophy and Phenomenological Research, LIII*(3), 577–598.

Fisher, L. D., & Van-Belle, G. (1993). *Biostatistics: A Methodology for the Health Sciences.* New York: John Wiley & Sons, Inc.

Franklin, K. A., Holmgren, K. P. A., Jönsson, F., Poromaa, N., Stenlund, H., & Svanborg, E. (2000). Snoring, Pregnancy-Induced Hypertension, and Growth Retardation of the Fetus. *Chest, 117,* 137–141

Friedman, G. D. (1994). *Primer of Epidemiology* (4th ed.). New York: McGraw-Hill Inc.

Friis, R. H., & Sellers, T. A. (1999). *Epidemiology for Public Health Practice* (2nd ed.). Gaithersburg, MD: An Aspen Publication.

Gordis, L. (1996). *Epidemiology.* Philadelphia: W. B. Saunders Company.

Hennekens, C. H., Buring, J. E., & Mayrent, S. L. (1987). *Epidemiology in Medicine.* Boston: Little, Brown, and Company.

Hopper, J. L., et al. (1999). Population-Based Estimate of the Average Age-Specific Cumulative Risk of Breast Cancer for a Defined Set of Protein-Truncating Mutations in BRAC1 and BRCA2. *Cancer Epidemiology, Biomarkers and Prevention, 8,*(a) 741–747.

Hubalek, Z., & Halouzka, J. (1999). West Nile Fever—A Reemerging Mosquito-borne Viral disease in Europe. *Emerging Infectious Diseases, 5*(5), 643–650.

Jacobs, E. J., Thun M. J., & Apicella, L. F. (1999). Cigar Smoking and Death from Coronary Heart Disease in a Prospective Study of US Men. *Archives of Internal Medicine, 159*(20), 2413–2418.

Lemaitre, R. N., Siscovick, D. S., Raghunathan, T. E., Weinmann, S., Arbogast, P., & Lin, D. Y. (1999). Leisure-Time Physical Activity and the Risk of Primary Cardiac Arrest. *Archives of Internal Medicine, 159,* 686–690.

Lilienfeld, D. E., & Stolley, P. D. (1994). *Foundations of Epidemiology* (3rd ed.). New York: Oxford University Press.

Lotufo, P. A., Chae, C. U., Ajani, U. A., Hennekens, C. H., & Manson, J. E.(2000). Male Pattern Baldness and Coronary Heart Disease. *Archives of Internal Medicine, 160,* 165–171.

Loy, T. (1998). Blood on the Axe. *New Scientist, 40,* 40–44.

Mandl, K. D., Tronick, E. Z., Brennam, T. A., Alpert, H. R., & Homer C. J. (1999). Infant Health Care Use and Maternal Depression. *Archives of Pediatric and Adolescent Medicine, 153,* 808–813.

Mausner, J. S, Kramer, S., Gann. P., Bowen S., & Morton, R. (1985), (2nd Ed.). *Epidemiology: An Introductory Text,* Philadelphia: W. B. Saunders Company.

Ming Wei, M., Kampert, J. B., Barlow, C. E., & Nichaman, M. Z. (1999). Relationship between low cardiorespiratory fitness and mortality in normal-weight, overweight, and obese men. *Journal of the American Medical Association, 282*(16), 1547–1553.

Moss, E. M., Lanphear, B. P., & Auinger, P. (1999). Association of Dental Caries and Blood Lead Levels. *Journal of American Medical Association, 281*(24), 2294–2298.

Nesse, R. M., & Williams, G. C. (1996). *Why We Get Sick: The New Science of Darwinian Medicine.* New York: Vintage Books.

Page, R. M., Cole G. E., &Timmreck, T. C. (1995). *Basic Epidemiological Methods and Biostatistics.* Boston: Jones and Bartlett Publishers.

Pearce, N. (1999). Epidemiology as a Population Science. *International Journal of Epidemiology, 28,* S1015–S1018.

Picciotto, I. H. (1999). What You Should Have Learned about Epidemiologic Data Analysis. *Epidemiology, 10*(6), 778–783.

Portney, L. G., & Watkins M. P. (2000). *Foundations of Clinical Research* (2nd ed.). Upper Saddle River, NJ: Prentice Hall Health.

Post, S. G. (1999). Future Scenarios for the Prevention and Delay of Alzheimer's Disease in High-Risk Groups. *American Journal of Preventive Medicine, 16*(2), 105–110.

Sarac, S., Ayhan, A., Hosal, A. S., & Kaya, S. (1999). Prognostic Significance of PCNA Expression in Laryngeal Cancer. *Archives of Otolaryngology, 124*(12), 1321–1324.

SEER. (2000). Survelliance, Epidemiology End Result Registery. Washington, DC: National Cancer Institute. Website Address: Http://www-seer.ims.nci.nih.gov

Selvin, T. (1996). *Statistical Analysis of Epidemiologic Data* (2nd ed.). New York: Oxford University Press.

Steffen, R., et al. (1999). Epidemiology, Etiology, and Impact of Traveler's Diarrhea in Jamaica. *Journal of the American Medical Association, 281*(9), 811–817.

Stone, D. B., Armstrong, W. R., Macrina, D. M., & Pankau, J. W. (1996). *Introduction to Epidemiology.* Madison, WI: Brown and Benchmark.

Susser, M. (1999). Should the epidemiologist be a social scientist or a molecular biologist? *International Journal of Epidemiology, 28*(5): S1019–S1022.

Timmreck, T. C. (1994). *An Introduction to Epidemiology.* Boston: Jones and Bartlett Publishers.

Tortora, G. J., Funke, B. R., & Case, C. I. (1998). *Microbiology* (6th ed.). Menlo Park, CA: Addison Wesley Longman Incorporated.

Walker, M. (2000). Invisible Enemies: Devastating Viruses Hitch a Life without Leaving A trace. *Science News, 165*(2223), 10.

WHO. (1999). *Infectious Disease Report.* Geneva, Switzerland: World Health Organization [Online] Available: Http://www.WHO.int/infectious-disease-report/

WHO. (2000). *Communicable Disease Surveillance and Response.* Geneva, Switzerland: World Health Organization [Online] Available: Http://www.who.int/emc/outbreak_news/

Zar, J. H. (1999). *Biostatistical Analysis.* Upper Saddle River, NJ: Prentice-Hall Inc.

9

The Future of International Health: Problems and Prognosis

Robert W. Buckingham and
Theresa H. Hollingsworth

The twentieth century saw a revolution in the modernization of health care, which inexorably led to major changes in the pattern of disease. This epidemiological transition resulted in a shift of the major causes of death and disability from infectious diseases to chronic noncommunicable diseases, especially in developed nations. Chronic noncommunicable diseases include cancer and heart disease (WHO, 2000). For example, in Chile in 1909, the major causes of death were respiratory infections; cancer took its toll on only 1.9% of the population, and cardiovascular diseases killed only approximately 12.9% of the people. However, in 1999, respiratory infections only killed 8.5% of the population, whereas cancer increased to 22.8% and deaths due to cardiovascular disease rose to 30.4% (WHO, 2000). It is important to note that Chile is not as developed as many other first world countries, where the situation is much more dire. Much of this shift from infectious to chronic disease is a direct result of the fact that life expectancies have risen by nearly 30 years in the last century; since cancers and cardiovascular diseases often strike in relatively older age groups, these data then makes sense. Despite this epidemiological transition, there remains a large discrepancy between the transition made by developed countries, and that of the progress made by third world countries. There still remains a huge inequality between first and third world countries' access to health care, and the subsequent ramifications that this imposes represent a large hurdle that the field of public health must overcome. The successes of healthy living that developing countries have enjoyed are not shared with the world's disadvantaged populations. Reducing the burden of this inequality is of utmost priority in international public health and is of major concern to the World Health Organization (WHO, 2000), along with countless other humanitarian organizations.

Not only have the major causes of death changed over the last century, as previously stated, the age of death has been steadily increasing. This directly results in a whole new host of challenges for health care systems. It appears that, in addition to the reemergence of infectious diseases in the twenty-first century, we will have to combat new and emerging epidemics of noncommunicable chronic diseases, neuropsychiatric disorders, and injuries. These are becoming more prevalent in developing and industrialized countries alike; thus, there is a double burden of disease that will have to be faced in the future—that of the noncommunicable diseases, and that of the infectious diseases that are once again gaining momentum. In addition, many other factors will also play a role in health in the twenty-first century. Though diseases themselves are of most obvious concern, it is imperative to look at the reasons behind their spread. Modern transportation is perhaps the biggest mediator. Any place on this Earth is at most only a 24-hour plane ride away. This means that any disease previously unknown to a region or country can be introduced within 24 hours, often with disastrous consequences. Examples of this intercontinental disease drift include HIV, Ebola, and hantavirus.

It is difficult to ascertain exactly what factors will most influence the future of international health. Infectious diseases (communicable), noncommunicable diseases, refugees, and poverty will all play a central role, as they do today. Further, it is necessary to understand their individual characteristics and their current roles in order to predict their future roles. These factors do not stand alone; in fact they are quite interwoven within the world's societies. Extinguishing one will not eradicate the other three; each one compounds the other. The priority of health care workers must then be to figure out a method to combat each of these problems in turn, while enabling developing countries to become more self-reliant in alleviating their problems. Each factor that was mentioned previously that contributes to our world's health must be individually assessed. People who live in poverty are at highest risk for communicable diseases, while those living in developed, technologically advanced societies are more at risk for chronic diseases. Refugees, who often live in overcrowded, unsanitary conditions, are at risk for communicable diseases as well.

The purpose of this chapter, then, is to illustrate the current and future role each of the four factors will play in the world's overall health status. It is only by understanding the present issues that we as humans face that any future predictions can be made, as well as solving any problems that the world faces today. We can understand the present only in terms of our past mistakes and victories; only through careful analysis of what has worked for different people in various nations can we begin to move in the direction necessary for the future well-being of the population of the planet. Before the era of mass transportation, it was much easier for people to ignore the problems that other nations were having. There was simply not much that we as a global community could do for each other. Now, however, it is not only possible, it is a moral obligation that we all as human beings must face: We must come together to bring all nations to a good, if not equal, health status.

Communicable Diseases

In 1998, the leading infectious killers around the world were diseases that generally infect people in developing countries; countries that are developed have effective means of combating these diseases. Often, these diseases are effectively transmitted through unsanitary water or other unhygienic conditions, through insects that serve as vectors, or a lack of immunization among children. These diseases include, but are not limited to, polio, cholera, dysentery, and malaria. In addition, one of the world's most disastrous infectious diseases, HIV, is taking its toll on millions of lives; and this disease, generally spread through body fluids, has currently cost billions of dollars.

Infectious diseases can be divided into emerging and reemerging diseases. Emerging infectious diseases can be defined as those whose incidence in humans has increased during the last two decades or which threatens to increase in the near future. The term includes newly appearing infectious diseases or those spreading to new geographical areas. Reemerging disease refers to those that were easily controlled by antibiotics but have developed antimicrobial resistance (WHO, 1996). It is important to note that not all infectious diseases necessarily fall into these categories. For instance, sexually transmitted diseases have been around for thousands of years, but as humans can traverse the globe quite easily, again, this provides quick means for their spread, as well as for the introduction of new diseases (see Table 9.1).

Sexually Transmitted Diseases (STDs)

Infectious diseases that are spread through sexual contact have shared much of their history with human evolution. Each year, approximately 333 million new cases of sexually transmitted diseases occur on a global basis (WHO, 1996). Obviously, this is an overwhelming health care burden that most countries cannot financially or diagnostically bear. Migration and rapid urbanization are major

TABLE 9.1   *Leading Infectious Disease Cause of Mortality*

Disease	Deaths
Acute lower respiratory	3,500,000
AIDS	2,300,000
Diarrhoeal diseases	2,200,000
Tuberculosis	1,500,000
Malaria	1,100,000
Measles	900,000
Neonatal tetanus	460,000

Source: World Health Organization (1996).

demographic factors that directly play a major role in sexual behaviors within a community. In large cities, rapid urbanization can produce a population that consists of more men than women; as a result, both casual and commercial sex are major modes of sexual expression. This adds to great increases in annual infections (WHO, 1996). In addition, high rates of poverty and gender inequality in many developing nations leave many women no choice but to turn to commercial sex as a means for their survival. These factors, along with political unrest, war, and the absence of diagnostic and treatment services for STDs, all exacerbate the growing STD problem in developing nations.

There is no doubt that sexually transmitted diseases produce serious health, social, and economic consequences; what is sobering is that all STDs are clearly preventable, and most are curable. This makes it crucial for governments and communities to come together to decrease—if not eliminate—the effect these diseases have on society. If progress can be made in decreasing STDs worldwide, then significant decreases in HIV infections, as well as in maternal and infant morbidity and mortality, will follow.

STDs can be classified as curable and incurable. STDs that are preventable, but not curable, include viral STDs such as the herpes simplex virus, the human immunodeficiency virus, hepatitis B, and the human papilloma virus. Curable and preventable STDs include gonorrhea, chlamydia, and syphilis. Of these STDs, it is projected that more than 2 million children and 19 million adults now carry HIV. It was estimated that, by the year 2000, there would be around 40 million cases of HIV on a worldwide basis (WHO, 1996) (see Tables 9.2 and 9.3).

As the tables illustrate, the amount of STDs is overwhelming. To combat the advent of new cases, we must design a multifaceted approach to controlling STDs that acknowledges each individual country's limitations. These limitations can include the behavioral and personal environments, the socioeconomic and sociodemographic environments, the political environments, and the technological environments of the country.

TABLE 9.2 *Estimated Yearly Global Incidence of STDs, Ages 15–49*

Region	Percentage of All STDs Worldwide
North America	2–3
Latin America and the Caribbean	7–14
Western Europe	1–2
Eastern Europe and Central Asia	3–8
East Asia and Pacific	1–2
South and Southeast Asia	9–17
Sub-Saharan Africa	11–35

Source: World Health Organization (1996).

TABLE 9.3   *Estimated Number of HIV-Infected Individuals by Region*

Region	Estimated Number of People with HIV
Australia	20,000
East Asia & Pacific	>50,000
Eastern Europe & Central Asia	>50,000
Latin America & the Caribbean	>1,500,000
North Africa & the Middle East	>100,000
North America	>750,000
Sub-Saharan Africa	8,500,000
South and Southeast Asia	3,000,000
Western Europe	450,000
Approximate Total	**14,420,000**

Source: World Health Organization (1996).

Current research in the field of STDs is focusing not only on preventative measures but on ways to treat them as well. It is thought that in the future there will be easier, more cost-effective methods of treatment. One that has been under careful scrutiny is that of the vaginal microcide. This entails a film, containing some sort of biocide, that is inserted into the vagina after sex. The antimicrobials in the biocide would be effective against viruses and bacteria alike; however, although the product is undergoing careful evaluation, it has not yet been approved for human use. Such a product would probably have high rates of patient compliance, since little knowledge, experience, or money would be necessary for its use.

Emerging Diseases

At least 30 new diseases have emerged in the last 20 years (WHO, 1996). Many different forces interact in their occurrence. Among these are poverty, poor water sanitation, population movement, and resistance to antibiotics. Ebola hemorrhagic fever, Dengue hemorrhagic fever, hantavirus, and human immunodeficiency virus are among the most dangerous and fatal emerging diseases.

Ebola.   Ebola hemorrhagic fever was retrospectively diagnosed from a nonfatal case in Tandala, Zaire, in 1972. Since then, outbreaks have occurred in Kikwit, Zaire, Plibo, Liberia, and Makokou, Gabon. This emerging disease causes between 60% to 90% fatality in all cases (WHO, 1996). Incubation of the disease lasts from 2 to 21 days, and it generally starts with a fever; within days, the victim will begin hemorrhaging from every orifice on the body. After the initiation of hemorrhaging, the patient will usually die within 48 to 96 hours (Fields, 1997). Unfortunately, there is no specific treatment or vaccine for Ebola; supportive care of the patient, such as intravenous fluids, is often the only recourse.

Little is known about the origin of Ebola hemorrhagic fever; however, there seems to be a natural reservoir. The World Health Organization is currently conducting research in Cote de'Ivoire, Gabon, and Zaire. Although the natural reservoir is unknown, the virus is known to be easily transmitted between humans, through an infected person's blood, secretions, or semen; there is also strong evidence of respiratory transmission (WHO, 1996).

Dengue.   Dengue fever is a mosquito-borne infection which manifests as a hemorrhagic fever, similar to Ebola. However, the disease does not share the alarming fatality rate, though it is potentially fatal. The disease is characterized by high fever, liver enlargement, and extreme bodily pain; hence the nickname "bonebreak fever". Circulatory failure, though not common, can be a fatal consequence of the disease.

Although Dengue has been a world health concern since it was first identified in the 1950s, the prevalence of Dengue hemorrhagic fever has increased dramatically in recent decades. It is now endemic in more than 100 countries in Africa, the Americas, the Eastern Mediterranean, South-East Asia, and the Western Pacific (WHO, 1996).

Hantavirus.   Hantavirus is another example of a deadly disease whose incidence is increasing at alarming rates. This disease occurs most often in the Southwestern United States, though different variants of the virus have caused disease in South America, as well as Korea. In the future, as more and more people move into areas not previously inhabited in the Southwest, the incidence of this disease will continue to increase unless careful preventative measures are taken. The disease is spread to humans by the urine or feces of infected deer mice, and it is estimated that 62% of its victims will succumb to the virus (Garrett, 1994). When humans inhale aerosolized particulates of the urine or feces, the virus gains entry into the respiratory tract. Flulike symptoms such as fever, muscle aches, and headaches typically herald the onset of hantavirus. After a period of two to four days, these symptoms escalate to coughing and irritation in the lungs; this irritation progresses to pulmonary edema within a matter of hours. Starving for oxygen, the heart can no longer keep up with the demands of maintaining life; death due to cardiac failure or pulmonary edema soon follows (Garrett, 1994).

HIV.   Of all infectious diseases, none has gained as much notoriety as HIV, the causative agent of AIDS. This disease is expected to take a major toll on the world's population, especially in developing countries. AIDS is now one of the most major infectious disease killers in the world (see Table 9.1)

Reemerging Diseases

As emerging diseases threaten the world's health, so to do many diseases that were once considered no longer a threat. Reemerging infections are those that had previously been nearly eradicated through the use of vaccines or antimicrobials.

Diseases such as tuberculosis, malaria, dysentery, cholera, and pneumonia are making a deadly comeback in many parts of the world, much of this due to the resistance of organisms to antimicrobials. Though antimicrobial resistance is not a new problem, it has steadily worsened over the last decade. All bacteria contain the genetic capability to evolve genes that render them resistant to other bacteria. By continually using antimicrobials, only the susceptible organisms are killed, leaving the resistant bacteria to spread their resistance on to other bacteria.

In the case of tuberculosis, poor patient compliance as well as poor prescribing practices have led to antibiotic resistant strains of Mycobacterium tuberculosis, the causative agent of TB. Malaria presents a double burden of resistance—both the *Plasmodium* parasites, which cause the disease, and the *Anopheles* mosquito, the vector of malaria, have evolved resistance to antimalarial drugs and insecticides, respectively. Today, more than 90% of Staphylococcus and pneumococci strains are resistant to penicillin (WHO, 2000).

Many factors may be cited in the growth of both emerging and reemerging diseases. Population growth is one such factor. The world's population is growing at an enormous rate. The increasing number of new births in many countries creates strain on health systems. Furthermore, as people move from the countryside to urban areas they increase the already poor sanitary conditions of the world's cities as they add to overcrowding. Still others seek land in areas never inhabited by people, putting millions at risk for unknown diseases. Population movement caused by wars, inner turmoil within the country, or natural diseases cause many people to relocate to new areas, with new diseases. These refugees often have not developed the resistance to diseases located in their new homes. As the world becomes smaller through international air travel, the routes for the spread of infectious disease increase. The future role that infectious diseases will play in the world's health will largely be determined by individual countries. Many resources are available for both the identification and eradication of disease. Unfortunately, many countries still face large internal struggles that divert their leaders' attention away from health concerns.

Noncommunicable Diseases

Noncommunicable diseases traditionally pose the most risk to people living in developed nations. The future risk of noncommunicable disease, however, lies in developing nations. Overall, the number of deaths from noncommunicable diseases is expected to climb from 28.1 million deaths in 1990 to 49.7 million in 2020, an increase of 77% in absolute numbers (WHO, 2000). In proportionate terms Group II [noncommunicable] deaths are expected to increase their share of the total from 55% in 1990 to 73% in 2020. These global figures, impressive as they are, mask the extreme nature of the change that is projected in some developing regions because they incorporate the projection for the rich nations, which show little overall change. In India, deaths from noncommunicable diseases are projected to almost double, from about 4 million to about 8 million a year, while Group I [communi-

TABLE 9.4 *Factors Involved in Certain Reemerging Diseases*

Disease/Agent		*Factors in Reemergence*
Viral	Rabies	Changes in land use, public health measures
	Yellow fever	Favorable conditions for mosquito vector; change in ecological conditions
	Dengue fever	Increased transportation, travel, migration, and urbanization
Bacterial	Plague	Economic development, land use changes, ecological imbalance
	Cholera	Travel, migration
	Tuberculosis	Changes in human demographics, human behavior
	Diphtheria	Lack of consistent immunizations due to political upheaval
Parasitic	Malaria	Drug and insecticide resistance; civil problems
	Schistosomiasis	Dam construction, irrigation, ecological changes

Source: WHO, 2000.

cable] deaths are expected to fall from almost 5 million to below 3 million a year. In the developing world as a whole, deaths from noncommunicable diseases are expected to rise from 47% of the total to almost 70 percent (Murray & Lopez, 1996).

It has been estimated that cardiovascular diseases will be the largest single disease burden globally by the year 2020 (WHO, 2000). Within this category fall stroke, ischemic heart disease, and heart attacks. However, there is substantiative evidence that current programs already in place for cardiovascular disease prevention offer the most feasible, cost-effective ways to reduce mortality and morbidity from this disease. Implementing these programs must then become a priority in both developed and underdeveloped nations.

Surprisingly, in developed countries, neuropsychiatric disorders are also in the top five causes of disability. Since these diseases have limited mortality consequences, not much emphasis has been placed on their prevention and treatment. However, the disease burden resulting from these disorders, especially depression, is estimated to increase in both developing and developed countries. Alcohol use is thought to be a major disease burden, and was globally the leading cause of disability for men in 1990 (WHO, 2000).

Malignant neoplasms (cancers) are the third largest cause of morbidity and mortality in developed nations. Lung cancer is by far the largest contributor to

TABLE 9.5   *Leading Causes of Death Worldwide from All Causes, 1998*

Type of Death	Disease	Total Deaths
Infectious diseases	Respiratory illness AIDS Tuberculosis Malaria Diarrheal diseases	13,300,000 (25%)
Chronic diseases	Cancers Cardiovascular diseases	7,000,000 (13%) 16,700,000 (31%)
Injuries	All types	5,900,000 (11%)
All others	Maternal/infant, others	10,780,000 (20%)

Source: World Health Organization (2000).

TABLE 9.6   *Deaths Rates of the Four Major Chronic Diseases of the United States, 1998*

Cause of Death	Number of Deaths	Percent of Total Population
Total cardiovascular disease	955,591	41.2%
Chronic obstructive pulmonary disease	102,899	4.5%
Diabetes	59,254	2.6%
All cancers	538,455	23.3%
All others	655,132	28.4%
Total Deaths	**2,312,132**	**100%**

Source: WHO, 2000.

this rate of disease, and it is expected to become even more prevalent over the next decades (WHO, 2000). This will be especially true if current smoking trends continue.

Refugees and Displaced Persons

As mentioned previously, refugees have increasing become an international health problem. The United Nations estimates that there are at least 30 million internally displaced people worldwide (UN, 1999). When people leave their homeland because of political or religious turmoil, they often find themselves in refugee camps, which are often the breeding grounds for diseases. Thus, poor sanitation and lack of clean food and water often plague the camps. Poor sanitation quickly leads to cholera, diarrheal diseases, and malaria. Without proper nutrition and water people quickly become dehydrated from these preventable diseases. Dehydration acts quickly in the very young, the elderly, and those already weakened by illness. This same scenario has been repeated worldwide, and although international health agencies are continually working to aid refugees, it is a continual struggle for survival. In addition, as mentioned earlier, political turmoil, wars, and the lack of consistent health care leave refugees at a much higher risk for STDs, especially HIV. In the future, if developing countries do not install health care systems for these displaced people, they will be the source of sobering numbers of new STDs and other diseases. The future fate of refugees will be determined not only by their governments, but also by the international community. Countries that are developed have many of the resources available to help prevent problems such as these. However, many countries have decreased their humanitarian spending, and in the general public, charitable contributions are down. It is in the best interest of the world community to support these displaced people.

Poverty

Despite the extraordinary advances of the twentieth century, a significant component of the global morbidity and mortality is due to the ill effects of poverty. The final factor influencing the future of international health is a silent and deadly killer. Dr. Nakajima on the World Health Organization's Executive board stated, "Poverty remains the main obstacle to health development. For millions of people, poverty implies lack of access to proper food, water, and shelter, and therefore greater vulnerability to disease. Poverty itself is often caused and perpetuated by ill-health" (WHO, 1996). Infectious diseases, undernutrition, and maternal and child disability and mortality are primarily concentrated in the poorest countries, and within those countries, they especially afflict those populations living in poverty. Within countries, those living in poverty have a five times higher probability of death between birth and the age of 5 years, and a 2.5 times higher probability of death between the ages of 15 and 59 years (WHO, 1996).

Poverty is the greatest indirect cause of ill health and suffering worldwide. The International Classification of Diseases codes this killer Z59.5—extreme poverty. Poverty's influence on the world's health is strong; moreover, combating the disease of poverty is extremely difficult and involves changing societies on many levels.

Worldwide poverty influences health from every direction. It is the main reason children aren't vaccinated. It hinders the development of clean water and sanitation measures. Poverty acts as a barrier between lifesaving curative drugs and millions of the world's people. Life expectancy is considerably lower in poverty-stricken countries. One of the biggest health problems associated with poverty is that of malnutrition, with vast and far-reaching effects.

Malnutrition

Undernourishment.   On a global basis, approximately 49% of the 10 million children who died in 1998 died of malnutrition. Nearly 30% of all humankind throughout the world are suffering from one or more forms of malnourishment (WHO, 2000). Unlike many diseases, malnutrition affects all age groups across the entire life span. Throughout different age groups, it manifests in many different ways. Fetuses are at risk for brain damage, intrauterine growth retardation, stillbirth, and low birth weight. Small children are perhaps the most at risk for the various malnutrition diseases, such as protein-energy malnutrition (PEM), vitamin A deficiency, iodine and iron deficiencies, and they often exhibit learning and developmental disabilities. Adults are at risk for these diseases also; in addition, they can have folate and calcium deficiencies. Sadly, overall progress in reducing the most common disease of malnutrition, protein-energy malnutrition, among infants and young children has been discouraging. The year 2000 goal of a 50% reduction in 1990 PEM prevalence levels around the world has been met at merely a 14.3% reduction (WHO, 2000). However, though progress has been slow, this still represents a significant decrease from the worldwide levels in 1980.

Overnourishment.   At the other end of the malnutrition spectrum lies the problem of overeating, which is very both common in developed countries and increasing in developing nations. In all actuality, recent evidence strongly suggests that the prevalence of overweight and obesity is becoming a problem of massive global proportions. Due to the current lack of consistency and agreement over the classification of obesity among children and adolescents, it is difficult to ascertain the true global prevalence for these age groups. However, in industrialized nations, an epidemic of obesity is occurring in children, adolescents, and adults. The true health consequences of the high rates of childhood obesity may not become fully apparent until years down the road. Obesity can coexist with undernutrition in many developing nations, though it is more common in the urban areas of the disadvantaged countries. More than half the adult population in many industrialized countries is affected by obesity, and with the subsequent consequences associated with overeating. Heart disease, hypertension, stroke, cancer, and diabetes are some of the ramifications of long-term obesity.

Diet is a major causative agent in many types of cancers and other chronic illnesses, especially in industrialized nations. Obesity is also one of the key risk factors for a range of serious noncommunicable diseases, such as diabetes mellitus, GI diseases, and other diseases, as well as accidents. Obesity is perhaps the most significant modifiable risk factor for noninsulin-dependent diabetes mellitus. By 2025, it is predicted that there will be a 122% increase in the number of adults affected by diabetes mellitus (WHO, 2000). Even though cancer is mostly a preventable disease, there are staggering numbers of people worldwide with various types of cancers. Diets with ample amounts of fruits and vegetables, decreased intake of alcohol, physical exercise, and maintaining an appropriate body weight will prevent between 30% and 40% of all cancers. Based on current scientific evidence, it should be fairly easy to manage our risk for cancers. Yet the global incidence of cancer is expected to rise from 10.3 million cases annually in 1996 to 15 million by 2020 (WHO, 2000). According to the World Cancer Research Fund, a feasible goal for the dietary prevention of cancer is reducing the global incidence by 10% to 20% within the next 10 to 25 years.

It is clear that public health strategies for the prevention and management of overweight and obesity must be developed and implemented. In fact, several industrialized nations have become so disturbed by escalating numbers of people entering the range of obesity that they are currently developing national prevention and management strategies. Indeed, if serious public health action is not taken now, the financial burdens on the health care systems of these countries will become staggering.

Life Expectancies

In the richest countries, life expectancy in the year 2000 reached 79 years. In some of the poorest it went backwards to 42 years. Thus the gap continues to widen between rich and poor, and by the year 2000 at least 45 countries were expected to have a life expectancy at birth of 60 years (WHO, 2000). Unfortunately, research shows that poverty will continue to be a major obstacle to the world's health. The fall of the former Soviet Union has placed millions of people below the poverty line with no government social system in place to support health care. In many former Soviet block countries there is no medication available to fight even the most curable of infections. The World Health Organization illustrated this point when it wrote:

> Although in the past 10 years there has been a global trend towards the democratization of political systems, the much anticipated "peace dividend" has failed to materialize. Poverty has continued, and will continue, to be a major obstacle to health development. The number of poor people has increased substantially, both in developing countries and among underprivileged groups and communities within developed as well as developing countries. (WHO, 2000)

Poverty will continue to be one of the world's leading influences on international health. It is necessary for developing countries and segments of the developed world to pursue lessening the gap between the world's rich and poor. Until that gap is narrowed and financial stability attained, poverty will continue to have a socially destabilizing effect.

Global Burden of Disease

In the next twenty years a dramatic change will occur in the health needs of the world's population. It is stated that in developing regions where four-fifths of the world's population currently live, noncommunicable diseases will replace infectious diseases and malnutrition as the leading cause of disability and death.

It is expected that by the year 2020, 7 out of 10 deaths will occur from non-communicable diseases. Currently noncommunicable diseases account for less than half of the deaths annually. Injuries, either intentional or unintentional, will rival infectious diseases as a worldwide source of health problems.

The theory of "epidemiologic transition" may explain the change in the world's health care problems. This theory holds that as a population's birth rate falls, the number of adults relative to children increases. Thus a population's most common health problems are those of adults rather than those of children. The study noted that this shift has already begun in China, some other parts of Asia, and Latin America.

Many governments worldwide are not prepared to handle this rapid change. Health care systems will fail to monitor and adjust because public health officials often lack the most basic data needed to make public health policies. The purpose of the researchers at the Harvard School of Public Health and the World Health Organization was to fill the gap between the actual state of world health and the information currently held by the world's health care policy makers. The result was a comprehensive, internally consistent, and comparable set of estimates of current patterns of mortality and disability from disease and injury for all regions of the world, including projections to the year 2020.

The researchers were able to develop a method that quantifies not merely the number of deaths but also the impact of premature death and disability on a population by combining these into a single unit of measurement of the overall "burden of disease" on a population. This particular study is unique in that it provided the first estimates of the proportion of mortality and disability that can be attributed to risk factors for diseases—such as tobacco use, alcohol use, poor water and sanitation, and unsafe sex.

The findings were reported in a 10-volume series. The first volume, *The Global Burden of Disease* (Murray & Lopez, 1996), contains information on the key concepts as well as methods and results. The second volume, *Global Health Statistics,* includes the mass of underlying epidemiology and demographic data. The remaining eight volumes deal with specific conditions and country-based analyses.

The researchers divided the world into eight demographic regions. These include: the established market economies (EME); the formerly Socialist economies of Europe (FSE); India (IND); China (CHN); other Asia and Islands (OAI); Sub-Saharan Africa (SSA); Latin America and the Caribbean (LAC), and the Middle Eastern Crescent (MEC). The information attained from each of these eight demographic regions was then analyzed by five age groups and by sex and cause.

The *Global Burden of Disease* (GBD) uses an approach to measuring the health status of the world that is different from other statistical measures because it does not suffer from the several limitations that reduce the practical value of most statistical information. The practical value of statistical information is usually reduced because of three main factors.

The first is that most information attained is partial and fragmented. Many countries are unable to attain even the most simple data—for example, the number of deaths from a particular cause each year. Mortality rates by nature do not allow for conceptualization of the impact of nonfatal outcomes of disease and injury. The second limitation of most analyses is that the estimates of numbers killed or affected by particular conditions or diseases may be exaggerated beyond demographically plausible limits. According to the researchers, epidemiologists become advocates for people afflicted by certain health problems. This advocacy, combined with competition for the limited resources of the world health systems, leads to epidemiology estimates for all conditions which are demographically impossible. It has been found that people in a given age group or region would have to die twice over to account for all the deaths that are claimed. Finally, traditional health statistics do not allow policy makers to compare the relative cost effectiveness of different interventions. This becomes increasingly important as funds for health services become increasingly scarce.

In order to accomplish their goal, the researchers had to find a currency that captured the impact of both premature death and disability. Historically, researchers have agreed that time is an appropriate currency; time (in years) lost throughout premature death, and time (in years) lived with a disability. Each country has developed its own time-based measures, many of them variants of the quality-adjusted life year or QALY. The researchers involved with *The Global Burden of Disease* developed an internationally standardized form of the QALY, called the DALY or disability-adjusted life year. The DALY is expressed in years of life lost to premature death—death that occurs before the age to which the dying person could have expected to survive if he or she were a member of a standardized model population with a life expectancy at birth equal to that of Japan. Japan has the world's longest-surviving population. In order to calculate a DALY for a condition of a given population, years life lost (YLLs) and years lived with disability of known severity and duration (YLDs) are each estimated and then the total summed.

In order to measure a burden, a society must make five value choices. The researchers asked these questions:

1. How long "should" people live?

2. Are years of healthy life worth more in young adulthood than in early or late life?

3. Is a year of health life now worth more to society than a year of healthy life in 30 years' time?

4. How do you compare years of life lost due to premature death and years of life lived with disabilities of differing severities?

The following is a brief outline of the egalitarian principles on which the DALY is based.

How long "should" people live?
- GBD assumes that a standard life table for all populations, with life expectancies at birth fixed at 82.5 years for women and 80 years for men.

- A standard life expectancy allows deaths in all communities at the same age to contribute equally to the burden of disease.
- Life expectancy is not equal for men and women.
- The difference between men and women is determined by men's higher exposure to various risks such as alcohol, tobacco, and occupational injury, rather than biological differences.

Are years of healthy life worth more in young adulthood than in early or late life?

- A range of studies confirms a broad social preference to "weight" the value of a year lived by a young adult more heavily than one lived by a very young child or an older adult.
- Adults are widely perceived to play a critical role in the family, community, and society.
- Age weighting was incorporated into the DALY.

Is a year of healthy life now worth more to society than a year of healthy life in 30 years' time?

- GBD researchers decided to discount future life years by 3% per year.
- A year of healthy life bought 10 years in the future is worth 24% less than one bought now. Thus the relative impact of a child's death compared to an adult death is reduced.
- GBD publishes alternative results based on DALYs without discounting.
- Discounting reduces the value of interventions, which pay off largely in the future.

How do you compare years of life lost due to premature death and years of life lived with disabilities of differing severities?

- All nonfatal health outcomes of disease are different from each other in their causes, nature, and their impact on the individual, and the impact on the individual is in turn mediated by the way the community responds.
- Surprisingly, there was wide agreement between cultures about what constitutes a severe or mild disability.

Using these basic principles, the researchers were able to design a study that amassed an enormous amount of information. This information is essential if proper planning of health services is to take place. The GBD study has show that noncommunicable diseases will soon become the dominant cause of ill health in the world. Many diseases such as mental illnesses have long been overlooked in developing regions. The GBD study has shown that this can no longer continue.

The study's researchers note that the impact of the GBD will be judged in two ways: first, by the degree to which it stimulates other researchers to apply the same rigorous methods of measuring disease burden in all regions; and second, to the extent that it changes priorities for public health in the decades ahead.

The Future of International Health

Communicable disease (including the sexually transmitted), noncommunicable disease, refugees, and poverty (including malnutrition) will all play an important role in the future of international health. As this chapter has illustrated, although these four factors can be named separately, they are in fact interwoven in the daily lives of the world's population. In the coming decade it should be expected that although the burden of infectious disease might decrease, new and more deadly diseases will arise for which we as humans have no cure. Growth of new diseases will be facilitated by the same factors that allow a reemergence of those once thought to be controlled. Resistance of disease-causing organisms to antimicrobial drugs and other agents will have a deadly impact on control. Increases in international travel, in trade food as well as other trade, and tourism all mean that disease-causing organisms can readily be transported from one continent to another. To counter such a threat, global health surveillance of infectious diseases must be instituted, as well as a global international information network. As the burden of infectious disease decreases, the burden of noncommunicable diseases will increase. This shift will occur in populations previously not associated with noncommunicable diseases. The state of the world's refugees will continue to influence international health by placing people in areas that contain diseases foreign to their immune systems. This, combined with poor sanitation and nutrition, will only lead to disaster if the world's community doesn't increase its humanitarian efforts. Poverty, the single most influential factor affecting the world's health, will continue to plague the next decade. Only very broad changes in the world's social structures will facilitate an end to the vicious cycle of poverty and ill health.

Though the overall outlook on the future of public health may seem bleak, it is important to remember the areas in which we have succeeded in making our lives healthier. The eradication of smallpox, a disease that ravaged the planet for centuries, is probably the most significant success of the twentieth century. When the global smallpox eradication program was launched in 1967, there were an estimated 10 to 15 million cases a year; of these, two million died and more than 10 million remained disfigured (WHO, 1996). However, the 12-year eradication campaign against smallpox was successful; the last naturally occurring case was in Somalia in 1977. The success of this campaign encouraged the decision by WHO to eradicate polio by the year 2000. Though the number of cases has become increasingly small, there are several differences between the viruses themselves that may cause more difficulty in eradicating polio. Unlike smallpox, polio does not always cause symptomatic disease, thus allowing a potential case to slip through the public health system. As a result, exhaustive surveillance work is required to ensure that low-level cases are detected and that any poliovirus circulating among healthy children is caught.

Predicting the future of international health accurately is nearly impossible. Predictions about health are difficult to make because health is about people, and human behavior is difficult to control, especially on a global basis. Although much research shows a bleaker picture for the world's health, all is not lost. Humanity will surely struggle and move forward. Collective action is required on the part of each individual country to address such tasks as global leadership and advocacy for health, generating and disseminating an information base for all countries to use, setting norms and standards, targeting specific global or regional health problems, helping to provide a voice for those whose health is neglected within their own country, and ensuring that critical research and development for the poor receive financing.

A global health perspective requires a worldwide surveillance system to identify new diseases that are cropping up, to monitor risk factors, and to find workable solutions for preventative measures. In most cases, surveillance of a disease by itself is not enough for successful prevention efforts. For example, trends in the occurrence of chronic diseases are usually related to some environmental exposure to predisposing risks, which can precede the outcome (the actual disease) by decades. Therefore, monitoring trends of deaths alone cannot be used to identify populations that are currently at risk for a chronic disease and in need of preventative actions (WHO, 2000). Surveillance of risk factors is necessary to track particular lifestyles associated with chronic or infectious disease. For example, well-known risk factors for chronic diseases include poor diet, low levels of activity, high blood cholesterol, high blood pressure, tobacco use, and obesity. Modification of these factors holds the potential to improve the health of targeted populations.

Despite intense efforts on the part of many nations, the development of a global surveillance system is still in its early stages. There are large data gaps that exist across populations; indeed basic information on populations, such as diet, weight, and physical activity, is still largely unavailable for many populations. In addition, it is essential that any global surveillance system of risk factors must incorporate a universal definition of social class. This is because health and disease are strongly patterned by social class, and there is a growing disparity in outcomes from around the world. In order to reverse current trends, more research in the field of social class for the purpose of worldwide comparisons of health status must become a high priority. In addition, there are five priorities identified at the World Health Assembly of 1998:

- Promoting social responsibility for health.
- Increasing community capacity and empowering the individual.
- Expanding and consolidating partnerships for health.
- Increasing investments for health development.
- Securing an infrastructure for health promotion.

The dawn of a new millenium offers an opportunity to reflect on future directions of public health and to celebrate past victories. No one should question the remarkable contribution that public health has provided the human species in the understanding of the causes and consequences of disease, illness, and death in our societies. With every decade that passes, we come to know more about ourselves, and to learn about what can make us potentially healthier people.

Discussion Questions

1. Explain why chronic, noncommunicable diseases will pose more of a threat in the future to developed nations than to underdeveloped ones.

2. What are the problems for a country that has high rates of STDs?

3. Explain the difference between emerging infections and reemerging infections.

4. What are the specific problems associated with overnutrition? Malnutrition?

5. Name ways in which public health policy can help prevent the outbreak of new diseases.

6. Overall, what is going to be the biggest threat to the health of humankind in the future? Explain.

References

ASM. (1999). *Infectious Disease Threats, A Congressional Briefing: As We Enter the New Century: What Can We Do?* American Society for Microbiology [Online] Available Http://www.asmusa.org/

Garrett, L. (1994). *The Coming Plague.* New York: Penguin Books.

Murray, C. J., & Lopez, A. D. (1996*). The Global Burden of Disease.* Geneva, Switzerland: World Health Organization.

WHO. (1996). *Infectious Diseases Kill Over 17 Million People a Year.* Geneva, Switzerland: World Health Organization.

WHO. (2000). *Infectious Disease Report.* Geneva, Switzerland: World Health Organization [Online] Available: Http://www.WHO.int/

Index

Abortions, 123, 132, 135–137, 149, 155
  complications from unsafe, 124, 125, 128, 129, 135
Accelerated aging of the skin, 54
Accident insurance, 153
Accidents, 139, 145, 152
  years of potential life lost to (YPLL), 185
Acid rain, 27, 33, 43
Acinetobacter, 71
Acquired Immunodeficiency Syndrome (AIDS), 62–63, 107, 185, 189. *See also* HIV/AIDS
  candida albicans and, 70
  as health system burden, 170, 172
  as leading infectious cause of death, 206, 209, 212
Acupuncture, 6, 150
Acute hemorrhagic colitis, 72
Acute otitis media, 70, 71
Acute respiratory infection, infant and child mortality, 131, 193
Adaptation and change
  human, 43, 44, 46, 75
  microbial, 63, 64, 67, 68, 69
Adjusted rates, 184
Aerosol propellants, 50, 54
Afghanistan, mortality rate, 33
Africa, 27, 35, 43, 86, 194
  disease environment, 9, 13, 51, 99, 207, 209
  Health for all Africans (HFA) 2000, 111–112, 115, 121
  HIV/AIDS pandemic, 62, 208
  regional food patterns, 98–99
African sleeping sickness, 13
Agent-host-environment triad, 192
Agents of disease transmission, 195, 197, 201
  definition, 193
Age of Degenerative and Man-Made Diseases, 38, 39
Age of Degenerative Diseases, 38, 39
Age of Pestilence and Famine, 38, 39
Age of Receding Pandemics, 38, 39
Age-specific mortality rate (ASMR), 183, 184, 185
  formula, 183
AGIS: Sisters of St. Elizabeth of Hungary, 74
Agriculture, 36, 42, 43, 55, 58. *See also* Fertilizer; Insecticides
  crops, 25, 50
  irrigation and water usage, 56, 60
  production and global warming, 49–51

Air pollution, 53, 64, 75, 77, 148
  global environmental health and, 33, 48–49, 53–56
Air pollution resources, 56
Air quality, epidemiology, 178
Alcohol use, 100, 139, 165, 211, 214
  chronic disease and, 38, 39, 77
  as disease risk factor, 216, 218
  maternal and child health and, 130, 131
Algeria, 114, 127
Allergens, 53, 55
Allergic rhinitis, 55
Alma-Ata Conference, 104, 111–113, 121
  key objectives of, 112–113
Alma-Ata, Declaration of, 104, 110, 112, 121
Aluminum exposure, 199
Alzheimer's disease, 38, 173, 199
American Cancer Society, 95, 96, 97
American Diabetes Association, 98
American trypanosomiasis, 52
Anemia, iron deficiency, 86, 89, 91, 98, 130
Aneurysm, 97
Angola, maternal mortality rates, 126
Anorexia nervosa, 95
Anthrax, 9, 24–25, 140, 191, 199
Antibiotic resistance, 65, 67–72, 78
Antibiotics, 68, 69–70, 72, 152, 206
Antimalarial drugs, 10, 114, 210
Antimicrobial resistance, 206, 208, 209, 210, 219
Antimicrobials, 67–69, 192
Antipyretic drugs, 6
Apgar birth outcome scores, 185
Apartheid, 171
Aquifer recharge rates, 58
Arbovirus infection, 13
Arterial revascularization, 168
Aryans, health history, 4
Ascorbic acid, 92
Asia, 51, 115, 126, 207–208, 216
  plague/epidemics in, 9, 13, 191
  population projection, 34, 35
Asian-Americans, diabetes and, 97
Aspirin, 114
Asthma, 53, 55, 72, 185
Atherosclerosis, 2, 93, 94
"Attack rate" (AR), formula, 197
Australia, 34, 128, 141–145, 208
Auto-immune diseases, 61, 74
Autolysin mechanism, 68
Azerbaijan, 36
AZT drug therapy, 62
Aztecs, history of medicine, 6–7

Baby boom generation, 36, 120, 169
Baby bust, 35
Bacteremia, 70, 71, 193
Bacteria, 58, 68–71, 192, 193, 208
Bacterial disease, reemerging disease factors, 211
Bacteriodes, 71
Bacteriology, 11
Bancroftian filariasis, 59
Bangladesh, 90, 100, 126, 128
Bantu blacks, 94
Barbados, 36
Behavioral risk, 130, 131, 133, 135, 139
Behavior-choice diseases, 139, 172
Behaviors, human, 177, 197, 211, 220
  sexual, 13, 207
Benin, 127
Beriberi, 92
Beringia, 43
Bhopal India, pesticide pollution, 181
Bias, types of, 179, 187, 189–190
Bills of Mortality, 200
Binge-purging behavior, 95
Biocide, 208
Biogenetic engineering, 74
Biological weapons, 24, 25
"Biomarkers", molecular, 199, 200
Biomass combustion, air pollution from, 53, 55
Biomolecular research, 173, 177, 199
Biopiracy, 24
Biotechnology, 24, 173
Bioterrorism, 24–25
Birth attendants, PHC training of, 113, 114–115
Birth defects, 130
Birth rate, 33, 78, 142, 145, 148
  of comparative health care systems, 152–153, 157, 161, 163, 170
  population dynamics and, 37, 38, 39, 41, 43
Black Death, 9, 85, 191–192
Blacks, incidence of diabetes, 97
Blindness, vitamin A deficiency, 89–90, 98
Blood clot, 97
Blood glucose levels, 97, 130
Blood pressure, 92, 94
Blue Cross and Blue Shield, 167
Body mass index (BMI), 94–95
Bolivia, 10
Bonebreak fever, 209
Bone deformity, 91
Bone mass measurement, 120
Botswana, HIV/AIDS in, 62
Botulinum toxin, 25

Bovine spongiform encephalopathy (BSE), 72
Brazil, 90, 127, 194
Breast feeding, 88–90, 132, 134, 136
British doctors' smoking study, 177
Broad-spectrum beta-lactam antibiotics (BSBL), 69, 73
Bubonic plague, 191, 192. *See also* Black Death
Bulimia, 95
Burden of disease, 215–218, 219
Bureau of Public Health (Japan), 158
Burundi, mortality rate, 33

Cache Valley fever, 67
Cairo conference, 40–42
Calcium, dietary, 91, 214
Campylobacter jujuni pathogen, 70, 71
Canada, 20, 48, 50, 127–128, 198
    health care system of, 141, 145–147
Canada Health Act (1984), 146, 147
Cancer, 23, 38, 73, 204, 212
    bladder, 96
    breast, 96, 97, 179, 200
    candida albicans and, 70
    colon, 85, 96, 97
    colorectal, 96, 120
    diet and, 95–98, 100, 214, 215
    endometrial, 96
    esophageal, 96
    gallbladder, 96
    kidney, 96
    laryngeal, 200
    as leading cause of death, 152, 157, 211, 212
    liver, 96
    lung, 77, 96, 152, 185, 211–212
    lung, causes of, 23, 53, 55, 177, 180
    mortality rates for, 14, 85, 96, 100, 102, 193
    obesity and, 87, 92, 94, 96, 214
    ovarian, 96
    pancreas, 96
    prostate, 96, 97, 120, 173, 179
    registries, 195
    risk factors, 96, 100, 186, 199, 214
    skin, 54, 179, 190
    stomach, 96
    testicular, 201
Candida albicans, drug resistance, 70
Capital flight, 32
Carbohydrates, Kwashiorkor and, 89
Carbon dioxide emissions, 46, 49, 50, 52
Carbon monoxide, as air pollutant, 53
Cardiorespiratory fitness, 185
Cardiovascular disease (CVD), 88, 100, 187, 193, 199, 211
    mortality rate, 204, 212
    obesity and, 87, 93
    risk reduction, 93–94
CARE. *See* Cooperative American Relief Everywhere

Career opportunities, in international health, 3
Caribbean, 99, 194, 207, 208, 216
"Carrying capacity," 36, 37, 45
Case-control design, 187, 197, 198
Case definition, 196–197
Case fatality rate (CFR), formula, 183
"Casemix" indicator, 144
Castlemans disease, 61
Catalytic converters, 53
Cataracts, 54
Catholic church, charitable health services, 161–162
Causality, analysis of, 178, 179–180, 187, 192, 197
"Cellular hijacking," 74
Cellular phones, 26
Center for Overpopulation, 42
Centers for Civilian Biodefense Studies, 29
Centers for Disease Control (CDC), 25, 29, 62, 66–67, 73
Centers for Disease Control, Morbidity, Mortality Weekly Report, 200
Central America, 97, 209
Central planning economy, 150, 151, 152, 163, 173
Cephalosporin, 69
Cerebral hemorrhage, 97
Cerebral palsy, 128
Cesarian sections, 5
Chad, 127
Chagas disease, 13
Chance, causality of, 180, 188
Chemotherapy, 96, 206
Chicken pox, 61
Childbed fever, 201
Childbirth, complications from, 124–125, 126, 129
Child health, 51, 107, 115, 123, 207
    effect of malnutrition on, 86, 214
    global perspective, 123–137
    health education and, 1, 76
    interventions, 113, 123 , 129
    political environment and, 123, 137
    primary health care, 105, 115
    preventive medicine, 149
    protein-energy malnutrition (PEM), 87–88, 98, 100, 214
    socioeconomic levels and, 123, 124, 137
    vaccination/immunization and, 12, 15, 22
    vitamin/mineral deficiency, 90, 91, 214
Child mortality, 99, 113, 115, 132, 218
    dehydration and, 213
    from infectious diseases, 160, 193
    malnutrition and, 85, 88–89, 133, 137, 214
    parasitic disease and, 160
    poverty levels, 131, 213
    rates, 12, 22

risk and influencing factors, 123, 132–134
    vitamin A deficiency and, 90
Children, 14–15, 23, 28, 77, 172
Children Worldwide, 16
Chile, shift in major causes of death, 204
Chimpanzee, HIV-1 transmission, 62–63
China (CHN), People's Republic of (PRC), 27, 48, 57, 185, 216
    abortion and contraception, 136
    birth/death rate, 33, 34, 100, 128
    environmental degradation, 75
    epidemiologic transition in, 46, 216
    family planning policies, 34, 36
    health care system of, 141, 148–152
    history of medicine in, 5–6, 7–8, 9, 10
    newly emerging influenza strains, 66–67, 78
    vitamin B deficiency, 92
China Epidemiology Net, 200
Chlamydia, 13, 192, 207
Chlorination, 51
Chlorine compounds, ozone depletion and, 54
Chlorofluorocarbons (CFC) emission, 49, 50, 54, 55
Chloroquine, 10, 70
Chlorotetracycline, 70
Cholera, 4, 11, 13, 191, 195
    antibiotics and, 67
    epidemic, 199
    epidemiology of, 177
    as reemerging disease, 210, 211
    research vaccines for, 73
    transmission of, 58, 206, 213
Cholera pathogen 0139, 63
Cholesterol, 92, 93, 94, 100, 220
Chronic disease, 14–15, 157, 172, 199–201, 220. *See also* Noncommunicable disease
    definition, 192
    mortality rates, 14, 38, 77, 212
    nutrition-related, 86–87, 92–98, 100, 102, 214
    population growth and, 33, 77
    shift from infectious diseases, 32, 79, 204, 205
Chronic fatigue syndrome, 61
Chronic obstructive pulmonary disease, 22, 38, 212
Christian Democratic Union, 154
Church, history of medicine and, 7, 8, 9
Ciprofloxacin, 24
Circulatory system diseases, 152, 160
Climate Change and Human Health Web, 52
Climatic change, 33, 43, 48–49, 78
Cocaine, 6
Cohort design, 186, 187, 190, 197

Colonization, spread of disease and, 10

Commissioner of Labor (PRC), 149

"Common cold," 71

Commonwealth Department of Health (Australia), 142

Communicable disease, 206–210, 219. *See also* Infectious disease

Communication, 26, 75, 98

Compensatory births, 77

Competition, globalization of world economy and, 19, 20, 76

Confidence intervals (CI), 188–189

Confounding variables, 179

Constitution of 1917, 160

Constitution of the Republic of South Africa, 171

Contagion, history of international health and, 9, 10

Contraception, 41, 123, 130, 132, 135–137, 149

Contractural network, 118

Cooperative for American Relief Everywhere (CARE), 15

COPLAMAR, 161

Coronary heart disease (CHD), 2, 93, 168, 185–186, 199

Cost-benefit analysis (CBA) model, 116–117, 121

Cost containment legislation, 153, 156

Cost-effective analysis (CEA) model, 116, 117, 118, 121

Cost effectiveness, 123, 137, 173, 208, 211, 217

Council for Scientific and Industrial Research (CSIR) (India), 24

Couple fecundity, theories of, 39–40

Cretinism, 90, 91, 100

Creutzfeldt-Jakob disease (CJD), 72

Croatia, 127

Crude mortality rate (CMI), formula, 182

Crusades, history of medicine and, 8, 9

Cryptosporidiosis, 51, 64

Cuba, 10, 113, 127, 136

Cultural influences, 101, 109, 115, 178, 192

maternal and child health and, 123, 129, 131, 133–134, 137

Cultural Revolution, 150

Culture, 19–20

Cumulative incidence (CI), formula, 182

Curare emetine, 6

Curative medicine, 115, 116, 121, 131, 213

Cyprus, 36

Cytokines, 55

Cytomegalovirus, 61

Cytotoxins, 58

Czech Republic, 127

Dam construction, 57, 211

Darwinian selection, 75

Data collection/analysis, 125–126, 178, 190, 197, 199. *See also* World Health Organization

DDT, 43

Death, 3, 100, 204–205, 212. *See also* Mortality; Mortality rates; Premature death

group I (communicable), 210–211

group II (noncommunicable), 210, 211

"Death of distance," 78

Debt "restructuring", 76

Decentralization of responsibilities, 18, 162

Deficiency diseases, 101

Deforestation, 43, 65

Dehydration, 47, 56, 58, 60, 213

Dementia, 14

Democracy, globalization and, 18

Democratic deficits, 18

Democratic Republic of Congo, 36, 195

Demographers, 37, 38, 43

Demographic factors, 11, 12, 173

change indicator for, 185, 197, 199

spread of infectious disease and, 207, 211, 216

"Demographic fatigue," 77

Demographic transition (DT) model, 37–38, 39, 41

Dengue hemorrhagic fever, 13, 59, 185, 194, 211

as emerging disease, 208, 209

global warming and, 51, 52

Department of National Health and Population Development (South Africa), 170, 171, 173

Dependency ratio (DR) of a given society, formula, 185

Depression, 1, 188, 189, 211

Developed countries, 26, 27, 75, 76, 135, 206

birth/death rates, 14, 21, 22, 33, 35, 38

diseases of, 1, 2–3, 23, 77, 205

health issues of, 3, 12, 17, 23, 91

leading causes of death, 102, 204

maternal and child mortality rates, 126, 131, 132

obesity, 85, 94–95, 214

Developing countries, 98, 117, 119, 135, 165

birth/death rates, 33, 35, 36, 76–77

cost of health care service, 106, 109

degradation of environment in, 21, 26, 32, 53, 77–78

education levels, 21, 23, 32, 76–77

health issues of, 2–3, 12, 15, 76–77, 124

infectious disease, 62, 193, 206, 207

international debt, 21, 75–76

knowledge generation and transfer, 24, 75, 105, 115, 173

malnutrition in, 85–86, 87–92, 101, 102

maternal and child mortality rates, 125–126, 130, 131, 132, 137

mortality rates, 12, 14, 21, 22, 32

noncommunicable disease in, 194, 199, 205, 214

population growth, 21, 32

poverty problems, 27, 161

safe water/sanitation, 23, 28

Deworming, 113

Diabetes mellitus, 5, 85, 100, 128, 172, 212

obesity and, 87, 92, 214

Type I insulin-dependent (IDDM), 97, 98

Type II noninsulin dependent, 38, 97, 185

Diagnosis of disease, 5, 6, 105, 128, 137, 196

Diagnostic Related Grouping, 150

Diarrhea, 89, 99, 113, 115, 213

bloody, 71

E. coli and, 72–73

in developing countries, 2, 15, 22

infant and child mortality, 22, 114, 131, 193

as leading infectious cause of death, 206, 212

oral rehydration therapy, 134

vitamin A and, 90

as water-related disease, 58–60, 76

Diesel exhaust particles, 55, 56

Diet, 5, 87, 89, 91, 220

cancer risk and, 96, 100, 214

cholesterol and, 93, 94, 116

deficiencies, 87, 101

definition, 95

disease control by, 93–94, 98, 100

high fats, 23, 93, 97–100, 185, 194, 199

in developed nations, 1, 2, 77

low-fat, 92, 100, 116

sodium intake, 94, 99, 100

variety and moderation, 96, 102

Dietary fiber, 96–97, 102

Dieting, 95

Digitalis, 6

Diphtheria, 9, 39, 105, 113, 133, 191

as reemerging disease, 211

Director of Medical and Health Services (PRC), 149

Director of Urban Services and the Urban Council (PRC), 149

Disability, 12, 178, 215

years lived with (YLD), 217, 218

Disability-adjusted life year (DALY), 217, 218

Disease, 37, 87, 101, 105, 213. *See also* Chronic disease; Communicable disease; Individual diseases;

Infectious disease; Noncommunicable disease; Parasitic disease
causality, 51, 178, 192, 204, 211
epidemiology of, 177, 178
gene-based, 139
globalization phenomena, 21, 195
newly emerging/reemerging, 63–64, 194–195, 206, 208–209, 219–220
prevention of, 104, 109, 120–121, 130, 133–134, 149
reemergence of, 63–64, 211, 219
risk assessment, 185–190, 197
risk factors, 133, 177–178, 182, 194, 199, 220, 216
spread of, 4, 8–9, 11, 205
water-related classifications, 4, 13, 58–60
Disease burden, 124, 215–218
Disease outbreaks, 196–197
Disease patterns, 194, 204
Disease vectors, 4, 51–52, 58, 62, 66–67, 105
black rats as, 192–193
insects as, 191, 192, 206, 209, 210, 211
Displaced persons, 212–213
Dissident groups, biological warfare, 25
Diuretics, 6
DNA adenine methylase (DAM) protein, 73
Doctor-patient loads, 168
Doctor's workshop, 118
Dominican Republic, 113, 136
Dracunculiasis (Guinea-worm disease), 13, 59
Drought, food production and, 101
Drug resistance, 63, 211
Drugs, 6, 36, 154, 158, 160
antibiotics/antimicrobials, 67–69
antimalarial, 10, 114, 210
curative, 12, 131, 213
generic, 24
health care funding for, 151, 152
placebo, 189
shortage of basic, 110, 114
Drug therapy, AZT therapy for HIV/AIDS, 62
Durba, 195
Dysentery, 71, 73, 195, 206, 210

Early childhood development programs, 28
East Asia, resource utilization, 27
Eastern equine encephalomyelitis, 67
Eastern Mediterranean, 98, 99–100, 127, 209
Eating disorders, 95, 130
Ebola hemorrhagic fever, 13, 64, 65, 205, 208–209
Ebola virus, 13, 63, 193
Eclampsia, maternal mortality, 125

Ecological disruption, newly emerging infectious disease and, 64, 65–67, 211
Ecology, science of, 44, 45
Economic analysis, of health care treatment, 116–117, 121
Economic growth/development, 26, 36, 107, 109–110, 151–152
disease and, 10, 21, 23, 27
globalization and, 19, 20–21, 29
sustainability, 28, 77
Economic patterns of living, 178
Ecosystem, planetary, 33, 37, 43–44, 75, 77
Ecuador, 10, 127
Education, 113, 135, 164, 172, 196. See also Knowledge transfer
family planning and, 33, 41, 149
lack of, 86, 87, 90, 107–108
levels, 76, 78, 79, 135
life expectancy and, 34, 35
maternal and child health and, 128, 130, 133, 134, 137
"Effect modifiers," 186
Egalitarian ideal of quality care, 117, 118, 119, 121
Egypt, 4, 7, 50, 100, 126–127
Elderly, 14, 51, 62, 172, 213
access to health care, 119–120, 144, 159, 167, 173
Elephantiasis, 13
El Nino, 52
Emerging Infectious Information Network, 74
Emigration, 3, 4, 29, 33, 34
"Emotional nucleation" theory, 40
Emphysema, 55
Encephalitis virus, 66
Endemic, 192, 194, 196, 198, 209
Endotoxins, 58, 193
Enteric diseases, 58
Enterobacteria, 71
Enterococci, 71
Entertainment deregulation, 18, 19–20
Environment, 18, 42, 47
disease causality, 178, 201
globalization of, 1, 2, 33, 48–53
human modification of, 43, 44, 45, 46, 75
risk to maternal and child health, 123, 130, 132
two sources of hazards for human life, 77–78
Environmental degradation, 44–47, 75, 77–79, 101, 152
globalization and, 20, 26, 27, 28, 33
industrialization pollution, 43, 53
lead contamination, 185, 199
Environmental health, 3, 11, 33, 74–78, 79
Environmental impact formula (IPAT), 45
models, 42–47

Environmental justice, 19, 26, 28, 47
Environmental protection, 19, 20, 32, 53
Environmental Protection Agency (EPA), air pollution studies, 53, 55, 56
Environmental resource managers, 44
Environmental studies, 177
Environment movement (1970s), 43, 44, 53
Epidemics, 8–11, 191–192, 194, 196, 198–199
of noncommunicable disease, 1, 85, 205
Epidemiologic Transition (ET), 38, 39, 78, 204, 216
Epidemiology, 1, 3, 15, 106, 177–201
adjusted rates, 184
age-specific mortality rate (ASMR), 183, 184, 185
analytical domain, 181, 199
assessing risk, 185–190, 195, 197
attack rate (AR), 197
basic concepts of, 178–180
basic measures, 181–185
case-control design, 187, 197
case fatality rate (CFR), 183
cohort design, 186, 187, 190, 197
confidence intervals (CI), 188–189
counts as measurement, 181, 197
crude mortality rates (CMR), 182, 184
cumulative incidence (CI), 182
definition, 177, 178
descriptive domain, 181
exposure odds ratio (EOR) calculation, 187–188, 189, 198
frequency rates, 181–182, 199
incidence rate (IR), 182, 186, 187, 194, 197
in history of international health, 9, 10
percentage formula, 181
percentages as measurements, 181
the practice of, 191–198
prevalence formula, 181, 182, 194
proportional mortality rate (PMR), 184
proportions as measurement, 181
relative risk (RR), 185, 186, 188, 189, 198
sources of error: bias, 189–190
standardized mortality rates (SMR), 184
statistical significance, 188
surveillance, 193–195, 219, 220
two-by-two contingency table, 185–186
Epidemiology Data Center: University of Pittsburgh, 200
Epidemiology Supercourse, University of Pittsburgh, 200

Epidemiology Virtual Library: University of California, San Francisco, 200
Epstein-Barr, 61
Ergotism, 9
Eritrea, 127
Escherichia coli (E. coli), 65, 70–73, 139, 196, 198
Established market economies (EME), 216
Ethics, 5, 7, 18, 168, 172
    in health care treatment, 117, 121
Ethiopia, 36, 99
Etiology (causality), 178, 192, 197, 199
Europe, 43, 48, 55, 198, 207–208
    historical spread of disease in, 9, 10, 191
    as major cultural region, 98, 100
    managed care in, 119
    maternal mortality rates in, 126, 127
    population projection, 34, 35
European Community, health insurance, 156
European Environmental Agency, 56
Exercise, 2, 92, 116, 157, 220
    levels and cardiac arrest risk, 187
    maternal health and, 130
    weight maintenance, 96, 98, 214
Exotoxins, 58, 193
Exposure odds ratio (EOR), 189, 198
    formula, 187–188
Extended-spectrum beta-lactamase (ESBL), 68

Famciclovir, 61
Family planning, 105, 115, 148
    education, 33, 34, 36, 41, 124
Family planning services, 41, 125, 129, 130, 136
Famine, 37, 38, 101
Famvir, 61
Fasting, 99
Federal Department of Health and Human Services (Germany), 153
Federal Ministry of Health (FMOH) (Russia), 163, 164, 165
Federal Ministry of Health (Sudan), 196
Fee-for-service health care, 117–120, 151, 153, 158–160, 165
Female genital mutilation, 124
Fertility rates, 37, 142, 145, 148, 153–154
    of comparative health care systems, 157, 159, 161–163, 166, 170
    declining, 33–35, 36, 40, 41, 78, 135
Fertilizers, 43, 50, 58, 77–78
Fetal death rate, 90, 128, 132
    formula, 183
Fire, as air pollutant, 42, 53
Flavivirus, 66, 194
Flesh-eating bacteria, 73

Floods, 51
Fluconazole, 24
Fluoride, 180
Fluorine poisoning, 100
Fluoroquinolone resistance, 70
Flu shot, 67
Folate, 86, 129, 133, 214
Food, 2, 14, 79, 88, 134
    access to, 213
    fortifying, 90, 91
    high-fat, 95–97, 99
    patterns by world regions, 98–101, 102
    poisoning, 139, 197
    production, technology and, 36, 37
    supply, 4, 36, 42, 87, 101, 105
Food and Agricultural Organization, 134
Food energy deficit, 86, 98
Formerly Socialist economies (FSE), 216
Formula feeding, 134
Fossil fuel burning, 37, 43, 49, 50, 53
France, 72, 119, 127, 128
Freshwater distribution, 56–57, 58
Future Health Care, 29

Gabon, Ebola in, 208, 209
"Gaming the system," 168
Gastrointestinal (GI) diarrheal diseases, 51, 71, 72
Gastrointestinal dysentery, 70
Gatekeepers, 168, 169
Gender equality, 41, 48, 78
Gender inequality, 207, 218
General Agreement on tariffs and Trade (GATT), 20, 21
Genetic engineering, 73, 200
Genetics, as epidemiological specialty, 177, 199, 200
Gene typing, 200
Genital herpes, 13
Geriatric Health Act, 159
German Hospital Association, 153
German spa rejuvenation centers, 154
German Supreme Court, 155
Germany, 56, 119, 127, 141, 152–157, 191
Germ theory, 198, 199
Ghana, 90, 141
Giardia, 58, 192
The Global Burden of Disease, 216, 217
Global burden of disease (GBD), 215–218
    standard life table, 217, 218
Global Environmental Epidemiology Network, 200
Global health, definition, 15
Global Health Cooperation, 16
Global Health Statistics, 216
Global international information network, 219
Globalization Action Center, 29

Globalization Studies Homepage, 29
Global surveillance system of risk factors, 220
Global warming, 27, 43, 44, 46, 48
    carbon dioxide emissions, 46
    causing global warming, 52
    consequences of, 49–51, 64
    hydrologic cycle and, 57
    impact on health, 51–53
    long-term forecasts, 49, 78
Goiter, 90–91, 100
Gonorrhea, 13, 207
Greece, history of medicine and, 7, 8, 9
Greenhouse effect, 43, 48
Greenhouse gases, 49, 50
Gross domestic product (GDP), proportion spent on health services, 141, 143, 147, 155, 157, 159–162, 170
Groundwater, as freshwater source, 57
Group A streptococcus pyrogenes (GAS), 73
Guatemala, 127
Guillain-Barre syndrome (GBS), 70, 71
Guinea-worm disease, 13

Habitat degradation cycle, 78
Habitat restoration, 78
Haemophilus influenza virus, 71
The Hague Forum (Operational Review and Appraisal of the Implementation of the Program of Action of ICPD), 41
Haiti, 10, 113, 127
Hand washing, 59, 72, 125, 201
Hansen's disease, 191
Hantavirus, 205, 208, 209
Hantavirus pulmonary syndrome, 64, 66
Hardening of the arteries, 94
Harvard School of Public Health, 216
Hay fever, 55
Hazardous waste, 26, 47
Health, 22, 116, 140
    definition, 1–2
    global warming impact on, 51–53
    poverty as main obstacle, 213, 215
Health care, 130, 165, 215. See also Health care, access to; Health care, public; Health care services; Primary health care
    administration, 158, 163, 167
    costs, 22, 32, 118, 121, 159, 160, 173
    economic analyses, 116–117, 121
    facilitating, 117–120
    managed approach, 39, 117
    poverty and, 11, 12
    universal, 141, 145, 146, 151, 153, 163, 173
    welfare system of, 153–154, 160
    Western model of, 109, 115

226

Health care, access to, 22, 24, 98, 139, 169
  abortion mortality rates, 135
  barriers to, 106, 107, 108–109, 114, 115, 124
  Canada Health Act (1984), 146
  deteriorating, 164
  equity/inequity of, 1–2, 117–119, 161, 170–173, 204
  for elderly, 120
  malnutrition and, 87
  maternal health, 124, 130
Health care financing, 98, 155–156, 158, 173
  agencies, 140
  by individuals, 139, 140–141, 146, 151, 154
  by private sector, 140, 142–143, 146–147, 151, 156, 161
  by public sector, 146–147, 150, 156, 166, 169, 172–173
  by state budgets, 164, 165
  cost-cutting strategies, 168, 173
  government subsidies, 162, 173
  payment process, 167, 169, 173
  private cost, 39, 107, 116–117, 167, 168–173
  underfunding, 164, 165
Health Care Financing Administration (HCFA), 167
Health care providers, 150, 151
  training, 108–109, 149, 161, 164, 172
Health care, public, 39, 88, 91–92, 131, 165
  Alma-Ata declaration and, 104, 112
  breakdown and disease, 64
  disease outbreak action, 197, 201
  epidemiology branch of, 178
  financing, 140–142, 146–147, 150–151, 153, 169
  future priorities, 218
  globalization and, 19, 21–24, 204
  immunization, 134
  Mali case study and, 114
  state-funded, 8, 11, 167
  surveillance of infectious diseases, 219
Health care reform, 151–152, 163, 165, 167, 173
Health care services (HCS)
  church-affiliated, 161, 162
  comparative world systems, 141–173
  costs, 140–141, 153, 158, 173
  cost shifting, 167
  economic goal of, 116, 121
  future planning for, 218
  government funding, 106–108, 117, 119–121, 139–142, 167
  Health for all Africans (HFA) 2000 and, 112
  maintenance, 106, 112, 120
  managing, 142, 163

  private, 139, 170–172
  public/professional support of, 106, 120
  scarce funding, 217
  and societal functioning, 139–141
  utilization of, 131
Health education, 1–3, 79, 100, 108, 114, 115
  maternal/child health, 1, 14, 76–77, 78
"Health for all Africans by 2000" (HFA 2000), 111, 112, 115, 121
Health indicators
  for Australia, 141, 142, 143
  for Canada, 145, 147
  for Germany, 153, 155
  for Japan, 157, 159
  for Mexico, 161, 162
  for Peoples Republic of China (PRC), 148
  for Russia, 162, 163
  for South Africa, 170
  for U.S., 166
Health insurance, 39, 150–151, 156, 168, 173
  employment-based system, 151, 156, 157, 158, 159, 167
  government employees, 151, 154, 156
  hospital care, 142, 145–146, 151
  Medicaid as, 167
  national health insurance plan, 157, 158, 159
  private, 142–144, 146–147, 152, 154, 156, 158, 169–170
  publicly financed, 146, 147, 153, 166, 169
  statutory, 154, 156
  uninsured, 169
  universal, 145–146, 149–151, 153, 157, 163, 166, 173
The Health Insurance Act (1883), 153
Health Maintenance Organization (HMO), 119, 167–169
Health promotion, 99, 100, 140, 150, 201
Health status
  by place, 105–106, 149, 150, 162, 178
  epidemiology of, 178
  global, 102, 115, 205, 216, 220
  of individuals, 110, 123–124, 137, 178, 183
Heart attacks, 94, 187, 211
Heart disease, 1, 23, 38, 77, 148
  as chronic noncommunicable disease, 92, 116, 139, 204, 214
  mortality rates, 14, 85, 97, 102, 145, 157
Heart failure, and vitamin B deficiency, 92
Helminthes (worms), 59, 65, 192
Hemorrhage, maternal mortality, 125, 129

Hendra virus, 64, 66
Hepatitis, 61, 128
Hepatitis A, 39
Hepatitis B, 13, 39, 192, 207
Hepatitis C, 64, 192
Hepatitis D, 64
Herbal medicine, 114, 150
"Herd immunity," 65
Herpes simplex virus, 13, 60–61, 62, 64, 199, 207
H5N1 Avian influenza, 64, 194
High blood pressure, 2, 220
High-density lipoprotein cholesterol (HDL), 93
Hispanics, incidence of diabetes, 97
Histology, 11
Hohokum, 37
Homelessness, rate in America, 3
Hong Kong, infectious disease surveillance, 194
"Honor-based" abuse, women and, 124
Hookworm, 13
Hospice services, 120
Hospital health care, 39, 144, 159, 164
  Medicare coverage, 120, 143, 144
  sectors of, 142–145, 147, 150, 155–156, 168, 171
Hospital Insurance Trust Fund, 120
Human adaptability, 43, 44, 46, 75
Human ehrlichiosis, 64
Human Genome Project, 200
Human health frailties, categories, 139
Human immune systems (HIS), 65, 68, 73–74, 78, 92
  compromised for refugees, 205, 210, 213, 219
  malnutrition effects on, 85, 88
Human immunodeficiency virus (HIV), 62–63, 70, 88–90, 170, 204–209, 213
Human immunodeficiency virus/acquired immunodeficiency virus (HIV/AIDS), 3, 13, 22, 62–63, 170, 172
  as chronic infectious disease, 33, 124, 192
  cryptosporidiosis and, 51
  treatment, 24, 73
Human monkeypox, 64
Human papilloma virus, 207
Human primary needs, 47–48
Human toxoplasmosis, 64
Human waste management, 4 47, 50, 57, 59, 160
Hungarian National Epidemiology Center, 195
Hungary, 127, 195
Hunger, as global problem, 85, 100, 101
Hydrologic cycle (HC), 56, 57

Hygiene, 58–59, 71–72, 88, 100, 206
  history of international health and, 4, 5, 7, 8, 10–11
  maternal and child mortality and, 125, 129, 131, 132, 137
Hyperplastic obesity, 95
Hypertension, 87–88, 93–94, 172, 185, 214
  mortality rates from, 85, 100, 125
Hypertrophic obesity, 95
Hypoalbuminemia, 89

Illiteracy, as health barrier, 101, 108, 115
Immigration, 3–4, 29, 33, 34, 65
Immune response inflammatory mediators, 55
Immunization, 76, 129, 134, 140, 179, 211, 213
  for influenza strains, 66–67
  in developing countries, 2, 15, 22
  primary health care (PHC) promotion of, 105, 113, 115
Immunocompetency status, 54, 179
Incas, history of medicine, 6, 7
Incidence rate (IR), 182, 186, 187, 197
  formula, 182
India (IND), 24, 33–34, 36, 75, 100, 216
  Bhopal pesticide pollution, 181
  cultural influences, 133, 192
  historical development of medicine, 4–5, 7–8, 9, 10
  mortality rates, 126, 128, 210
  reemergence of cholera, 63
  vitamin A supplement studies, 90
  water-usage rates, 58
Indian Council of Medical Research, 100
Indonesia, 33
Industrialization, 10–11, 26, 33, 46, 152
  environmental pollution, 14, 43, 50, 53, 55–56
Industrial Revolution, 10–11, 38, 43, 49, 153
Infant health, 87, 115, 123–137, 172, 207, 214
Infant mortality, 76–77, 115, 123, 178, 212
  causes, 91, 131, 133, 137, 207
  decreases in, 41, 99, 100
Infant mortality rate (IMR), 2, 12, 41, 113–114, 119, 131–134
  comparative health care systems, 141–142, 148–149, 153–154, 157, 159, 163, 170
  comparative health care systems of the Americas, 145, 161, 166
  demographic transition (DT) model, 38
  formula, 183
  in developing countries, 22, 32, 76–77

Infection, specific periods of, 193
Infectious agents, characteristics of, 193
Infectious Control and Hospital Epidemiology, 200
Infectious disease, 1, 11, 33, 54, 65, 77, 140
  acute, 192, 200
  chronic, 192, 199, 201, 204
  comparative health care systems and, 148, 152, 160
  control of, 3, 23, 38, 39
  emerging diseases, 206, 208–209, 219–220
  epidemiology and, 177, 191, 204
  global environmental health and, 33, 60–74
  global health surveillance of, 219, 220
  in comparative health care systems, 148, 152, 160, 161
  infant mortality rate, 131, 132, 137
  latent or quiescent, definition of, 193
  leading causes of death, 206, 212, 215, 216
  malnutrition and, 89, 100
  mortality rates, 12–15, 21–23, 32, 193
  poverty and, 213
  properties of, 192–193
  reemerging/newly-emerging, 63–67, 70–75, 78, 205–206, 209–210, 219
  transmission, 59, 60, 61, 62, 63
  world wide web sites, 74
Infectious Disease Links, 74
Infectivity, definition, 193
Infertility, 130, 135
Influenza, 9, 65, 67, 73, 78, 196
Influenza A (H5N1) flu virus, 64, 194
Injuries, 177, 193, 197, 199, 218
  as leading cause of death globally, 205, 212, 216
Insecticides, resistance to, 210, 211
Insulin, 97
Insulin-resistance syndrome, 38
Intensive care unit (ICU), nosocomial infections, 70
Interactive Fertility Transition Model (IFT), 40
Interactive World Population Counter, 42
Intercontinental disease drift, 205
International Classification of Diseases-10, 124, 213
International Clinical Epidemiology Network, 200
International Conference on Population and Development (ICPD), 40, 41
International debt, of developing countries, 21, 75–76
International development, 19, 28

International disease control, 9
International Epidemiological Association, 200
International Forum on Globalization, 29
International Fund for Agriculture Development, 134
International health, 2–11, 15
  future of, 204–221
International health organizations, 14–15, 16
The International Institute for Sustainable Development, 29
International Monetary Fund (IMF), 29
International salmonellosis outbreak, 197–198
International trade, and spread of infectious disease, 20, 219
International travel, and spread of infectious disease, 64, 65, 195, 210, 211, 219
Internet, 19, 26, 32, 197
Intersectional coordination, 162
Interventions, 123–124, 129–130, 134–135, 172, 217–218
Intrauterine device (IUD), 136
Iodine deficiency, 86, 87, 89, 214
  diseases (IDD), 90–91, 98, 100
  supplementation, 129, 133
Iodization programs, 89, 91, 100
IPAT formula. See Environmental impact formula
IPAT model, 45
Iran, 100, 127
Iraq, 33, 127
Ireland, and mad cow disease, 72
Iron deficiency, 86, 87, 214
  diseases, 91, 98
  supplementation, 91, 129, 133
Irrigation, 56, 58, 75, 211
Israel, 127
Italy, 72, 119

Jamaica, 194, 198
Jamaica Ministry of Health, 198
Japan, 10, 27, 34, 48, 73, 97, 128
  food patterns, 100–101
  health care system of, 141, 157–160, 166, 173
  life expectancy in, 217
Japanese encephalitis (JE), 66, 67
Johns Hopkins HIV Service, 74
Johns Hopkins Population Information Program, 57
Johns Hopkins School of Public Health: Department of Epidemiology, Center for Epidemiology and Policy, 200
Joint United Nations Program on HIV/AIDS, 74
Journal of Emerging and Infectious Diseases, 74
Journals of Epidemiology, 200

228

Kala-azar, 13
Kaposi's sarcoma, 61
Kazakhstan, 36, 104, 127
Kenya, 38, 51, 127
Klebsiella, 71
Knowledge transfer, to Poverty-Quagmire countries, 75–77, 79
Korea, Democratic People's Republic of, 27, 48, 100, 209
Korean hemorrhagic fever, 66
Krankenkasse (sickness funds), 154, 155–156
Kuwait, 127
Kwashiorkor, 88, 89
Kyoto Protocol, 49
Kyrgyzstan, 36, 127

Land use modification, 49, 50, 211
Language, process of dominant, 19, 20
Larsen B ice shelf, 48
Lasa fever, 64
Latin America, 13, 15, 27, 35, 207–209, 216
    food patterns, 99
    health care model, 115
    public health expenditure, 113
Laxatives, 6
Lead, blood levels and disease risk, 185, 199
Lebanon, 100
Legionnaire's disease, 64, 195
Leishmaniasis, 13, 52
Leprosy, 9, 114, 191
Leptospirosis, 4
Leukemia, 61
Liberia, 36, 208
Life expectancy, 8–9, 34, 38, 99–100, 204, 217–218
    comparative health care in North America, 145, 166
    comparative health care systems and, 141–142, 148–149, 152–153, 157, 159–163, 169–170
    decline in, 107, 162, 169
    Mali case study, 114
    poverty and, 12, 213, 215
    primary health care (PHC) study, 113
Lifestyle related disease, 23, 77, 177, 199, 220
Lifestyles, 3, 95–96, 99, 116, 124
    changes from globalization, 27, 28, 29
    healthful habits, 92, 94, 96
    in developed nations, 1, 23, 38, 77
Lifetime Health Cover Program, 145
Listeria, 74
Literacy, universal primary education and, 108
Living standards, sustainability, 28
Logistic regression analysis, 199
Low-density lipoprotein cholesterol (LDL), 93

Lyme disease, 64, 66, 195
Lymphatic filariasis (elephantiasis), 13, 52
Lymphoadenopathy, 61
Lymphocytosis, 61
Lymphomas, 61

Macronutrient deficiency, 89
Madagascar, 127, 195
Mad cow disease, 72
Malaria, 4, 10, 70, 86, 128–129, 191
    mortality rates, 13, 114–115, 131, 193, 212
    as reemerging disease, 210, 211
    transmission of, 51, 52, 59, 67, 206, 213
Malaysia, emergence of Nipah virus, 66
Mali, primary health care (PHC) case study, 114–115
Malnutrition, 1, 3, 64, 133, 161, 214–215, 219
    child mortality, 133, 134, 137
    global forms of, 85–87, 100, 101
    illness as consequence of, 85, 86, 99
    primary health care program and, 113
    water-related diseases and, 58, 60
Mammography, 120, 168, 179
Managed health care, 117–121, 168, 169
Marasmus, 88–89
Marburg hemorrhagic fever, 195
Marburg virus, 78
Market-driven economy, 18, 38, 151, 152, 173
    formula vs. breastfeeding, 134
    in Russia, 165
Market ideology, globalization and, 18
Massachusetts Bay Colony, vitamin C deficiency, 92
Mass consumption, 18, 32, 79
Mass/cultural media, 19
Maternal conditions, as a leading cause of adult disease burden, 124
Maternal health, 1, 14, 15, 28, 76
    cultural influences and, 123, 124, 137
    a global perspective, 123–137
    in Mali case study, 114
    mortality rates, 12, 32, 41
    nutritional deficiencies, 90, 91, 99, 124
    prenatal care, 160
    preventive medicine, 149
    primary health care (PHC) promotion of care, 105, 115
    rights to care, 172
    risk status, 185, 186–187, 188–189
    socioeconomic levels and, 12, 123, 137
Maternal morbidity, 123–126, 129, 130, 135, 207

Maternal mortality, 124–130, 135, 137, 212, 213
    due to childbed fever, 201
    etiology of, 199
    in Africa, 98
    iron deficiency and, 91
    STD and, 207
    vitamin A supplement and, 90
Maternal mortality rate (MMR), 126–129, 130, 135
    formula, 183
Mauritius, abortion and contraception, 136
Mayans, history of medicine, 6
MD disease, 72
Measles, 9, 13
    immunization, 15, 105, 179
    infant and child mortality, 114, 131, 133, 193, 206
Medicaid, 119, 121, 166, 167
"Medical arms race," 118
Medical priority, 147
Medical scheme coverage, 170, 171
Medical service providers, 141
Medical staff shortages, 147
Medicare, 119–121, 143, 167
    Australian, 142, 143–144
Medicinal herbs/plants, 5–7, 10, 24
Medicine, historical development of, 4, 5, 6, 11
Meningitis, 24, 71, 73, 195, 196
Meningococcal disease, 195, 196
Mental health services, 142, 144
Mental illness, 12, 140, 218
Mental retardation, 90, 98
Mesopotamia, 4, 7, 42
Metabolic disorders, 97
Metabolism, cholesterol and, 93
Methane emission, 49
Methyl chloroform, 53
Mexican Institute of Social Security, 161
Mexico, 20, 51, 99, 127
    health care system of, 141, 160–162
Microbial toxins, 193, 198
Microbiology, 11, 24, 67, 69
Micronutrient deficiency, 87, 89
    diseases, 89–92
Middle Ages, 8, 9, 85, 183, 191
Middle East, 9, 42, 194, 208
Middle Eastern Crescent (MEC), 216
Midwives, 113, 114, 150, 172
Migration patterns, 29, 43, 206, 211
Military conflicts, 33, 64
Millenium Institute of Water, 60
Ministry of Health (Hungary), 195
Ministry of Health (Mexico), 161
Ministry of Health (Sierra Leone), 195
Ministry of Health and Welfare (Japan), 158, 160
Ministry of Public Health, Mali, 114, 115

Ministry of Public Health (PRC), 151, 152
Minnesota Department of Health, 70
Minoans, 7
Miscarriage, 132
Missionaries, 3
Molecular epidemiology, 199
Mongolia, global warming in, 48
Mononucleosis, 61, 192
Morbidity, 55, 58, 59, 77, 87, 113, 121
current cardiovascular programs to reduce, 211
etiology (causality), 178, 179, 194, 197, 198, 199, 213
infant and child, 115, 131–133
maternal health and, 123, 124–126, 129, 130, 135
Morbillivirus, 64
Morocco, food patterns, 99
Mortality. *See also* Deaths
current cardiovascular programs to reduce, 211
effects of poverty, 213
etiology (causality) of, 178, 194, 199
infant and child, 131–133
infectious diseases and, 58, 59, 77, 148
maternal health, 123–130, 135
nutrition-related chronic disease and, 87
Mortality rates, 121, 166, 170
abortion, 135
child, priority and, 115
of comparative health care systems, 142, 145, 148, 153, 157, 161, 163
crude mortality rate (CMR), 182–183
crude mortality rate formula, 182
for emerging diseases, 208–209
from heart disease, 85
global, 12–14, 21–22, 32–34
HIV/AIDS, 62
infant, priority and, 115
population dynamics and, 37, 38, 39, 41
SPM exposure levels, 55
Mosquito, as disease vector, 10, 51, 66, 67, 194, 196, 209–211
Multiple drug resistance (MDR), 69
Multiple regression analysis, 199
Multiple sclerosis, 72, 74
Multivariate statistical analysis, 199
Mumps, 179, 191
Municipal incinerators, 26
Muslim belief, food patterns and, 100
Myaloma, 61
Mycobacteria, 71
Mycobacterium tuberculosis, 210
Mycoses (fungi), 192
Myocardial infarction, blood cholesterol and, 93

National Cancer Institute (US), 195
National Center for HIV, STD and TB Prevention, 74
National Center for Infectious Diseases, 74
National Environment Satellite Data and Information Service, 48
National Headquarters for Negative Population Growth, Inc., 42
National Health Amendment Act, 145
National Health Insurance System (Japan), 157–158
National Health Ministers Benchmarking Working Group, 144
National Institute for Virology (NIV) (South Africa), 195
National Institutes for Water Resources (NIWR), 60
National Institutes of Health (NIH), 51
National Ozone Organization, 52
National Snow and Ice Data Center (NSIDC), 48
National Wildlife Fund International Population and Environment Site, 42
Natural resources, 27, 33, 37, 45, 47, 56–60
fossil-fuel energy reserves, 37, 43
in developed/developing country contrast, 2–3, 76, 78
Natural selection, 44
Necrotizing fasciitis (NF), 73
Negative radiative forcing, 49
Neiching, 6
Neoclassical Microeconomics Theory, 39, 40
Neonatal mortality, 12, 131–132, 183, 206
Neonatal to post-neonatal death ratio, 132
Nepal, 100, 126, 136
Nerve gas, 25
Netherlands, 41, 198
Net present value (NPV) model, 116, 117, 121
Neuropsychiatric disorders, emerging epidemic of, 205, 211
New economic mechanism (NEM), 165
Nicotine addiction, 23, 139
Niger, 90
Nigeria, 33, 36, 58, 127
Night blindness, 89, 90, 99
Nipah Virus, 64, 66
Nitrogen oxide reaction formula, 54
Nitrogen oxides, 53, 54
Nitrous oxide emission, 49, 50
Noncommunicable diseases, 79, 100, 193–194, 199, 210–212, 214–216, 218–219. *See also* Chronic disease
in developed countries, 1, 23
Nonindifferent misclassification, 189

North America, 35, 43, 48, 70, 198
incidence of disease in, 207–208, 209
North American Free Trade Agreement (NAFTA), 20
North American Indians, 6, 97
Nosocomial infections, 70, 71–72
Nuclear waste, 26
Nurses, primary health care, 172
Nursing homes, 120, 142, 143
Nursing school (NS), 164
Nutrient deficiencies, 86, 87, 101, 102, 148
malabsorption of, 58, 60
supplementation, 22, 90–91, 129
Nutrition, 3, 11, 15, 22, 28, 45, 177
cancer risk and, 96
deficiency, 45, 132, 133, 213, 219
life expectancy and, 35, 77
maternal and child health and, 76, 124, 128, 130–131, 132–134, 137
primary health care (PHC) education on, 105, 113, 115
Nutrition counseling, 88, 95, 101

Obesity, 1, 2, 38, 94–95, 98
disease risk, 185, 220
epidemic of, 85, 87
overnutrition and, 92
undernutrition and, 88, 214
Obstructed labor, maternal mortality, 125, 128
Oceania, population projections, 35
Ocean pollution, 27, 50
Occupational injuries, 14, 218
safety provisions, 152
Occupational studies, 177, 184
Occupational toxins, 11
Oman, dependency ratio (DR) for, 185
Onchocerciasis (river blindness), 13, 52, 59
One-child policy, 148
Oral rehydration therapy (ORT), 22, 58, 77, 113, 115, 134
Osteoarthritis, 38
Osteoporosis, 14, 120
Other Asia and Islands (OAI), 216
Otitis media, 70, 71
Outbreak, 196
Outbreak News, 74
Overnutrition, 86–87, 92, 214–215
diseases of, 93–98
Overpopulation, 148–149
Ozone depletion, 27, 33, 43, 44, 53–54

Pakistan, 33, 36, 100, 126
Palliative care, 172
Panama Canal, 10
Pan American Health Organization (PAHO), 23
Pandemics, 62, 191, 192
Parasitic disease, 38, 58, 63, 152, 211
mortality rates, 12, 13, 21, 22, 131, 160

Patent procedure, in U.S., 24
Path analysis, 199
Pathogenicity, 7, 193, 198
Pathogens, 65, 193
Patient rights charter, 171–172
PCB, 43
Peace Corps, 3, 15, 16
Pellagra, 47
Pelvic inflammatory disease, 130
Penicillin, 67, 68, 70
Perinatal conditions, mortality rates of, 12, 131, 132, 183
Person-years, 182
Pertussis, 105, 113, 133
Peru, 6, 10
Pesticides, 43, 58, 77–78, 181
Pfizer pharmaceuticals, 24
Pharmaceuticals, 24, 32, 68, 72, 73 *See also* Drugs
  costs, 117, 143, 144, 147, 152
Pharmacoeconomics, 117
Pharmacology, early history of, 7
PHC. *See* Primary health care
Phenylketonuria, 130
Photokeratitis, 54
Physicians, 4, 7, 118, 144, 171
  fee-for-service payment, 144, 149, 154, 159, 160, 165
  government employed, 149–150, 154, 164
  hospital-based, 159
  number of practicing, 150, 154–155, 159, 162, 164–166, 171, 173
  per-session payment, 144
  publicly financed payment, 146, 147
  salaries, 144, 164
  specialists, 169, 170, 171
Physiology, 11
Pilgrims, vitamin C deficiency and, 92
Pityriasis rosea, 61
Placebo drugs, 189
Plague, 8–9, 67, 73, 191, 192, 211
Plague bacillus, 192
Plaque deposits, 93
Plasmid gene transfer, 69
Plasmodium parasites, 51, 70, 210
PM 10, 46
Pneumococci, penicillin resistant, 210
Pneumocystis carinii, 62
Pneumonia, 62, 67, 70, 71, 193, 210
Pneumonitis, 71
POET model, 45, 46
Point-of-service (POS) plan, 119
Poland, 127
Poliomyelitis, 59, 105, 113, 133, 140, 206, 219
Poliovirus, 219
Political change, 4, 18–21, 32, 45
Political environment, 19, 32
  maternal and child health and, 123, 124, 137

Political ideology, 178
  health care costs and, 141, 142, 173
Political power structures, international health and, 2, 3, 32
Political systems, democratization of, 215
Political upheaval, 32
  and spread of infectious disease, 207, 211, 212, 213
Polyaromatic hydrocarbons, 55
Pooling fund, 159
Poor/rich gap, 113
Population and environment connection: impact models, 42–47
Population at risk, -based aggregate occurrences, 178, 181, 182, 189, 190, 201
Population change, global environmental health and, 33–47
Population control
  Cairo conference, 41
  China family planning program, 34, 36
Population Council, 14, 16
Population coverage, 107
Population demographics, 14, 131, 152
Population density, 33
Population dynamics, theories of, 36–39, 40, 43
Population ecologist, 44
Population-environment-food trap, 45
Population growth, 2–3, 4, 29
  by population momentum, 78
  degradation of world environment, 21, 27, 28, 33, 78
  environmental impact formula, 45
  food production rate and, 101
  future projection, 124
  historical ebbs and surges, 9, 10, 11, 12
  minimum water needs, 57, 58
  newly emerging infectious disease, 64, 65
  reemerging diseases, 210
  slowing of, 33
  sustainability, water and, 60
  unlimited, 37
Population growth rate, 148
  of comparative health care systems, 142, 145, 153, 157, 161–163, 166, 170
  reduction in, 140
Population Index Office of Population Research, 42
Population momentum, 34, 35, 36
Population movement
  emerging diseases and, 206, 208
  reemerging diseases, 210, 211
Population Reference Bureau (USAID), world Internet address, 42

Population size, global environmental health concerns and, 75, 77–78
Population stability, 78
Populism, globalization and, 19
"Porous borders," 65
Portugal, 72
Post-neonatal mortality, 131–132
  rate formula, 183
Postpartum care, maternal health and, 129
Poverty, 20, 27–28, 78, 161, 205, 213–215, 219
  Americas, food patterns and, 99
  basic health care and, 11, 12, 105, 107–108, 120, 167
  cycle of, 60
  in developed countries, 86, 101
  in developing countries, 2, 3, 99
  infectious disease and, 205, 207, 208
  malnutrition and, 86, 101
  maternal and child health and, 124, 126, 131, 133
  WHO focus and, 22
Poverty line, 215
Poverty-Quagmire countries, 32, 36, 47, 53, 60, 75–78
PRC. *See* China, Peoples Republic of
Precipitation, 51, 56, 57
Preferred provider organization (PPO), 119
Pregnancy, 35, 124–125, 126, 128, 129, 130
  register, 132
  unwanted, 41, 125, 129, 136
Premature death, 3, 45, 46, 133, 216, 217
  nonpotable water, 57
  Russian society and, 165
  unprocessed solid fuel use and, 53
  of women/children, 22
  years of life lost (YLL), 217, 218
Prenatal care, 124, 128–130, 132, 145, 160
Prescription drugs, 154, 158, 160
Preservationists, 44
Pre-Technophile countries, 32, 36, 46, 47, 78
Prevalence rates, formula, 182, 194
Prevention
  of disease, PHC and, 104, 109, 111, 113, 120–121, 211, 220
  levels of, 178–179, 194
  maternal and child disease, 140
  of STDs, 207–208
Preventive medicine, 116, 117, 120
  HMO and, 168
  in Germany, 154, 155
  in PRC, 149
  maternal and child health and, 130, 131
  primary care, 169
Preventive strategies
  for disease, 177, 197, 201
  for injury, 177

Primary health care (PHC), 1, 23, 35
  benefits of, 109–110, 121
  community utilization rates, 111
  comparative health care systems
    and, 149
  core components, 105, 110, 113, 120
  costs of, 106, 109, 110–114,
    120–121
  definition, 104, 112, 120
  evaluation of, 110
  financing sources, 151
  for developing countries, 22
  global policy of, 115
  main focus of, 104, 110
  national health care system sup-
    port for, 105–106, 108, 112
  nurse-oriented, 172
  primary accessibility, 104–107, 109,
    112, 120–121
  population coverage, 107
  problems, 110–111, 120, 121
  services, 105, 120
  sociopolitical role of workers, 111,
    113
Primary prevention, 178–179
Primordial prevention, 178, 179
Prions, 192
Private-for-profit system, 141
Project Concern International (PCI),
  14, 16
The Project Sante Rurale (PSR), 114
Proliferating cell nuclear antigen
  (PCNA), 200
Proportional mortality rate (PMR),
  formula, 184
Protectionism, globalization and, 19
Proteinaceous infectious particles
  (prion), 72
Protein deficiency, Kwashiorkor, 89
Protein-energy malnutrition, 86, 87,
  88, 98, 105, 214
  diseases, 87–89
Protozoa, 51, 70, 192
Pseudomonas aeruginosa, 71
Psychiatric care, 142, 168, 172
Psychiatric studies, as epidemiologi-
  cal specialty, 177
Psychological counseling, 95
Psychosocial care, 88
Publishing bias, 190
Pueblo Grande, 37
Puerperal fever, 201
Purulent meningitis, 70, 71
p-value, 188, 189
Pyrolysis, as air pollutant, 53

Quality-adjusted life year (QALY),
  117, 217
Quality of care, 163, 164, 165, 170,
  172
Quality of goods and services, 76
Quality of life, 37, 172
Quarentine, 9, 10, 25, 197
Quinine, 6, 10

Rabies, as reemerging disease, 211
Rabies virus, 193, 199
Radiation therapy, 96
Radioactive contamination, 27
Radon gas, 53
Rain, as freshwater source, 56
Recall bias, 179, 187, 199
Reforestation, emergence of new dis-
  ease and, 65
Refugees, 98, 205, 210, 212–213, 219
The Regimen Sanitatis Salernitarium, 8
Relative risk (RR), 185, 186, 188, 189,
  197, 198
  formula, 185, 186
Renal disease, 167
Reproductive freedom, 34
"Reservoir" of disease, 192, 209
Resources, 1, 23, 78, 170, 173
  depletion of natural, 27, 43
  financial, 109–111, 115, 116, 141
  population and, 3, 14, 21, 27
  water, 33, 47, 56–60
Respiratory disease, 12, 55, 77, 90, 148
  infections, 204, 206, 212
Rheumatoid arthritis, 14, 38, 74, 179
Rhinovirus colds, 186
Rickets, 92
Rickettsia, 192
Rift Valley fever, 64
River blindness, 13
Romania, 127, 135–137, 194
Rotavirus, 58, 198
Rubella, 179, 191
Rubeola, 191
Russia, 38, 39, 100, 107, 127
  health care system of, 141,
    162–165, 173
Russian Academy of Medical Sci-
  ence, 163
Russian Health Ministry, 165
Rwanda, mortality rates, 33, 127

Safe Motherhood and The World Bank,
  129
Safe Motherhood Initiative, 129
Saint Jude Children's Research Hos-
  pital (Memphis), 68
Salination, of water source, 56
Salmonella, 70, 198
Salmonella enterica serotype New-
  port, 197
Salmonella enteritis PT-4, 64
Salmonella typhi, 192
Salmonellosis, 198
Sanitation, 4, 8–11, 87, 99, 114, 135,
  140, 161, 210
  Alma-Ata declaration concerning,
    104
  in developing countries, 22, 23, 28,
    79
  poverty and, 12, 131, 213, 219
  primary health care promotion of
    basic, 105, 113, 115
  water usage needs, 2, 56, 57, 59

Scabies, 9
Schistosomiasis, 4, 13, 52, 59, 211
Sclerosing panencephalitis, 192
Screening tests, 120, 128, 179
"Scrubber" technology, 53
Scurvy, 47, 92, 201
Secondary prevention, 178, 179
Secretary for the New Territories
  (PRC), 149
Security deficits, 18, 19
Semen, as HIV/AIDS vector, 62
Senegal, 51
Sepsis, 71, 125, 128, 129
Septicemia, 71, 193
Severely bald males study, 186
Sewage treatment facilities, 28
Sex education, 135
Sexual behavior, safe/unsafe, 139
Sexually transmitted diseases
  (STDs), 10, 13, 62–63, 71, 129,
    172, 219
  epidemiology of, 177, 197, 206–208,
    213
Seychelles, 36
Shanghai, sanitation infrastructure,
  57, 58
Shelter, access to, 213
Shiga, 58
Shigella dysteria, 71
Shigella flexneri, 195
Shigellosis, 195
Siberia, 43, 48
Sickness fund, 154, 156
Sierra Leone, infectious disease sur-
  veillance, 195
Silicon chip, 32
Singapore, resource utilization, 27
Skin depigmentation, 89
Slovakia, 127
Slovenia, 127
Smallpox, 9, 25, 63, 140, 191, 219
Small suspended particulate matter
  (SPM), as air pollutant, 53,
    55–56, 77
Smoking. See Tobacco use
Snacking, 95
Social barriers, 108, 111
Social-behavioral epidemiology, 177,
  178, 182, 197, 201
Social change/development, 21, 23,
  45, 150, 165, 173
Social class, 11, 220
Social consumption, theory of, 27–28
Social Democratic Party (SDP), 154
Socialized medicine, 119, 160
Social Security, 120, 161
Social support systems, 131, 134, 137,
  219
Social-technological level of sophisti-
  cation, 46, 78
Socioeconomic development, 123,
  124, 129, 131, 135, 136, 137
Sodium, dietary, 93, 94, 99, 100
Soil pollution, 75, 78

Somalia, 219
Sooty Mangabey monkey, and HIV-2 transmission, 63
South Africa, 24, 51, 94, 127, 195
  health care system of, 141, 169–173
South America, 43, 51, 52, 194, 209
South American Indians, history of medicine and, 6–7
South Asia, resource utilization, 27
Southeast Asia, 36, 97, 98, 100–101, 128, 209
South Korea, 38
Soviet Union, 38, 162, 163, 165, 215
Species, interdependence of, 43, 44, 45
Splenomegaly, 61
Sri Lanka, 36, 100
Standardized mortality ratio (SMR), formula, 184
Staphylococcus, penicillin resistant, 210
Staphylococcus aureus, 70, 71
Staphylococcus pneumoniae, 71
Starvation, 12, 88, 95, 102
State Administration of Traditional Chinese Medicine, 151
State Committee for Sanitary and Epidemiological Surveillance (SCSES) (Russia), 163, 164
Statistical significance criterion, 188, 189
Sterilization, 136
Stillbirth, 214
Strep throat, 73
Streptococcal pneumonococcus, 70
Stress, 12, 157, 165
Stroke, 14, 94, 148, 152, 211, 214
  mortality rates from, 85, 97, 102
Structural equation modeling, 199
Sub Saharan Africa (SSA), 216
Substance abuse, poverty and, 12
Sudan, 196
Sudden death, vitamin C deficiency and, 92
Suicide, poverty and, 12
Sulfa drugs, 67
Sulfate aerosols, 49
Sulfur dioxide, as air pollutant, 46, 53
Superstition, history of medicine and, 7, 9
Supplementation, 113, 129
Surplus production, 42–43
Surveillance of disease, 193–195, 219, 220
Surveillance Epidemiology End Result (SEER), 195
  Cancer Registry, 200
  Cancer Registry web site, 200
Sustainability, 22, 60, 79, 134
  international development and, 18–19, 27–28, 41, 43, 77
Suzhou Creek, and water pollution, 57

Sverdlovsk, Russia, 25
Swaziland, HIV/AIDS pandemic, 62
Sweden, 100, 119, 185
Swine flu influenza (1918, 1919), 67
Switzerland, 22, 72, 127, 166, 195
Syphilis, 10, 13, 63, 67, 73, 191, 193
  curable/preventable, 207

Taiwan, 38
Tariff barriers, GATT and, 20
Technology, 36, 45
  access to advanced medical, 140, 142, 147, 160, 165, 170, 173
  cooperation among countries, 109, 112, 115, 173
  health care advances and, 104–105, 108, 116, 119, 121, 139
  revolution/innovation, 18–19, 21, 26, 29, 32–33, 43
Technophile countries, 32, 34–35, 38, 47, 77–78
Telecommunication, global, 26
Tertiary prevention, 178, 179
Tetanus, 105, 113, 129, 133
Thailand, 100, 128
Thiamin, 92, 133
Third Reich, 153
Third World countries. See Developing countries
30th World Health Assembly (1977), 111
35th World Health Assembly (1982), 112
Three Gorges Dam, 57
Time, as epidemiological dimension, 178, 187, 196, 217
Tobacco industry, targeting developing nations, 23, 24
Tobacco production, 23
Tobacco use, 22–24, 185, 199, 212, 216, 220
  chronic disease and, 38–39, 77, 139, 148, 152, 157, 165
  lung cancer causality, 179, 180
  maternal and child health and, 130, 131
  mortality rates from, 193, 194, 199, 218
Tobago, 36
Togo, 127
Toxemia, 193
Toxic shock syndrome, 73
Toxigenicity, 193
Trachoma, 9, 59
Trade, 43
  international, as disease spreaders, 20, 21, 27, 64, 67
Trade-Related Aspects of Intellectual Property Rights (TRIPS), 24
Traditional Chinese medicine (TCM), 149, 150, 151, 152
Traditional healers, 114
Training, of medical personnel, 149, 161, 164, 169, 172

Training programs for primary health care providers, 108–109, 110, 114, 121, 130, 137
Transmissible spongiform encephalopy (TSE), 72
Transportation, 98, 205, 211
  inaccessible health care and, 107, 110, 121, 126, 133
  and pollution, 49, 50, 53, 55, 56, 75
Traveler's diarrhea (TD), 198
Trichomoniasis, 13
Trichuris, 13
Trinidad, 36
Tritaeniorhynchus, 66
Trypanosomiasis, 59
Tuberculosis, 9, 11–13, 24, 65, 191–192
  as leading infectious cause of death, 124, 206, 212
  maternal and child mortality and, 128, 129, 133
  primary health care program and, 113, 114, 172
  resistant strains of, 39, 65, 67, 69, 71, 78, 210–211
Tunisia, food patterns, 100
Turkey, and abortion and contraception, 136
Two-by-two contingency table, 185–186, 187
Typhoid fever, 4, 191, 192, 195

Ukraine, 127, 194
Ultraviolet B spectrum (UV-B) radiation, 54
Ultraviolet sun radiation (UVR) exposure, 179
Underactivity, obesity and, 95
UNESCO. See United Nations Educational, Scientific, and Cultural Organization
UNICEF. See United Nations International Children's Emergency Fund
Uninsured, 169
Union Carbide pesticide factory explosion, 181
United Kingdom, 11, 72, 157, 198
United Nations, 15, 29, 34, 123
  Alma-ATA conference representation, 112
  Food and Agricultural Organization, 134
  World Food Programme, 134
United Nations Convention on Climate Change, 52
United Nations Educational, Scientific, and Cultural Organizations (UNESCO), 14, 16
United Nations General Assembly, 41
United Nations International Children's Emergency Fund (UNICEF), 3, 14, 23, 29, 90, 112, 123, 196

United Nations Population Division, 33

United States (U.S.), 20, 25–27, 49–50, 55, 198, 209
  birth/death rate, 33–34, 36
  eating habits in, 86–87, 92, 95, 99, 100
  environment movement, 44
  health care system of, 118, 141, 160, 166–169
  leading causes of death in, 23, 212
  maternal and child mortality, 127–128
  poverty in, 86, 107

United States Agency for International Development (USAID), 14, 16, 42, 114

United States Bureau of the Census, 33, 34, 42

United States Customs, 72

United States Department of Agriculture, 25

United States Environmental Protection Agency: Office of Air and Radiation, 56

United States Environmental Protection Agency: Office of Water, 60

United States National Oceanic and Atmospheric Administration (NOAA), 48, 52, 54

United States Patents and Trademarks Office, 24

United States Supreme Court, 168

Universal health care, 119, 141, 143, 145, 146, 166, 173
  in Germany, 153
  in Japan, 157
  in Peoples Republic of China, 149–151
  in Russia, 163

Universal medical care insurance, 145, 146

Universal primary education, cost of, 108

University of Mississippi Medical Center, 24

Urbanization, rapid, disease and, 206, 207, 210, 211

Urinary tract infections, 71

Uruguay, 24

USAID. *See* United States Agency for International Development

Vaccination, 12, 25, 131

Vaccines, 23, 25, 73, 76, 105, 134, 186
  disease control and, 51, 63, 66, 140, 196, 198–199, 209

Vaginal microcide, 208

Valaciclovir-Hcl, 61

Valtrex, 61

Varicella-Zoster, 61, 193

Vedas, 4–5

Venereal disease, 10, 149

Vibrio cholera, 139

Vietnam, 128

Viral bronchitis, 71

Viral polymorphism, 63

Virulence, 193

Virus, 25, 58, 192, 208, 211

Visceral leishmaniasis (Kala-azar), 13

Vitamin A, 133
  deficiency, 87, 89–90, 98–99, 214

Vitamin B, 133
  deficiency, 87, 99

Vitamin C, 133
  deficiency, 86, 87, 92, 201

Vitamin D deficiency, 87, 91–92

Vitamin deficiency, diseases, 89–92

Vitamin supplements, 89, 90

Volatile organic compounds (VOC), 53

War, 4, 22, 32
  reemerging diseases and, 210, 213

Waste dumping, 26, 27, 43, 46

Wasting, 88, 133

Water, 57–60, 213
  clean supply and, 2, 4, 12, 13, 14
  contamination of, 43, 45, 51, 177
  minimal needs, 56, 58, 79
  potable, 57–58, 63, 76, 104, 131, 140, 160
  potable, in developing countries, 23, 28, 78, 113, 114
  potable, malnutrition and, 87, 99, 101
  potable, primary health care promotion of adequate, 105, 115
  -related disease classifications, 58
  unpotable, 57, 58, 59, 75, 134, 160
  unpotable, disease transmission and, 64, 192, 197, 206, 208, 213, 216

Waterborne diseases, 4, 13

Water-scarce classification, 57

Water-stressed classification, 57, 58

Water usage patterns, 56, 58

Wealth Flows Theory, 40

Weather changes, 52–53

Web of Causation model, 198–199

Weimar Republic, 153

Welfare system, of health care, 160

Western Europe, 27, 34

Western Pacific area, 98, 100–101, 128, 209

Western-style medicine, 149, 150, 152, 170

West-Nile-like virus, 194

Wheat smut fungus, 25

Wilkens ice shelf, 48

Women, 23, 41, 76, 78, 124

World Bank, 28, 29, 123

World Cancer Research Fund, 215

World Food Programme, malnutrition and, 134

World Food Summit (1996), 134

World Health Assembly (1998), 220

World Health Organization (WHO), 3, 44, 55, 62, 86, 204
  Alma-ATA health conference, 104, 111, 112
  Communicable Disease Surveillance and Response Center, 74
  data collection/analysis, 97, 195, 216
  disease outbreak expertise, 196, 197, 209
  Expanded Program on Immunization, 15
  goals of, 90, 99, 104–105, 112, 115, 120
  health definition, 1–2
  main objective, 14, 15, 22, 23
  maternal and child health data, 123, 131, 134, 140
  mortality rates of member states, 127–128
  poverty stand, 215
  Promotion of Environmental Health program, 22
  regional food patterns, 98–101
  World Health Report (1995, 1999), 12, 23, 111, 124, 126, 128, 131
  world wide web address, 16, 29, 74

World Health Organization's Executive Board, 213

World Health Report (1995), 131

World Health Report (WHO, 1999), 12, 111, 124, 126, 128

World No Tobacco Day, 24

World population, world Internet connection sites, 42

World Population Council, 42

World population projections, 34, 35

World Trade Organization (WTO), 20, 21, 24, 29

Years life lost (YLL), 217, 218

Years lived with disability of differing severities (YLD), 217, 218

Years of potential life lost (YPLL), 184

Yellow fever, 4, 10, 52, 67, 73, 195, 211

Yemenites, incidence of diabetes, 98

Yugoslavia, food patterns, 100

Zaire, Ebola in, 208, 209

Zimbabwe, 51, 62

Zinc deficiency, 87, 89